PROTEASES IN GASTROINTESTINAL TISSUES

PROTEASES IN BIOLOGY AND DISEASE

SERIES EDITORS:

NIGEL M. HOOPER, *University of Leeds, Leeds, United Kingdom*

UWE LENDECKEL, *Otto-von-Guericke University, Magdeburg, Germany*

Volume 1
PROTEASES IN TISSUE REMODELLING OF LUNG AND HEART
Edited by Uwe Lendeckel and Nigel M. Hooper

Volume 2
AMINOPEPTIDASES IN BIOLOGY AND DISEASE
Edited in Nigel M. Hooper and Uwe Lendeckel

Volume 3
PROTEASES IN THE BRAIN
Edited by Uwe Lendeckel and Nigel M. Hooper

Volume 4
THE ADAM FAMILY OF PROTEASES
Edited by Nigel M. Hooper and Uwe Lendeckel

Volume 5
PROTEASES IN GASTROINTESTINAL TISSUES
Edited by Uwe Lendeckel and Nigel M. Hooper

PROTEASES IN GASTROINTESTINAL TISSUES

Edited by

UWE LENDECKEL

Otto-von-Guericke University,
Magdeburg, Germany

and

NIGEL M. HOOPER

University of Leeds, United Kingdom

Springer

A C.I.P. Catalogue record for this book is available from the Library of Congress.

ISBN-10 1-4020-4482-8 (HB)
ISBN-13 978-1-4020-4482-3 (HB)
ISBN-10 1-4020-4483-6 (e-book)
ISBN-13 978-1-4020-4483-0 (e-book)

Published by Springer,
P.O. Box 17, 3300 AA Dordrecht, The Netherlands.

www.springer.com

Printed on acid-free paper

Printed in the Netherlands.

Contents

Contributing Authors

Agarwal, Atul
Achillion Pharmaceuticals
300 George Street
New Haven, CT 06511, USA
e.mail: aagarwal@achillion.com

Alfalah, Marwan
Department of Physiological Chemistry
School of Veterinary Medicine Hannover
Bünteweg 17
D-30559 Hannover, Germany
e.mail: malfalah@biochemie.tiho-hannover.de

Bunnett, Nigel W.
Departments of Surgery and Physiology
University of California San Francisco
521 Parnassus Ave
San Francisco, CA 94143-0660
e.mail: nigelb@itsa.ucsf.edu

Charnley, Richard M.
Department of Surgery
University of Newcastle upon Tyne
HPB Surgical Unit, Freeman Hospital
Newcastle upon Tyne, NE7 7DN, UK
e.mail: Richard.Charnley@nuth.nhs.uk

Cottrell, Graeme S.
Departments of Surgery and Physiology
University of California San Francisco
521 Parnassus Ave
San Francisco, CA 94143-0660, USA
e.mail: graemec@itsa.ucsf.edu

Freker, Nadine
Dept. Functional and Applied Anatomy
Hannover Medical School
OE 4120,
Building I03, Level H0, Room 3110
Carl-Neuberg-Str. 1
30625 Hannover, Germany
e.mail: Nadinefreker@gmx.de

French, Jeremy J.
Department of Surgery
The Medical School
University of Newcastle upon Tyne
Newcastle, NE2 4HH, UK
e.mail: jeremyjfrench@doctors.org.uk

Gemeinhardt, Anja
Institute of Physiological Chemistry
Faculty of Veterinary Medicine
University of Leipzig
Leipzig, Germany
e.mail: Anja-schneide@gmx.de

Huang, Mingjun
Achillion Pharmaceuticals
300 George Street
New Haven, CT 06511, USA
e.mail: mhuang@achillion.com

Jaroszewicz, Jerzy
Department of Infectious Diseases
Medical University of Bialystok
Zurawia 14 Str.
15-540 Bialystok, Poland
e.mail: jerzyj@medprakt.pl

Khushalani, Nikhil I.
Department of Medicine
Veterans Affairs Medical Center
3495 Bailey Ave, 111H
Buffalo, NY 14215, USA
e.mail: Nikhil.Khushalani@med.va.gov

Krahn, Michael
Department of Physiological Chemistry
School of Veterinary Medicine Hannover
Bünteweg 17
D-30559 Hannover, Germany
e.mail: Michael.Krahn@tiho-hannover.de

Kuyvenhoven, Johan P.
Leiden University Medical Center
Department of Gastroenterology and Hepatology
PO Box 9600
2300 RC Leiden, The Netherlands
e.mail: kuyvenhoven@kg.nl

Leung, Po Sing
Department of Physiology
Faculty of Medicine
The Chinese University of Hong Kong
Shatin, New Territories, Hong Kong
The People's Republic of China
e.mail: psleung@cuhk.edu.hk

Magro, Fernando
Gastrorenterology Department and
Institute of Pharmacology and Therapeutics
Faculty of Medicine,
Rua José da Silva passos 48-52
4200-319 Porto, Portugal
e.mail: fm@med.up.pt

Malfertheiner, Peter
Department of Gastroenterology, Hepatology and Infectious Diseases
Otto-von-Guericke Unversity
Leipziger Str. 44
D-39120 Magdeburg, Germany
e.mail: peter.malfertheiner@medizin.uni-magdeburg.de

Moniuszko, Anna
Department of Infectious Diseases
Medical University of Bialystok
Zurawia 14 Str.
15-540 Bialystok, Poland
e.mail: aputamento@poczta.onet.pl

Naim, Hassan
Department of Physiological Chemistry
School of Veterinary Medicine Hannover
Bünteweg 17
D-30559 Hannover, Germany
e.mail: hassan.naim@tiho-hannover.de

Parfieniuk, Anna
Department of Infectious Diseases
Medical University of Bialystok
Zurawia 14 Str.
15-540 Bialystok, Poland
e.mail: anya_p79@o2.pl

Phadke, Avinash
Achillion Pharmaceuticals
300 George Street
New Haven, CT 06511, USA
e.mail: aphadke@achillion.com

Pasricha, Pankaj J.
Enteric Neuromuscular Disorders and Pain Group
Division of Gastroenterology and Hepatology
Department of Internal Medicine
University of Texas Medical Branch
Galveston, TX 77555-0764, USA
e.mail: jpasrich@utmb.edu

Ramnath, Nithya
Department of Medicine
Roswell Park Cancer Institute
Elm and Carlton Streets
Buffalo, NY 14263, USA
e.mail: Nithya.Ramnath@RoswellPark.org

Schwab, Dennis
Department of Physiological Chemistry
School of Veterinary Medicine Hannover
Bünteweg 17
D-30559 Hannover, Germany
e.mail: Dennis.Schwab@tiho-hannover.de

Sewpaul, Avinash
Department of Surgery
Medical School
University of Newcastle upon Tyne
NE1 7RU, United Kingdom
e.mail: avinash.sewpaul@ncl.ac.uk

Sier, Cornelis F.M.
Leiden University Medical Center
Department of Gastroenterology and Hepatology
PO Box 9600
2300 RC Leiden, The Netherlands
e.mail: C.F.M.Sier@lumc.nl

Slesiona, Silvia
Department of Physiological Chemistry
School of Veterinary Medicine Hannover
Bünteweg 17
D-30559 Hannover, Germany
e.mail: Silvia Slesiona@tiho-hannover.de

Vaday, Gayle
Northport Veterans Affairs Medical Center
Dept. of Research
79 Middleville Rd.
Northport, NY 11768, USA
e.mail: Gayle.Vaday@med.va.gov

van Hoek, Bart
Leiden University Medical Center
Department of Gastroenterology and Hepatology
PO Box 9600
2300 RC Leiden, The Netherlands
e.mail: B.van_Hoek@lumc.nl

Verspaget, Hein W.
Leiden University Medical Center
Department of Gastroenterology and Hepatology
PO Box 9600
2300 RC Leiden, The Netherlands
e.mail: H.W.Verspaget@lumc.nl

von Hörsten, Stephan
Dept. Functional and Applied Anatomy
Hannover Medical School
Building I03, Level H0, Room 3110
Carl-Neuberg-Str. 1
30625 Hannover, Germany
e.mail: Hoersten.Stephan.von@mh-hannover.de

Wei, Yao Hong
Department of Pharmacology
School of Medicine, Zhejiang University
353 Yan'an Road
Hangzhou 310031, The People's Republic of China
e.mail: yhgwei_215@yahoo.com.cn

Wex, Thomas
Department of Gastroenterology, Hepatology and Infectious Diseases
Otto-von-Guericke Unversity
Leipziger Str. 44
39120 Magdeburg, Germany
e.mail: thomas.wex@medizin.uni-magdeburg.de

Wiercinska-Drapalo, Alicja
Department of Infectious Diseases
Medical University of Bialystok
Zurawia 14 Str.
15-540 Bialystok, Poland
e.mail: alicja@poczta.onet.pl

Zack, Michael
Department of Gastroenterology, Hepatology and Infectious Diseases
Otto-von-Guericke Unversity
Leipziger Str. 44
39120 Magdeburg, Germany
e.mail: zacki137@gmx.de

Zucker, Stanley
Department of Medicine
State University of New York
Stony Brook, NY 11794
Northport Veterans Affairs Medical Center
Dept. of Research and Medicine
79 Middleville Rd.
Northport, NY 11768, USA
e.mail: s_zucker@yahoo.com

Preface

This, the fifth volume in the *Proteases in Biology and Disease* series, is devoted to Proteases in Gastrointestinal Tissues. Of course, proteases play an important role in the digestion and utilization of ingested proteins, but besides that they elicit a wide range of physiological and pathological effects. Proteases have been recognized as essential regulators, acting both locally and systemically, of normal development, growth and functioning. Dysregulation of protease expression and/or enzymatic activity is often associated with the onset or progression of disease and, thus, proteases represent interesting targets for the pharmacological therapy of e.g. cancer, chronic inflammation, graft rejection, fibrosis, diabetes, vascular disease, and viral or bacterial infections. In addition, changes in the localization, abundance or activity of proteases may serve as informative diagnostic or prognostic markers. This volume focuses on stomach, gut, pancreas, and liver and highlights the role of proteases in normal physiology and disease processes involving these tissues.

The first chapter by Nigel W. Bunnett and Graeme S. Cottrell reviews the current knowledge about the protease-activated receptors (PARs) in gastrointestinal tissues. Starting with the mechanisms of activation, signal transduction, and regulation of PAR, their role in controlling gastrointestinal functions and the possible involvement in gastrointestinal diseases are summarized. In Chapter 2, Nikhil I. Khushalani and Nithya Ramnath review the role of matrix metalloproteases (MMPs) and their natural inhibitors, TIMPs, in different types of gastric cancer. Current therapeutic options based on the pharmacological inhibition of MMPs and prospects of

MMP-inhibitor development are discussed. The role of host- and pathogen-derived proteases in the development of Helicobacter pylori-mediated diseases of the stomach is covered by Thomas Wex, Michael Zack, and Peter Malfertheiner in Chapter 3. In the next chapter, Avinash Sewpaul, Jeremy J. French, and Richard M. Charnley review the recent advances in the understanding of the crucial role that proteases and their inhibitors play in the development of acute and chronic diseases of the exocrine pancreas. Multiple proteases, including MMPs, cathepsin B, trypsin, and elastase, all have been implicated in the mechanism underlying pancreatic disease. In chapter 5, Pankaj J. Pasricha discusses the pathogenesis of pain in pancreatic disease and highlights the role that PARs play in pancreatic nociception. In Chapter 6 by Po S. Leung, the regulation and importance of the local renin-angiotensin system (RAS) for the function of both endocrine and exocrine pancreas is reviewed. Therapeutic strategies based on angiotensin II receptor blockade or inhibition of angiotensin-converting enzyme (ACE) are discussed.

In Chapter 7, Mingjun Huang, Avinash Phadke, and Atul Agarwal discuss hepatitis C virus (HCV) proteases, focusing on the functions and structures of the proteases, and the development of highly effective inhibitors of the viral proteases. In the next chapter, Yao H. Wei reviews the role of dysregulated ACE in the pathophysiology of liver fibrosis and the beneficial effects resulting from blocking the RAS by ACE inhibitors or angiotensin II receptor blockers for the prevention of hepatic fibrosis and subsequent liver cirrhosis. In Chapter 9, Hein Verspaget, Johan Kuyvenhoven, Cornelis Sier, and Bart van Hoek discuss the potential contribution to and role of MMPs in liver fibrosis, hepatocellular carcinoma, ischemia/reperfusion injury and acute rejection after liver transplantation. In Chapter 10, Alicja Wiercinska-Drapalo, Jerzy Jaroszewicz, Anna Parfieniuk, and Anna Moniuszko outline the recent evidence for the involvement of MMPs, TIMPs, and members of the family of 'a disintegrin and metalloproteases' (ADAMs) in the pathogenesis of inflammatory bowel disease (IBD). The focus of the next chapter by Gayle G. Vaday and Stanley Zucker are both MMPs and chemokines as two important regulatory factors in the tumor microenvironment that cooperatively regulate one another. Thereby, they promote tumor progression, dissemination and metastasis as outlined for colorectal cancer. MMP inhibitors and chemokine antagonist may be applied in the treatment of cancer. In Chapter 12, Fernando Magro describes the role of ACE and some of its major substrates in the development and progression of inflammatory disease of the gut. The last chapter by

Stephan von Hö rsten, Hassan Naim, Marwan Alfalah and colleagues reviews the current knowledge about cellular transport mechanisms that are required for proper expression at the cell surface of ecto-peptidases. The consequences of mistrafficking for the development of disease are discussed, as exemplified for sucrose isomaltase and dipeptidyl peptidase IV (DPIV), as is the role of DPIV in diabetes.

We hope that, like the previous volumes in the Proteases in Biology and Disease series, this fifth volume will prove to be a timely and valuable source for both newcomers to the field and clinicians and researchers interested in protease function and/or disease of gastro-intestinal tissues. Finally, we would like to thank all the authors for their scholarly contributions and apologize to them for editorial changes in the interest of consistency and clarity.

Uwe Lendeckel and Nigel M. Hooper

September 2005

Chapter 1

Protease-Activated Receptors in Gastrointestinal Function and Disease

Nigel W. Bunnett and Graeme S. Cottrell
Departments of Surgery and Physiology, University of California San Francisco, 521 Parnassus Ave, San Francisco CA 94143-0660

1. INTRODUCTION

The gastrointestinal tract is the richest source of proteases of any tissue. Proteases are a vital component of digestive secretions from exocrine glands such as the pancreas and glands within the stomach and intestine. The vast numbers of bacteria in the colon produce and secrete large amounts of proteases. Coagulating proteases arise from the circulation, and proteases are produced by immune cells, epithelial tissues and the nervous system. The principal function of some of these enzymes is to degrade dietary proteins in the lumen of the gastrointestinal tract. However, certain proteases can directly regulate cells by cleaving and activating protease-activated receptors (PARs). Some digestive enzymes may also regulate intestinal epithelial cells under physiological circumstances by cleaving PARs. However, many of the enzymes that activate PARs, such as the coagulation factors and proteases from inflammatory cells and epithelial tissues, are generated and secreted during injury and inflammation, and PARs control critically important responses to these insults, namely hemostasis, inflammation, pain and repair. Thus, proteases and PARs are important in the gastrointestinal tract under normal and pathological conditions, and protease inhibitors and PAR antagonists may be useful for the treatment of certain gastrointestinal diseases.

Here we briefly summarize the mechanisms of activation, signal transduction and regulation of PARs, to discuss the role of PARs in controlling particular gastrointestinal functions, and to summarize their

U. Lendeckel and Nigel M. Hooper (eds.), Proteases in Gastrointestinal Tissue, 1-31.

possible involvement in gastrointestinal diseases. There are several comprehensive reviews of the proteases and PARs in many systems (Coughlin 2000; Vergnolle 2000; Macfarlane *et al* 2001; Ossovskaya and Bunnett 2004).

2. PROTEASE-ACTIVATED RECEPTORS (PARs): ACTIVATION, SIGNALING AND REGULATION

2.1 PARs are a family of G-protein coupled receptors

PARs are G-protein coupled receptors (GPCR) with a seven trans-membrane topology. Currently there are four members of this receptor family, which are activated by the proteolytic cleavage of their extracellular amino terminus. This action reveals a new N-terminus, which acts as a tethered ligand to bind and activate the receptor (Figure 1).

The first member of this family of receptors is PAR1, which responds to thrombin. Using mRNA from cells responding to thrombin to transfect *Xenopus* oocytes, the cDNA for human (Vu *et al* 1991) and hamster (Rasmussen *et al* 1991) PAR1 were isolated. Analysis of the cDNA for human PAR1 revealed a protein of 425 residues, with a potential signal sequence, five potential glycosylation sites and an unprocessed molecular mass of 47 kDa. The protein was predicted to have the seven transmembrane topology of a typical GPCR. The activation of this receptor is a two-stage process. Firstly, thrombin binds to PAR1 either side of the proteolytic cleavage site. One of these sites ($D^{51}KYEPF^{56}$) is similar to that of hirudin, an anticoagulant found in the saliva of leech. This binding increases the affinity of the action by thrombin. Following binding of the protease, cleavage occurs between Arg^{41} and Ser^{42} to expose the new N-terminus starting with $S^{42}FLLRN^{47}$. This tethered ligand domain then interacts with residues on the second extracellular loop of the receptor and presumably induces a conformational change, which activates the receptor.

PAR2 is the second member of this receptor family and is activated by the proteolytic cleavage performed by trypsin. This receptor was initially cloned from a mouse genomic library using degenerate primers to the bovine neurokinin-2 receptor (Nystedt *et al* 1994; Nystedt *et al* 1995a) and then in humans (Nystedt *et al* 1995b; Bohm *et al* 1996b). The human cDNA for PAR2 encoded a protein of 397 amino acids, with a potential signal sequence, two potential glycosylation sites and an unprocessed molecular mass of 44 kDa. Human PAR2 shares 31% sequence identity with human PAR1. Unlike PAR1 and thrombin, activation of PAR2 by trypsin does not require binding of the enzyme prior to cleavage. Tryptic cleavage of PAR2 occurs between Arg^{36} and Ser^{37} to reveal the tethered ligand and new amino terminus of $S^{37}LIGKV^{42}$.

PAR3 is a second receptor for thrombin. The observation that platelets from PAR1 knockout mice still responded to thrombin gave evidence of another receptor for this protease (Connolly *et al* 1996). The cloning of PAR3 was first accomplished for humans (Ishihara *et al* 1997; Scase *et al* 1997). The open reading frame of the human cDNA encodes a seven transmembrane receptor of 374 residues, with a signal sequence, three potential glycosylation sites and an unprocessed molecular mass of 43 kDa. PAR3 shares 28% and 31% sequence identity with PAR1 and PAR2 respectively. This receptor also contains a downstream hirudin-like domain ($F^{48}EEFP^{52}$), which facilitates binding to and cleavage of the receptor by the protease. Thrombin cleaves PAR3 between K^{38} and T^{39} to unmask its tethered ligand of $T^{39}FRGAP^{44}$. However, unlike other members of this receptor family, which can be activated by synthetic peptides corresponding to their tethered ligand domains, PAR3 cannot. The reason for this has yet to be elucidated but could be explained by differences in structure and the unavailability of the binding site for the required interaction in the absence of proteolytic cleavage.

PAR4 cloned in 1998, is the last member of this proteolytically activated receptor family and responds to both thrombin and trypsin (Kahn *et al* 1998; Xu *et al* 1998). It is a protein of 385 amino acids, with a potential signal sequence, one potential glycosylation site and a molecular mass of 41 kDa. PAR4 shares 27% sequence identity with PAR1 and PAR3 and 28% with PAR2. Trypsin and thrombin cleave the receptor between residues Arg^{47} and Gly^{48}. Activation is similar to that of PAR2 in that there are no binding sites for the proteases and so cleavage occurs directly. The tethered ligand exposed is $R^{47}GYPGQV^{53}$ and synthetic peptides corresponding to this sequence activate the receptor in a similar fashion to PAR1 and PAR2.

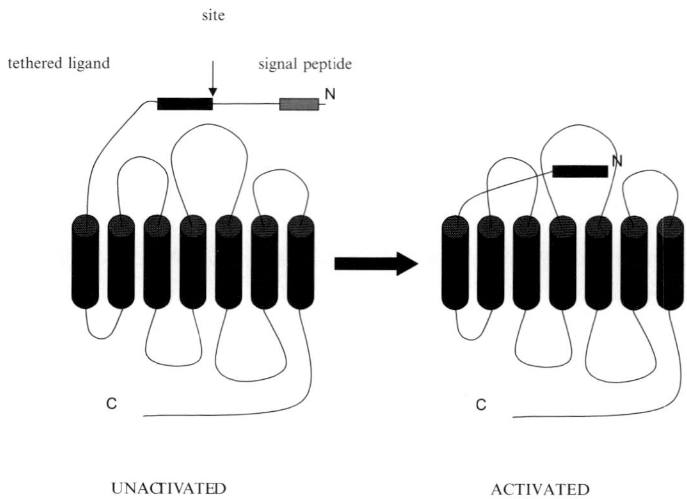

Figure 1: Structure and mechanism of proteolytic cleavage and activation of PARs. The protease cleaves the extracellular domain to expose a new amino terminus, which interacts with the second extracellular loop to initiate signal transduction.

2.2 Multiple proteases can cleave PARs

PAR1, PAR3 and PAR4 are receptors for thrombin, whilst PAR2 and PAR4 can be activated by trypsin. However, there has been much work focusing on the ability of other serine and non-serine proteases to either activate or disable these receptors. The widespread expression of these receptors lead to the belief that other activating or disabling proteases must exist. A summary of the potential activators is given in table 1.

Table 1. Summary of activating or disabling proteases and peptide agonists of PARs

	PAR1	PAR2	PAR3	PAR4
Tethered Ligand	SFLLRN	SLIGKV	TFRGAP	GYPGQV
Selective Peptide Agonist	TFLLRN	SLIGKV	None	AYPGKF
Activating Proteases	Thrombin Factor Xa APC	Trypsin Tryptase Factor VIIa, Xa Proteinase 3	Thrombin	Thrombin Trypsin Cathepsin G
Disabling Proteases	Plasmin	Elastase Cathepsin G Proteinase 3 Pseudolysin	Cathepsin G Elastase	None known

2.2.1 Coagulation and anticoagulation proteases

Thrombin can exist in at least two distinct forms. γ-thrombin is formed by the proteolytic cleavage of α-thrombin. Studies have shown that α-thrombin activates PAR1 with a 100-fold higher affinity than γ-thrombin (Bouton *et al* 1995). This difference can be explained due to the lack of the anion-binding site in γ-thrombin. The potency with which γ-thrombin and α-thrombin cleave PAR4 is similar as PAR4 lacks the thrombin-binding site (Xu *et al* 1998).

As described, thrombin (also known as factor IIa) can cleave and activate PAR1, PAR3 and PAR4, although all with differing potencies. Factor VIIa and Xa are also serine proteases of the coagulation pathway and they can also activate PARs. However, the ability of these enzymes to activate the PARs is heavily influenced by the availability of membrane bound anchoring proteins. Tissue factor (TF) is a single transmembrane protein, which is upregulated during inflammation. TF serves as a membrane-binding partner for factor VIIa, which can in turn cleave PAR2 (Camerer *et al* 2000). In the absence of TF even high concentrations of factor VIIa do not cleave PAR2 efficiently. In the presence of factor X the factor VIIa/TF complex efficiently cleaves factor X to its activated form (factor Xa), which in turn can activate PAR2. The same mechanism occurs during the cleavage of PAR1 by factors VIIa and Xa. On vascular endothelial cells another anchoring protein effector cell protease receptor-1 provides a high affinity site for factor Xa, thereby facilitating cleavage of PAR2 (Bono *et al* 2000). Further, a study using mice expressing a mutant of TF (lacking the cytoplasmic domain) indicates a role for TF in the negative regulation of PAR2, with mutant mice showing enhanced PAR2-dependent angiogenesis (Belting *et al* 2004).

Activated protein C (APC) is considered an anticoagulant protease as it cleaves and inactivates factors Va and VIIa. However, thrombin when partnered with thrombomodulin (a modulator of thrombin function) converts protein C to APC and when the APC itself is anchored to the membrane can cleave PAR1 (Riewald *et al* 2002).

2.2.2 Trypsins

Trypsin is normally considered to be an enzyme involved in the digestive process. Three isoforms of trypsin have now been cloned from human pancreas (Emi *et al* 1986; Nyaruhucha *et al* 1997). Trypsinogen I and II are the major isoforms secreted from the pancreas constituting 23% and 16% of the total secretory proteins respectively (Scheele *et al* 1981), with mesotrypsinogen constituting less than 0.5% (Nyaruhucha *et al* 1997). Trypsinogen IV is a splice variant of mesotrypsin, differing only at the N-terminus and was cloned from human brain (Wiegand *et al* 1993). Both mesotrypsin and trypsin IV have identical catalytic units and are resistant to proteinaceous inhibitors such as soybean trypsin inhibitor (Nyaruhucha *et al* 1997; Cottrell *et al* 2004) and further it has been demonstrated that mesotrypsin actually cleaves and inactivates these inhibitors (Szmola *et al* 2003).

There is increasing evidence that trypsins are not only produced in the pancreas, but are also expressed in the nervous system and in extrapancreatic epithelial and endothelial tissues (Koivunen *et al* 1989; Koshikawa *et al* 1998; Cottrell *et al* 2004). Extrapancreatic trypsins I and II derived from T84 and COLO-205 cells respectively have been shown to cleave and activate PAR2 (Ducroc *et al* 2002; Alm *et al* 2000). Further, it has been shown that trypsin IV is expressed in epithelial cell lines derived from the lungs, prostate and colon, and in normal colonic mucosa (Cottrell *et al* 2004). Trypsin IV cleaves and activates both PAR2 and PAR4.

2.2.3 Inflammatory cell proteases

Tryptase released from mast cells and cathepsin G, elastase and proteinase 3 from neutrophils all influence signaling through PARs.

The tryptase content of human mast cells can comprise up to 25% of their total cellular proteins (Schwartz *et al* 1981). Many of the mitogenic and inflammatory effects of tryptase can be mimicked by the selective peptide agonists of PAR2. After the cloning of PAR2, tryptase was the second enzyme reported to cleave and activate this receptor (Molino *et al* 1997). However, the efficiency with which tryptase activates this receptor is much lower than trypsin and many purified, recombinant forms of tryptase fail to activate PAR2 (Huang *et al* 2001). To further complicate issues, it has been suggested that the glycosylation state of human PAR2 influences its sensitivity to activation by tryptase (Compton *et al* 2001). Mutation of a potential N-terminal glycosylation site (N30A) dramatically increases the potency with which tryptase can activate PAR2. This effect was mimicked by treating cells with *Vibrio cholerae* neuraminidase, which removes oligosaccharide moieties (Compton *et al* 2001) and by expressing PAR2 in glycosylation defective cells (Compton *et al* 2002).

The azurophil granules of neutrophils contain cathepsin G, elastase and proteinase 3. Cathepsin G causes the aggregation of platelets, an effect that is blocked by a neutralizing PAR4 antibody (Sambrano *et al* 2000). This study also demonstrated PAR4 signaling by cathepsin G in transfected fibroblasts, *Xenopus* oocytes, and washed human platelets. It has also been reported that cathepsin G and elastase can cleave and activate PAR2 leading to the release of cytokines in human gingival fibroblasts (Uehara *et al* 2003). In contrast, the effect of cathepsin G and elastase on human alveolar and bronchial cells is not to activate but to cleave PAR2 in such a manner that it become unresponsive to trypsin, but can still be activated by activating peptides (Dulon *et al* 2003). Proteinase 3 has been shown to activate human oral epithelial cells (Uehara *et al* 2002) and that anti-proteinase 3 antibodies lead to the secretion of interleukin-8, monocyte chemoattractant protein-1 and aggregation of proteinase 3 on the cells (Uehara *et al* 2004).

2.2.4 Membrane proteases

It has been demonstrated that membrane-spanning proteases can also cleave and activate PARs. A solubilized form of membrane-type serine protease-1 was engineered by removing the transmembrane domain, and the unanchored form of this protease activated PAR2 expressed in *Xenopus* oocytes (Takeuchi *et al* 2000). This protease is expressed together with PAR2 in a human prostate cell line (PC-3) and could be its endogenous activator (Takeuchi *et al* 1999).

2.2.5 Microbial proteases

Of importance to other human diseases are the observations that proteases from bacteria, fungi and mites are also capable of cleaving PARs. The allergens produced by the dust mites *Dermatophagoides pteronyssinus* and *Dermatophagoides farinae* include two proteases, Der P3 (cysteine) and Der P9 (serine), which have been suggested as possible activators of PAR2 (Sun *et al* 2001).

Two arginine-specific proteases from *Porphyromonas gingivallis* (RgpB and HRgpA) have been found to exert effect through cleavage of PARs. *P. gingivallis* is implicated as a major contributor of periodontitis in humans. RgpB cleaves PAR2 (Lourbakos *et al* 1998), whilst HRgpA and RgpB both cleave PAR1 and PAR4 to release the proinflammatory cytokine interleukin-6 (Lourbakos *et al* 2001). Further, the release of the proinflammatory peptides substance P (SP) and calcitonin gene-related peptide (CGRP) was stimulated in human pulp cells by RgpB in a PAR2-dependent manner (Tancharoen *et al* 2005).

Finally, a metalloprotease (pseudolysin) from *Pseudomonas aeruginosa* whilst cleaving PAR2 does not lead to its activation, but yields a receptor unresponsive to further proteolytic activation (Dulon *et al* 2005). This may alter host innate defense mechanisms and respiratory functions, thus contributing to pathogenesis in the setting of a disease like cystic fibrosis.

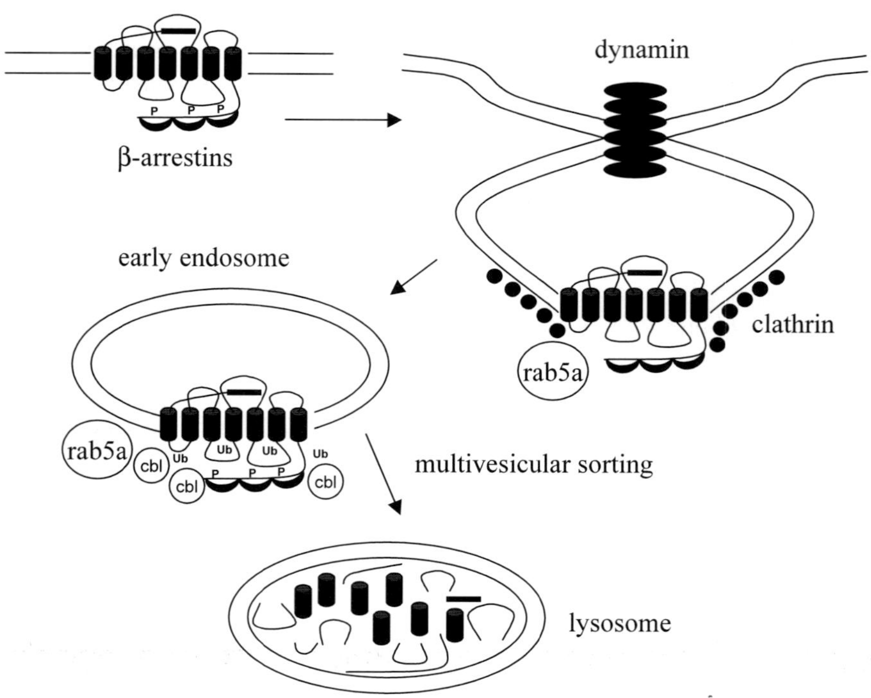

Figure 2: Internalization and trafficking of PAR2. Upon activation PAR2 is phosphorylated (P) by GRKs, which promotes translocation of β-arrestins from the cytosol. β-arrestins act as scaffolding proteins recruiting clathrin, and internalization proceeds via a dynamin-dependent mechanism. Rab5a mediates trafficking to early endosomes. PAR2 is ubiquitinated (Ub) on multiple lysine residues by the ubiquitin ligase, c-Cbl. This ubiquitination targets the receptor through multi-vesicular bodies for destruction in lysosomes.

3. ROLE OF PROTEASES AND PARs IN CONTROLING THE GASTROINTESTINAL TRACT

3.1 Expression and localization of PARs in the gastrointestinal tract

All PARs are widely expressed throughout the gastrointestinal tract, although the majority of research has focused on PAR2, which plays important roles in the control of transport, motility, permeability and secretion.

PAR1 is found on the endothelial cells of the lamina propria and submucosa as well as on the epithelial cells of the intestine, smooth muscle cells and on neurons within the enteric nervous system. PAR2 is very highly expressed and has been observed on both the apical and basolateral membranes of enterocytes, endothelial cells, myocytes in the muscularis externa and muscularis mucosa and on immune cells including mast cells, neutrophils and lymphocytes. Expression of both PAR1 and PAR2 has been observed in neurons within the enteric nervous system (Bohm *et al* 1996a; Corvera *et al* 1999).

Less is known about the expression of PAR3 except that mRNA has been detected in the stomach and small intestine. The exact cell types expressing functional receptors have yet to be determined. As with PAR3, PAR4 expression in the gastrointestinal tract is not yet clearly defined other than that expression has been observed in the small intestine and colon (Mule *et al* 2004).

3.2 Effects of PAR agonists on gastrointestinal functions

Given the widespread expression of PARs in the gastrointestinal tract, and considering the abundance of proteases under physiological and pathophysiological conditions, it is not surprising that proteases and PARs regulate almost all digestive functions. The roles of PARs in different cell types are summarized in figure 3.

3.2.1 Intestinal ion transport

PAR1 and PAR2 have been reported to play a role in the control of ion transport within the intestinal mucosa. Activation of these receptors stimulates the secretion of chloride ions. During intestinal inflammation this secretion may play a protective role, promoting the removal of bacterial toxins from the mucosa and presenting as symptomatic diarrhea. Evidence for this role in the modulation of electrolyte transport comes from experiments involving the use of Ussing chambers and the recording of short-circuit currents as an indicator of ion movement.

PAR1 expression has been confirmed on SCBN cells, a non-transformed human duodenal epithelial cell line derived from the crypts of the small intestine. Previous studies have proven this cell line to be capable of vectorial chloride ion secretion (Pang *et al* 1996). Basolateral application of either thrombin or a selective PAR1 activating peptide, Ala-parafluoro-Phe-Arg-cyclohexyl-Ala-Citrulline-Tyr (Cit-NH_2) to monolayers of these cells induced an increase in short-circuit current, indicative of chloride secretion (Buresi *et al* 2001; Buresi *et al* 2002). Although it is known that these cells also express functional cystic fibrosis transmembrane conductance regulator (CFTR) it is unlikely that the activation of PAR1 modulates its action since PAR1 is not known activate the cAMP cascade. More likely it is the transactivation of the epidermal growth factor (EGF) receptor and activation of the MAP kinase cascade, which phosphorylate cytoplasmic phospholipase A_2 and leads to stimulation of cyclooxygenase-1 and -2 and production of prostaglandins, which then enhance chloride ion secretion. Thus, PAR1 modulates intestinal chloride secretion via a Ca^{2+} dependent mechanism.

The study of a non-transformed rat small intestine cell line, hBRIE indicated that activation of PAR2 using either trypsin or activating peptide increased the mobilization of intracellular calcium and resulted in the release of arachidonic acid and prostaglandins E_2 and $F_{1\alpha}$ (Kong *et al* 1997). Prostaglandins are known modulators of chloride secretion. Further, Ussing chamber experiments using jejunal slices of rat intestine revealed that activation of PAR2 leads to an increase in short-circuit current, indicative of chloride ion secretion (Vergnolle *et al* 1998). This effect was dependent on prostaglandins since pretreatment of slices with indomethacin, an inhibitor of cyclooxygenase function abolished the effect on the short-circuit current.

A study on porcine ileal segments revealed that the effect of PAR2 activation on chloride secretion was due to modulation of opioid-sensitive neurons (Green *et al* 2000). Inhibitors of neuronal conduction (saxitoxin), the cyclooxygenase inhibitor (indomethacin) and the $Na^+/K^+/Cl^-$ cotransporter inhibitor furosemide and all attenuated the responses on chloride secretion evoked by application of PAR2 agonists. Delta-opioid receptor agonists prevented the action of trypsin, whilst antagonists of this receptor prevented this inhibitory effect (Green *et al* 2000). Supporting these findings are the observations that PAR2 agonists lead to the release of the neuropeptides, SP and CGRP from cultured neurons. Both these peptides have well-established roles in the modulation of ion transport. Thus, this may be the mechanism by which PAR2 agonists exert their effects in intestinal ion transport.

3.2.2 Control of paracellular permeability

The epithelial cells of the intestine form a protective barrier in front of the mucosa to prevent translocation of bacteria and macromolecules, which may contribute to inflammation. The permeability of this barrier is controlled by the number of tight junctions (TJ) present between each epithelial cell. The association of the proteins forming a TJ is controlled by agonists of PARs.

Agonists of PAR1 have been shown to induce apoptosis in intestinal epithelial cells and lead to a loss of TJ (Chin *et al* 2003). This increase in apoptosis together with the loss of TJs contributes to an increased paracellular permeability which can be prevented by inhibitors of caspase-3, tyrosine kinases and a myosin light chain kinase inhibitor, whilst being potentiated by an inhibitor of src.

PAR2 also regulates this protective epithelial barrier by controlling the formation of the TJs. Agonists of PAR2 reduced the transepithelial resistance and increased transport of macromolecules across colonocytes grown in a monolayer (Jacob *et al* 2005). These effects were dependent on β-arrestins and ERK1/2, as determined by downregulation of β-arrestins by siRNA and the use of an ERK1/2 kinase inhibitor. The association of internalized PAR2 with ERK1/2 is dependent on the protein scaffold formed by β-arrestins. The complex retains activated ERK1/2 in the cytosol where they may function to control the integrity of the epithelial cytoskeleton and TJs (Ge *et al* 2003; Jacob *et al* 2005).

3.2.3 Gastrointestinal motility

PARs are also reported to play a critical role in the modulation of gastrointestinal smooth muscle causing either contraction or relaxation. In rat both PAR1 and PAR4 are expressed in the oesophageal mucosa. These two receptors play opposing roles, with PAR1 leading to contraction and PAR4 inducing relaxation (Kawabata *et al* 2000b). However, the effective concentration of thrombin may determine the overriding effect as PAR1 is activated by much lower concentrations. Similar to PAR1, PAR2 also induces contraction of gastrointestinal smooth muscle. However, if the muscle is precontracted with carbachol, PAR1 agonists result in further contraction where as PAR2 and PAR4 agonists lead to relaxation (Kawabata *et al* 2000b). The PAR1 and PAR2 induced contraction of gastric smooth muscle is via a prostaglandin-dependent mechanism, as determined by the inhibitory effect of indomethacin.

In mice the effects of PAR1 and PAR2 activation are biphasic. Isolated gastric fundus first relaxes and then contracts following their activation. The relaxation responses caused by PARs are mediated through apamin-sensitive K^+ channels (Cocks *et al* 1999).

Using isolated primary cultures Corvera and coworkers showed that the PAR2 agonists tryptase and activating peptide caused a transient increase in intracellular calcium, and that PAR2 agonists influenced the rhythmic contractions of rat colonic tissue (Corvera *et al* 1997). They also demonstrated that this was caused by a mechanism independent of both cyclooxygenase and neuronal activity.

More recently, there is emerging evidence of a role for PAR4 in the colon of the rat. Molecular and immunohistochemical techniques have provided evidence for the expression of PAR4 on epithelial surfaces and submucosa (Mule *et al* 2004). Synthetic peptides induced a concentration dependent contraction of longitudinal muscle. These responses were significantly reduced by the use of tetrodotoxin, atropine and by prolonged pretreatment with capsaicin, indicating the contraction occurs at least in part via a neurogenic pathway.

3.2.4 Gastrointestinal secretion

PARs regulate secretions from the pancreas, stomach and salivary glands. The intravenous injection of PAR2, but not PAR1, selective activating peptides induces secretion of mucus and amylase from the acinar cells of mice and rats (Kawabata *et al* 2000a). The amylase secretion induced by PAR2 in mice occurs partially via a mechanism dependent on the formation of nitric oxide (Kawabata *et al* 2002) and in rats the mucin secretion is attenuated by genistein, an inhibitor of tyrosine kinases. Amylase release from the pancreas is also stimulated in response to PAR2 activation (Kawabata *et al* 2000a).

In the stomach, PAR2 activation leads to the secretion of mucus (Kawabata *et al* 2001), which may serve to protect the stomach from damage. The antagonism of CGRP type 1 receptors and neurokinin-2 receptors inhibits this secretion indicating it occurs through the release of neuropeptides (Kawabata *et al* 2001). This is in contrast to the salivary secretion of mucus and amylase, which are not dependent on sensory nerves (Kawabata *et al* 2002). The PAR2 receptors present on the chief cells in the stomach are responsible for the release of pepsinogen/pepsin (Kawao *et al* 2002). This enzyme release is a direct effect of PAR2 activation and is not reliant upon sensory neurons or nitric oxide formation.

3.2.5 Regulation of the intrinsic and extrinsic nervous system

Digestive tract function is not only controlled by nerves that connect the gastrointestinal tract to the central nervous system (CNS), but also by the enteric (intrinsic) nervous system (ENS).

The enteric nervous system is a locally controlled network of nerves, which functions independently from the CNS. The ENS comprises of two networks (plexuses) of neurons, which are embedded within the digestive tract and extend from the oesophagus to the anus. The myenteric plexus is located between the circular and longitudinal layers of muscle and its primary function is the control of digestive tract motility. The submucosal plexus is buried in the submucosa. Its principal role is in sensing and controlling the luminal environment, regulating blood flow and epithelial cell function. Sections of the submucosal plexus may be missing in areas where these functions are minimal, such as the oesophagus. Each of the plexuses contains three types of neurons, sensory neurons, motor neurons and interneurons. PAR1, PAR2 and PAR4 are expressed by a large subset of these neurons indicating possible roles for these receptors in the neuronal control of gastrointestinal functions.

Treatment of myenteric neurons from the ileum of a guinea pig with agonists of PAR2 (trypsin, activating peptide) induced a prolonged depolarization, which was often accompanied by an increased excitability (Linden *et al* 2001). This observation was expanded using other enzymatic activators of PARs (thrombin, tryptase) and using selective peptide agonists for PAR1, PAR2 and PAR4 (Gao *et al* 2002). Thus, modulation of neurons by agonists of PARs may play an important role in the motility of the intestine during normal and diseased states.

PARs are also expressed on nerves found within the submucosa of the guinea pig small intestine. The exact agonists of PARs in these sites are as yet unidentified. One potential candidate for the agonist of PAR2 is tryptase derived from mast cells within the submucosa. Mast cells are known to contain several mediators that can cause neuronal hyperexcitability (histamine, prostaglandins, serotonin). Mast cells also release proteases, one of which, tryptase, is an agonist of PAR2. Application of tryptase to these neurons induced a transient depolarization, which was followed by a long (several hours) hyperexcitability (Reed *et al* 2003). This leads to the hypothesis that agonists of PAR2 acting directly on submucosal nerves can alter fluid and electrolyte secretion and intestinal motility.

The extrinsic nervous system of the gut connects the gastrointestinal tract to the CNS via dorsal root ganglia (DRG). The primary spinal afferent neurons express SP and CGRP and play a major role in the sensing of pain and neurogenic inflammation, through a combination of GPCRs, receptor tyrosine kinases and ion channels, resulting in the release of these neuropeptides. Neurogenic inflammation is characterized by plasma extravasation, neutrophil migration, and vasodilatation. In the spinal cord SP and CGRP are important in the transmission of pain. Neurons in the rat DRG are known to express mRNA for all PARs (Zhu *et al* 2005) and PAR1 and PAR2 are expressed together in neurons containing SP and CGRP. Activation of these PARs is known to stimulate neuropeptide release (Steinhoff *et al* 2000; de Garavilla *et al* 2001). Thus, the proteases which cleave PARs signal through these neurons to control nociception and inflammation.

Much work has focused on the role of PAR2 within the extrinsic nervous system of the gastrointestinal tract and may have implications for the enteric nervous system. Activation of PAR2 in rat hind paw by intraplantar injection of PAR2 agonists leads to the formation of edema, which may last for hours (Vergnolle *et al* 1999). If lower doses of PAR2 agonists are given there is no inflammation but there is sustained thermal and mechanical hyperalgesia and associated expression of c-fos in the dorsal horn (Vergnolle *et al* 2001). This hyperalgesia is not seen in mice lacking the neurokinin-1 receptor or lacking the preprotachykinin A gene (encoding for both SP and neurokinin A).

Antagonism of the neurokinin-1 receptor also suppressed the level of hyperalgesia, suggesting that PAR2 mediated hyperalgesia occurs through the release and action of SP. The physiological activator of PAR2 in this setting is unknown, but a good candidate is the tryptase released upon degranulation of mast cells. Mucosal mast cells are found within close proximity of sensory nerves in normal and inflamed tissues (Stead *et al* 1987; Barbara *et al* 2004). Degranulation of mast cells with an intraplantar injection of compound 48/80 has been shown to induce hyperalgesia, which was absent in PAR2 knockout mice (Vergnolle *et al* 2001). The exact mechanism by which PAR2 induces inflammation and hyperalgesia has yet to be fully delineated. However, progress is being made and it has been shown that PAR2 activation sensitizes ion channels present on neurons. One such channel is the transient receptor potential vanilloid-1 (TRPV1), which is activated by heat, protons, ethanol and capsaicin (Caterina *et al* 1997; Julius and Basbaum 2001). Activation of PAR2 causes a sensitization of TRPV1 induced by phosphorylation of the ion channel by a PKC-dependent mechanism (Amadesi *et al* 2004; Dai *et al* 2004). Further, PAR2 mediated hyperalgesia was not seen in mice lacking TRPV1 or by treatment with the TRPV1 antagonist, capsazepine and the release of SP and CGRP in response to TRPV1 activation was also enhanced by pretreatment with PAR2 agonists (Amadesi *et al* 2004).

In contrast to the activation of PAR2, PAR1 activation causes an increase in the pain threshold to thermal and mechanical stimuli (Asfaha *et al* 2002). The mechanism by which this occurs is poorly understood and much work needs to be completed before the pathway is fully elucidated.

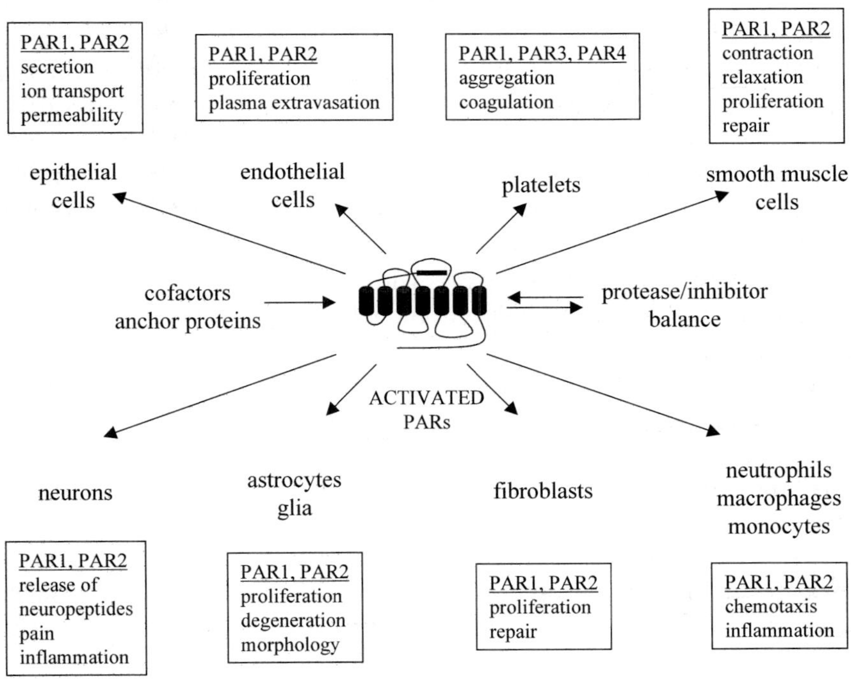

Figure 3: Summary of the potential roles of PARs in the cell types within the gastrointestinal tract.

4. CONTRIBUTIONS OF PROTEASES AND PARs TO GASTROINTESTINAL DISEASES

4.1 Protease expression in the diseased gastrointestinal tract

The gastrointestinal tract is awash with proteases from many different sources including the lumen, bacteria, mast cells, immune cells and from the circulation. The balance between the release, activation and inhibition of these proteases is at the heart of many disease states. A brief summary of the roles of PARs in gastrointestinal disease is given in Figure 4.

4.1.1 Proteases in pancreatitis

There are many causes of pancreatitis although alcoholism and biliary tract disease account for greater than 80% of all hospital admissions for acute cases. Whatever the cause of the disease, it is characterized by the uncontrolled release and activation of enzymes and proteases in the inflamed pancreas.

Tissue necrosis is caused by the elevated levels of trypsins and phospholipase A_2 (Mossner *et al* 1992; Kimura *et al* 1993). Trypsins can activate other enzymes within the pancreatic juice, whilst the phospholipase destroys lipids. Mesotrypsin, whilst only a minor component of pancreatic secretion is resistant to naturally occurring protease inhibitors and also neutralizes these molecules by cleaving them (Szmola *et al* 2003). The rat form of trypsin (trypsin V, p23) with similar inhibitor resistance is upregulated in a caerulein-induced model of pancreatitis (Fukuoka and Nyaruhucha 2002). Potentially, this enzyme can clear the level of inhibitors, signal through PARs and activate other forms of trypsin allowing uncontrolled signaling and destruction. Initially however, as PAR2 induces secretion of electrolytes and fluid the effect may be protective (Alvarez *et al* 2004). Mutations in trypsin genes can contribute to the premature activation of the enzyme and play a major role in hereditary pancreatitis (Whitcomb *et al* 1996; Gorry *et al* 1997).

Pancreatic elastase is responsible for the damage caused to vasculature within and outside of the pancreas. The elastase has been shown to breakdown the elastic fibres present within blood vessels, removing the barriers that prevent it entering the bloodstream to damage other tissues, such as the lung (Lungarella *et al* 1985).

4.1.2 Luminal proteases

Trypsins are expressed by the epithelial cells which protect the submucosa of the intestine and may also be expressed with natural activator of the enzyme, enteropeptidase. Trypsin IV is expressed by both normal and cancerous cell types originating from the intestine (Cottrell *et al* 2004). Trypsin IV has an identical catalytic domain to mesotrypsin and as such is also resistant to proteinaceous inhibitors and does not degrade itself. The function and regulation of this unique form of trypsin still remains to be elucidated.

Other proteases such as those from mast cells and neutrophils are also found in the inflamed intestine, many of which can signal through PARs.

4.1.3 Coagulation proteases

Endotoxemia is a condition where endotoxins from bacteria enter the bloodstream. The body's defense system then releases inflammatory compounds and causes fever to help fight the infection. Endotoxemia can be induced in mice by giving a high dose of lipopolysaccharide (Pawlinski *et al* 2004). When compared to mice expressing normal levels of TF, mice expressing low levels of TF showed reduced signs of coagulation, inflammation and mortality. This effect was mimicked by the inhibition of thrombin in mice lacking PAR2, indicating the importance of PAR signaling in a model of endotoxemia.

PAR signaling is increased following radiation therapy and is characterized by an upregulation of thrombin, TF, PAR1 and the down-regulation of thrombomodulin. The increased activity results in an increased deposition of fibrin and mucosal damage (Wang *et al* 2002a; Wang *et al* 2004). The damage was ameliorated by the use of hirudin as an inhibitor of thrombin. An earlier study also implicated an upregulation of PAR2 and participation of mast cell proteases (Wang *et al* 2003). Thus, uncontrolled protease activity and PAR1 and PAR2 signaling may contribute to complications surrounding radiation therapy.

4.1.4 Proteases generated during inflammation

In rats, a dinitro-benzene-sulphonic acid model of ulcerative colitis increased serine protease activity by up to 10-fold (Hawkins *et al* 1997). They observed that untreated rats had little inherent protease activity but treated rats had serine protease activity that was abolished by the use of serine protease inhibitors (Bowman-Birk inhibitor and diisopropylfluoro-phosphate). They postulated that the activity may have come from a number of sources including mast cells or other immune cells and that candidate enzymes included elastase and cathepsin G. Studies have confirmed this to be true in human patients with ulcerative colitis. Fecal samples were shown to exhibit increased levels of protease activity, including trypsin, chymotrypsin and elastase (Bustos *et al* 1998). The authors concluded that this activity contributes to some of the pathophysiology. Indeed, Kuno and colleagues concluded that neutrophil elastase activity negatively regulates cells reducing proliferation thereby impeding mucosal healing (Kuno *et al* 2002).

Mast cells and their inflammatory mediators are becoming increasingly important in the search for the mechanism involved in intestinal inflammation. Cultured mast cells from patients with ulcerative colitis secrete increased levels of histamine compared to normal patients (Raithel *et al* 1999). Indeed, this was also found to be true of tryptase release (Raithel *et al* 2001). In patients with irritable bowel syndrome, there are elevated numbers of mast cells, which spontaneously secrete more active tryptase and histamine than in control patients (Barbara *et al* 2004).

Cystic fibrosis (CF) is a condition associated with mutations in a chloride channel and improper salt balance in the cells and thick, sticky mucus. Inflammation of the gastrointestinal tract occurs in many patients suffering from CF (Raia *et al* 2000). Symth and coworkers, reported increased levels of elastase and that many patients exhibited increased levels of bacterial flora with bacterial proteases perhaps also playing a role in the emergence of the inflammation (Smyth *et al* 2000).

4.2 PARs in gastrointestinal disease

PARs potentially play a major role in the physiology and pathophysiology of the gastrointestinal tract. PARs have been implicated in a variety of diseases affecting the intestine including inflammatory bowel disorders, allergies, pancreatitis and cancer.

4.2.1 Inflammatory bowel disease

There are reports that there is an upregulation of certain proteases in patients suffering from inflammatory bowel disorders (Bustos *et al* 1998; Kjeldsen *et al* 1998). Many of these proteases are capable of cleaving PARs and so contribute to the pathogenesis of the disorders.

It has been demonstrated that intracolonic administration of agonists of PAR2 in mice causes an inflammatory response characterized by granulocyte infiltration, increased wall thickness, tissue damage, and elevated T-helper cell type 1 cytokine (Cenac *et al* 2002). These inflammatory markers were not seen in mice lacking PAR2.

A further study indicated that this inflammation caused by PAR2 activation occurs through a mechanism involving neurons, the generation of nitric oxide and an increased paracellular permeability (Cenac *et al* 2003). This increased paracellular permeability is brought about by disruption of tight junction proteins which occurs following PAR2 dependent activation of MAP kinase pathway (Jacob *et al* 2005b). The increase in the paracellular permeability could then have a detrimental effect on the submucosa allowing proteases from bacteria and the lumen to enter. These proteases could then cause aberrant PAR signaling leading to inflammation and pain.

However, PAR2 is also reported have a protective role in the intestine, where stimulation results in prostaglandin formation in enterocytes and mucus secretion from the stomach but not in the duodenum (Kawabata *et al* 2001).

The induction of intestinal inflammation using 2,4,6-trinitrobenzene sulphonic acid (TNBS) is a widely used and well-characterized model of hapten-induced colitis. Following such treatment in mice, activation of PAR2 using synthetic peptides actually reduces the markers associated with inflammation (Fiorucci *et al* 2001). The use of an antagonist of the CGRP type 1 receptor and suppression of sensory neurons via treatment with capsaicin prevents this protective effect and indicates that PAR2 works through a neurogenic pathway (Fiorucci *et al* 2001).

A recent report demonstrated upregulation of PAR1 in the colon of patients suffering from inflammatory bowel disease (IBD). Patients with both ulcerative colitis and Crohn's Disease exhibited higher mRNA levels for PAR1 when compared to healthy control patients (Vergnolle *et al* 2004). Immunohistochemical staining of the muscularis mucosae from human colon confirmed that the message was translated into protein. Further, TNBS induced colitis in mice also induced an increase in PAR1 expression. Intracolonic administration of PAR1 agonists led to the appearance of inflammatory markers such as edema and granulocyte infiltration. TNBS failed to induce similar symptoms when administered in mice lacking PAR1 or when PAR1 function was compromised with the use of antagonists (Vergnolle *et al* 2004).

Bacterial infections of the intestine can cause inflammation and lead to diarrhea and hemorrhagic colitis (Kaper *et al* 2004). Enterohemorrhagic *Escherichia coli* infection in human can be mimicked by the introduction of *Citrobacter rodentium* in mice (Donnenberg *et al* 1993). When such bacteria are introduced, they stimulate the release of granzyme A and trypsins by the host and induce damage to tissues (Hansen *et al* 2005). The addition of soybean trypsin inhibitor, a known inhibitor of granzyme A and trypsins reduced the macroscopic damage associated with infection, as did the removal of PAR2 in knockout mice.

These results suggest that attenuation both PAR1 and PAR2 function may be important in the context of chronic intestinal inflammation.

4.2.2 Irritable bowel syndrome

A hallmark symptom of irritable bowel syndrome (IBS) is abdominal pain and discomfort and the mechanisms by which these occur are poorly understood. In patients with IBS, there are elevated numbers of mast cells, which spontaneously secrete more active tryptase and histamine compared to control patients (Barbara *et al* 2004). The activated mast cells were also in closer proximity to nerve endings with could express PAR2. When PAR2 is activated on these neurons by tryptase released from mast cells there is release of SP and CGRP. These neuropeptides are important in the transmission of pain to the CNS and thus abnormal PAR2 signaling may contribute to the pain and dysfunction of the intestine in these patients.

4.2.3 Pancreatic inflammation and pain

Treatment of isolated rat DRG neurons with a PAR2 activating peptide induces an increase in currents evoked by capsaicin and KCl, as determined by release of the CGRP, suggesting a role for PAR2 in the pain pathway (Hoogerwerf *et al* 2001). Injection of peptide into the pancreatic duct of rats induced dorsal horn expression of c-fos, a recognized marker for pain. Further studies using rats analyzed the effect of injection of subinflammatory doses of trypsin. Elevated expression of c-fos and behavioral pain responses were observed (Hoogerwerf *et al* 2004). However, recent work has indicated that activation of PAR2 in acute pancreatitis is protective (Sharma *et al* 2005). This protective effect may be due to the retention of ERK1/2 in the cytosol rather than translocating to the nucleus. Therefore the function of these cytosolic ERKs may be reflected in the protective nature associated with PAR2 activation.

4.2.4 Fibrosis

Fibrotic disorders are associated with the overproduction and deposition of extracellular matrix proteins such as collagens and with persistent coagulation factor activity. Both thrombin and factor Xa induced activation of PAR1 on primary human lung fibroblasts increased the expression of connective tissue growth factor (Chambers *et al* 2000). Dependency on the PAR1 signaling pathway was demonstrated by lack of such upregulation in fibroblasts isolated from knockout mice.

The fibrosis caused by radiation treatments of rat intestine resulted in a marked upregulation of PAR1 expression and the loss of thrombomodulin (Wang *et al* 2002a). Thrombomodulin is an integral membrane glycoprotein, which binds to and alters the substrate specificity of thrombin. Thrombin when bound to thrombomodulin is unable to cleave and activate PAR1, nor can it cleave fibrinogen to fibrin. The PAR1 overexpression was seen in smooth muscle cells and the degree of upregulation correlated with the severity of the fibrotic damage.

4.2.5 Colon cancer

The expression of PARs, typically PAR1 and PAR2 and their potential proteolytic agonists in tumours has been well documented.

Studies using HT-29 cells as models of colon cancer have shown that activation of endogenously expressed PAR1 either with thrombin or specific activating peptides, induce cellular proliferation (Darmoul *et al* 2003), migration and matrix adhesion (Heider *et al* 2004). Proliferation induced by thrombin acts firstly by cleaving and activating PAR1. Then there is the release of a matrix metalloprotease, which acts to release transforming growth factor-alpha. This is a potent agonist of the EGF receptor, which in turn switches on the MAP kinase pathway and leads to the subsequent increase in cell number (Darmoul *et al* 2004). Using the selective peptide agonist, TFLRRN to activate PAR1 in HT-29 cells it was observed that two isoforms of protein kinase C (PKC) were activated (Heider *et al* 2004). Using selective inhibitors of these isoforms the authors deduced that PKCε was a crucial component in the signaling pathway leading to the increased motility and adhesion.

The expression of PAR2 in many human colonic cancerous cell lines has been demonstrated. Activation of PAR2 using either trypsin or synthetic peptides has been shown to induce calcium mobilization and to promote cell proliferation in serum-starved cells (Darmoul *et al* 2001). Further studies showed that these cells also contain transcripts for trypsinogen I, a potent agonist of PAR2 (Ducroc *et al* 2002). The authors demonstrated that trypsin was present in the medium at concentrations consistent with that necessary for PAR2 activation and suggested that an autocrine or paracrine regulation of PAR2 may occur. The potent effects on cellular proliferation following PAR2 activation have been demonstrated to be dependent on the transactivation of the EGF receptor and stimulation of the MAP kinase pathway (Darmoul *et al* 2004).

4.2.6 Stomach disease

Stomach diseases such as gastritis are associated with damage to the mucosal lining due to excessive acid secretion. Activation of PAR2, which stimulates mucus secretion may be beneficial in this setting to protect the epithelium from acid damage. It has also, been shown that PAR-2 agonists strongly suppress carbachol-induced gastric acid secretion, which would also contribute to the cytoprotective effect (Nishikawa *et al* 2002).

Helicobacter pylori was first linked to gastritis by Marshall and Warren (Marshall 1983; Marshall and Warren 1984) and subsequently linked to associated coronary heart disease (Mendall *et al* 1994). Patients with *H. pylori* positive gastritis were found to have an increased level of circulating thrombin (Consolazio *et al* 2004). This may lead to aberrant PAR1 signaling or excessive coagulation activity and may provide the link between gastritis and coronary disease. In similar patients, Bergin and colleagues observed increased levels of matrix metalloproteases (MMP-9 and MMP-2). Increased levels of these enzymes may contribute to tissue damage exacerbating inflammation (Bergin *et al* 2004).

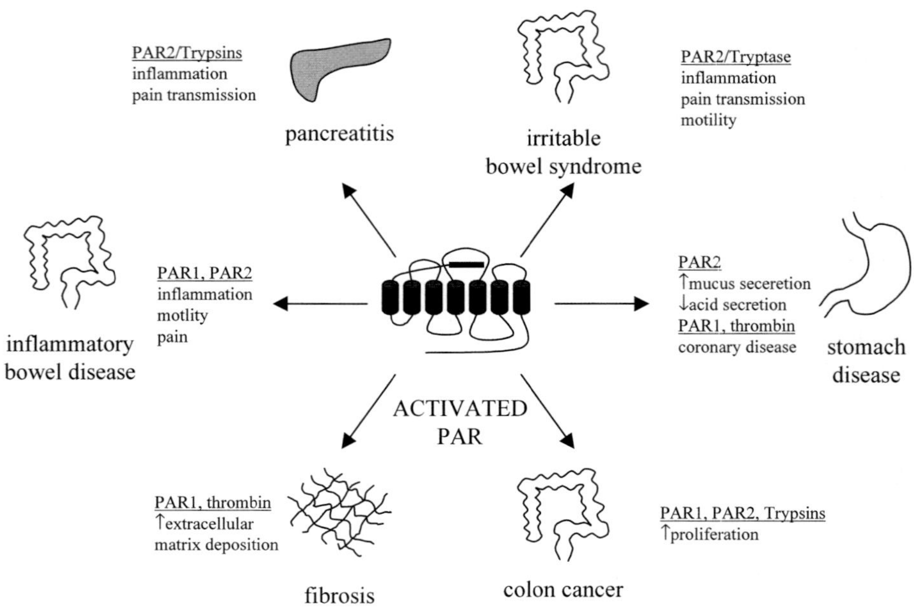

Figure 4: Summary of the potential roles of PARs in gastrointestinal diseases.

5. CONCLUSIONS

Major advances in identifying the endogenous and exogenous activators of PARs, the mechanisms by which the receptors are activated, trafficked and destroyed and the physiological functions of the receptors in physiological and pathophysiological settings have been made in recent years. However much remains to be learned.

It seems likely that yet more proteases, which either activate or disable PARs will be discovered as the mechanisms of activation get more and more complicated, especially with the discovery of anchoring proteins and cofactors. The development and use of selective peptide agonists too has aided much of this progress. These peptides allow the stimulation of single types of PAR to allow investigation of function when studying cell types expressing more than one PAR. The generation of knockout mice for PARs has proved very helpful in providing insights into human disease. Using these animals as models of intestinal diseases we now have insights into the role of PARs. However, care must be taken when interpreting these results as PARs may have different functions in different species, such as the differences between human and mouse platelets. Antagonists of PARs would prove very useful pharmacologic tools, but there have been very few reported and some are not fully characterized and as such are not widely used. Thus, as the functions of PARs are probed, the need for antagonists, not only in research but also in the potential treatment of human disease grows. Inhibition of the proteases which activate PARs could also prove beneficial. Work in animal models shows that protease inhibitors can ameliorate some of the symptoms of intestinal diseases. Indeed, inhibitors of tryptase have been used in the treatment of human disease, and inhibitors of trypsin help to reduce symptoms in animal models.

So, by using agonists, antagonists, knockout and animal models of disease we are beginning to understand the role of PARs in the gastrointestinal tract and how best we can use this knowledge to treat human disease.

REFERENCES

Alm AK, Gagnemo-Persson R, Sorsa T, Sundelin J, 2000, Extrapancreatic trypsin-2 cleaves proteinase-activated receptor-2. *Biochem Biophys Res Commun.* **275**: 77-83.

Alvarez C, Regan JP, Merianos D, Bass BL, 2004, Protease-activated receptor-2 regulates bicarbonate secretion by pancreatic duct cells in vitro. *Surgery* **136**: 669-676.

Amadesi S, Nie J, Vergnolle N, Cottrell GS, Grady EF, Trevisani M, Manni C, Geppetti P, McRoberts JA, Ennes H, Davis JB, Mayer EA, Bunnett NW, 2004, Protease-activated receptor 2 sensitizes the capsaicin receptor transient receptor potential vanilloid receptor 1 to induce hyperalgesia. *J Neurosci.* **24**: 4300-4312.

Asfaha S, Brussee V, Chapman K, Zochodne DW, Vergnolle N, 2002, Proteinase-activated receptor-1 agonists attenuate nociception in response to noxious stimuli. *Br J Pharmacol.* **135**: 1101-1106.

Barbara G, Stanghellini V, De Giorgio R, Cremon C, Cottrell GS, Santini D, Pasquinelli G, Morselli-Labate AM, Grady EF, Bunnett NW, Collins SM, Corinaldesi R, 2004, Activated mast cells in proximity to colonic nerves correlate with abdominal pain in irritable bowel syndrome. *Gastroenterology* **126**: 693-702.

Belting M, Dorrell MI, Sandgren S, Aguilar E, Ahamed J, Dorfleutner A, Carmeliet P, Mueller BM, Friedlander M, Ruf W, 2004, Regulation of angiogenesis by tissue factor cytoplasmic domain signaling. *Nat Med.* **10**: 502-509.

Bergin PJ, Anders E, Sicheng W, Erik J, Jennie A, Hans L, Pierre M, Qiang PH, Marianne QJ, 2004, Increased production of matrix metalloproteinases in Helicobacter pylori-associated human gastritis. *Helicobacter* **9**: 201-210.

Bohm SK, Khitin LM, Grady EF, Aponte G, Payan DG, Bunnett NW, 1996a, Mechanisms of desensitization and resensitization of proteinase- activated receptor-2. *J Biol Chem.* **271**: 22003-22016.

Bohm SK, Kong W, Bromme D, Smeekens SP, Anderson DC, Connolly A, Kahn M, Nelken NA, Coughlin SR, Payan DG, Bunnett NW, 1996b, Molecular cloning, expression and potential functions of the human proteinase-activated receptor-2. *Biochem J.* **314**: 1009-1016.

Bono F, Schaeffer P, Herault JP, Michaux C, Nestor AL, Guillemot JC, Herbert JM, 2000, Factor Xa activates endothelial cells by a receptor cascade between EPR-1 and PAR-2. *Arterioscler Thromb Vasc Biol.* **20**: E107-112.

Bouton MC, Jandrot-Perrus M, Moog S, Cazenave JP, Guillin MC, Lanza F, 1995, Thrombin interaction with a recombinant N-terminal extracellular domain of the thrombin receptor in an acellular system. *Biochem J.* **305**: 635-641.

Buresi MC, Buret AG, Hollenberg MD, MacNaughton WK, 2002, Activation of proteinase-activated receptor 1 stimulates epithelial chloride secretion through a unique MAP kinase- and cyclo-oxygenase-dependent pathway. *FASEB J.* **16**: 1515-1525.

Buresi MC, Schleihauf E, Vergnolle N, Buret A, Wallace JL, Hollenberg MD, MacNaughton WK, 2001, Protease-activated receptor-1 stimulates Ca(2+)-dependent Cl(-) secretion in human intestinal epithelial cells. *Am J Physiol Gastrointest Liver Physiol.* **281**: G323-332.

Bustos D, Negri G, De Paula JA, Di Carlo M, Yapur V, Facente A, De Paula A, 1998, Colonic proteinases: increased activity in patients with ulcerative colitis. *Medicina (B Aires)* **58**: 262-264.

Camerer E, Huang W, Coughlin SR, 2000, Tissue factor- and factor X-dependent activation of protease-activated receptor 2 by factor VIIa. *Proc Natl Acad Sci U S A.* **97**: 5255-5260.

Caterina MJ, Schumacher MA, Tominaga M, Rosen TA, Levine JD, Julius D, 1997, The capsaicin receptor: a heat-activated ion channel in the pain pathway. *Nature* **389:** 816-824.

Cenac N, Garcia-Villar R, Ferrier L, Larauche M, Vergnolle N, Bunnett NW, Coelho AM, Fioramonti J, Bueno L, 2003, Proteinase-Activated Receptor-2-Induced Colonic Inflammation in Mice: Possible Involvement of Afferent Neurons, Nitric Oxide, and Paracellular Permeability. *J Immunol.* **170**: 4296-4300.

Cenac N, Coelho AM, Nguyen C, Compton S, Andrade-Gordon P, MacNaughton WK, Wallace JL, Hollenberg MD, Bunnett NW, Garcia-Villar R, Bueno L, Vergnolle N, 2002, Induction of intestinal inflammation in mouse by activation of proteinase-activated receptor-2. *Am J Pathol.* **161**: 1903-1915.

Chambers RC, Leoni P, Blanc-Brude OP, Wembridge DE, Laurent GJ, 2000, Thrombin is a potent inducer of connective tissue growth factor production via proteolytic activation of protease-activated receptor-1. *J Biol Chem.* **275**: 35584-35591.

Cocks TM, Sozzi V, Moffatt JD, Selemidis S, 1999, Protease-activated receptors mediate apamin-sensitive relaxation of mouse and guinea pig gastrointestinal smooth muscle. *Gastroenterology* **116**: 586-592.

Compton SJ, Renaux B, Wijesuriya SJ, Hollenberg MD, 2001, Glycosylation and the activation of proteinase-activated receptor 2 (PAR(2)) by human mast cell tryptase. *Br J Pharmacol.* **134**: 705-718.

Compton SJ, Sandhu S, Wijesuriya SJ, Hollenberg MD, 2002, Glycosylation of human proteinase-activated receptor-2 (hPAR2): role in cell surface expression and signalling. *Biochem J.* **368**: 495-505.

Connolly AJ, Ishihara H, Kahn ML, Farese RV, Jr., Coughlin SR, 1996, Role of the thrombin receptor in development and evidence for a second receptor. *Nature* **381**: 516-519.

Consolazio A, Borgia MC, Ferro D, Iacopini F, Paoluzi OA, Crispino P, Nardi F, Rivera M, Paoluzi P, 2004, Increased thrombin generation and circulating levels of tumour necrosis factor-alpha in patients with chronic Helicobacter pylori-positive gastritis. *Aliment Pharmacol Ther.* **20**: 289-294.

Corvera CU, Dery O, McConalogue K, Bohm SK, Khitin LM, Caughey GH, Payan DG, Bunnett NW, 1997, Mast cell tryptase regulates rat colonic myocytes through proteinase-activated receptor 2. *J Clin Invest.* **100**: 1383-1393.

Corvera CU, Dery O, McConalogue K, Gamp P, Thoma M, Al-Ani B, Caughey GH, Hollenberg MD, Bunnett NW, 1999, Thrombin and mast cell tryptase regulate guinea-pig myenteric neurons through proteinase-activated receptors-1 and -2. *J Physiol.* **517**: 741-756.

Cottrell GS, Amadesi S, Grady EF, Bunnett NW, 2004, Trypsin IV, a novel agonist of protease-activated receptors 2 and 4. *J Biol Chem.* **279**: 13532-13539.

Coughlin SR, 2000, Thrombin signalling and protease-activated receptors. *Nature* **407:** 258-264.

Dai Y, Moriyama T, Higashi T, Togashi K, Kobayashi K, Yamanaka H, Tominaga M, Noguchi K, 2004, Proteinase-activated receptor 2-mediated potentiation of transient receptor potential vanilloid subfamily 1 activity reveals a mechanism for proteinase-induced inflammatory pain. *J Neurosci.* **24**: 4293-4299.

Darmoul D, Gratio V, Devaud H, Laburthe M, 2004, Protease-activated receptor 2 in colon cancer: trypsin-induced MAPK phosphorylation and cell proliferation are mediated by epidermal growth factor receptor transactivation. *J Biol Chem.* **279**: 20927-20934.

Darmoul D, Marie JC, Devaud H, Gratio V, Laburthe M, 2001, Initiation of human colon cancer cell proliferation by trypsin acting at protease-activated receptor-2. *Br J Cancer* **85**: 772-779.

Darmoul D, Gratio V, Devaud H, Lehy T, Laburthe M, 2003, Aberrant expression and activation of the thrombin receptor protease-activated receptor-1 induces cell proliferation and motility in human colon cancer cells. *Am J Pathol.* **162**: 1503-1513.

de Garavilla L, Vergnolle N, Young SH, Ennes H, Steinhoff M, Ossovskaya VS, D'Andrea MR, Mayer EA, Wallace JL, Hollenberg MD, Andrade-Gordon P, Bunnett NW, 2001, Agonists of proteinase-activated receptor 1 induce plasma extravasation by a neurogenic mechanism. *Br J Pharmacol.* **133**: 975-987.

DeFea KA, Zalevsky J, Thoma MS, Dery O, Mullins RD, Bunnett NW, 2000, beta-arrestin-dependent endocytosis of proteinase-activated receptor 2 is required for intracellular targeting of activated ERK1/2. *J Cell Biol.* **148**: 1267-1281.

Dery O, Corvera CU, Steinhoff M, Bunnett NW, 1998, Proteinase-activated receptors: novel mechanisms of signaling by serine proteases. *Am J Physiol.* **274**: C1429-1452.

Dery O, Thoma MS, Wong H, Grady EF, Bunnett NW, 1999, Trafficking of proteinase-activated receptor-2 and beta-arrestin-1 tagged with green fluorescent protein. beta-Arrestin-dependent endocytosis of a proteinase receptor. *J Biol Chem.* **274**: 18524-18535.

Donnenberg MS, Tzipori S, McKee ML, O'Brien AD, Alroy J, Kaper JB, 1993, The role of the eae gene of enterohemorrhagic Escherichia coli in intimate attachment in vitro and in a porcine model. *J Clin Invest.* **92**: 1418-1424.

Ducroc R, Bontemps C, Marazova K, Devaud H, Darmoul D, Laburthe M (2002) Trypsin is produced by and activates protease-activated receptor-2 in human cancer colon cells: evidence for new autocrine loop. *Life Sci.* **70**: 1359-1367.

Dulon S, Cande C, Bunnett NW, Hollenberg MD, Chignard M, Pidard D, 2003, Proteinase-activated receptor-2 and human lung epithelial cells: disarming by neutrophil serine proteinases. *Am J Respir Cell Mol Biol.* **28**: 339-346.

Dulon S, Leduc D, Cottrell GS, D'Alayer J, Hansen KK, Bunnett NW, Hollenberg MD, Pidard D, Chignard M, 2005, Pseudomonas aeruginosa Elastase Disables Proteinase-Activated Receptor 2 in Respiratory Epithelial Cells. *Am J Respir Cell Mol Biol.* **32**: 411-419.

Emi M, Nakamura Y, Ogawa M, Yamamoto T, Nishide T, Mori T, Matsubara K, 1986, Cloning, characterization and nucleotide sequences of two cDNAs encoding human pancreatic trypsinogens. *Gene* **41**: 305-310.

Fiorucci S, Mencarelli A, Palazzetti B, Distrutti E, Vergnolle N, Hollenberg MD, Wallace JL, Morelli A, Cirino G, 2001, Proteinase-activated receptor 2 is an anti-inflammatory signal for colonic lamina propria lymphocytes in a mouse model of colitis. *Proc Natl Acad Sci U S A.* **98**: 13936-13941.

Fukuoka S, Nyaruhucha CM, 2002, Expression and functional analysis of rat P23, a gut hormone-inducible isoform of trypsin, reveals its resistance to proteinaceous trypsin inhibitors. *Biochim Biophys Acta* **1588**: 106-112.

Gao C, Liu S, Hu HZ, Gao N, Kim GY, Xia Y, Wood JD, 2002, Serine proteases excite myenteric neurons through protease-activated receptors in guinea pig small intestine. *Gastroenterology* **123**: 1554-1564.

Gorry MC, Gabbaizedeh D, Furey W, Gates LK, Jr., Preston RA, Aston CE, Zhang Y, Ulrich C, Ehrlich GD, Whitcomb DC, 1997, Mutations in the cationic trypsinogen gene are associated with recurrent acute and chronic pancreatitis. *Gastroenterology* **113**: 1063-1068.

Green BT, Bunnett NW, Kulkarni-Narla A, Steinhoff M, Brown DR, 2000, Intestinal type 2 proteinase-activated receptors: expression in opioid- sensitive secretomotor neural circuits that mediate epithelial ion transport. *J Pharmacol Exp Ther.* **295**: 410-416.

Hansen KK, Sherman PM, Cellars L, Andrade-Gordon P, Pan Z, Baruch A, Wallace JL, Hollenberg MD, Vergnolle N, 2005, A major role for proteolytic activity and proteinase-activated receptor-2 in the pathogenesis of infectious colitis. *Proc Natl Acad Sci U S A.* **102**: 8363-8368.

Hawkins JV, Emmel EL, Feuer JJ, Nedelman MA, Harvey CJ, Klein HJ, Rozmiarek H, Kennedy AR, Lichtenstein GR, Billings PC, 1997, Protease activity in a hapten-induced model of ulcerative colitis in rats. *Dig Dis Sci.* **42**: 1969-1980.

Heider I, Schulze B, Oswald E, Henklein P, Scheele J, Kaufmann R, 2004, PAR1-type thrombin receptor stimulates migration and matrix adhesion of human colon carcinoma cells by a PKCepsilon-dependent mechanism. *Oncol Res.* **14**: 475-482.

Holler D, Dikic I, 2004, Receptor endocytosis via ubiquitin-dependent and -independent pathways. *Biochem Pharmacol.* **67**: 1013-1017.

Hoogerwerf WA, Shenoy M, Winston JH, Xiao SY, He Z, Pasricha PJ, 2004, Trypsin mediates nociception via the proteinase-activated receptor 2: A potentially novel role in pancreatic pain. *Gastroenterology* **127**: 883-891.

Hoogerwerf WA, Zou L, Shenoy M, Sun D, Micci MA, Lee-Hellmich H, Xiao SY, Winston JH, Pasricha PJ, 2001, The proteinase-activated receptor 2 is involved in nociception. *J Neurosci.* **21:** 9036-9042.

Hoxie JA, Ahuja M, Belmonte E, Pizarro S, Parton R, Brass LF, 1993, Internalization and recycling of activated thrombin receptors. *J Biol Chem.* **268**: 13756-13763.

Huang C, De Sanctis GT, O'Brien PJ, Mizgerd JP, Friend DS, Drazen JM, Brass LF, Stevens RL, 2001, Evaluation of the substrate specificity of human mast cell tryptase beta I and demonstration of its importance in bacterial infections of the lung. *J Biol Chem.* **276**: 26276-26284.

Ishii K, Hein L, Kobilka B, Coughlin SR, 1993, Kinetics of thrombin receptor cleavage on intact cells. Relation to signaling. *J Biol Chem.* **268**: 9780-9786.

Ishihara H, Connolly AJ, Zeng D, Kahn ML, Zheng YW, Timmons C, Tram T, Coughlin SR, 1997, Protease-activated receptor 3 is a second thrombin receptor in humans. *Nature* **386**: 502-506.

Jacob C, Cottrell GS, Gehringer D, Schmidlin F, Grady EF, Bunnett NW, 2005a, c-Cbl mediates ubiquitination, degradation, and down-regulation of human protease-activated receptor 2. *J Biol Chem.* **280**:16076-16087.

Jacob C, Yang PC, Darmoul D, Amadesi S, Saito T, Cottrell GS, Coelho AM, Singh P, Grady EF, Perdue M, Bunnett NW, 2005b, Mast cell tryptase controls paracellular permeability of the intestine: Role of protease-activated receptor 2 and beta-arrestins. *J Biol Chem* in press

Julius D, Basbaum AI, 2001, Molecular mechanisms of nociception. *Nature* **413**: 203-210.

Kahn ML, Zheng YW, Huang W, Bigornia V, Zeng D, Moff S, Farese RV, Jr., Tam C, Coughlin SR, 1998, A dual thrombin receptor system for platelet activation. *Nature* **394**: 690-694.

Kaper JB, Nataro JP, Mobley HL, 2004, Pathogenic Escherichia coli. *Nat Rev Microbiol.* **2**: 123-140.

Kawabata A, Nishikawa H, Kuroda R, Kawai K, Hollenberg MD, 2000a, Proteinase-activated receptor-2 (PAR-2): regulation of salivary and pancreatic exocrine secretion in vivo in rats and mice. *Br J Pharmacol.* **129**: 1808-1814.

Kawabata A, Kuroda R, Kuroki N, Nishikawa H, Kawai K, 2000b, Dual modulation by thrombin of the motility of rat oesophageal muscularis mucosae via two distinct protease-activated receptors (PARs): a novel role for PAR-4 as opposed to PAR-1. *Br J Pharmacol.* **131**: 578-584.

Kawabata A, Kinoshita M, Nishikawa H, Kuroda R, Nishida M, Araki H, Arizono N, Oda Y, Kakehi K, 2001, The protease-activated receptor-2 agonist induces gastric mucus secretion and mucosal cytoprotection. *J Clin Invest.* **107**: 1443-1450.

Kawabata A, Kuroda R, Nishida M, Nagata N, Sakaguchi Y, Kawao N, Nishikawa H, Arizono N, Kawai K, 2002, Protease-activated receptor-2 (PAR-2) in the pancreas and parotid gland: Immunolocalization and involvement of nitric oxide in the evoked amylase secretion. *Life Sci.* **71**: 2435-2446.

Kawao N, Sakaguchi Y, Tagome A, Kuroda R, Nishida S, Irimajiri K, Nishikawa H, Kawai K, Hollenberg MD, Kawabata A, 2002, Protease-activated receptor-2 (PAR-2) in the rat gastric mucosa: immunolocalization and facilitation of pepsin/pepsinogen secretion. *Br J Pharmacol.* **135**: 1292-1296.

Kimura W, Secknus R, Fischbach W, Mossner J, 1993, Role of phospholipase A2 in pancreatic acinar cell damage and possibilities of inhibition: studies with isolated rat pancreatic acini. *Pancreas* **8**: 70-79.

Kjeldsen J, Lassen JF, Brandslund I, Schaffalitzky de Muckadell OB, 1998, Markers of coagulation and fibrinolysis as measures of disease activity in inflammatory bowel disease. *Scand J Gastroenterol.* **33**: 637-643.

Koivunen E, Huhtala M-L, Stenman U-H, 1989, Human ovarian tumor-associated trypsin. Its purification and characterization from mucinous cyst fluid and identification as an activator of pro-urokinase. *J Biol Chem.* **264**: 14095-14099.

Kong W, McConalogue K, Khitin LM, Hollenberg MD, Payan DG, Bohm SK, Bunnett NW, 1997, Luminal trypsin may regulate enterocytes through proteinase-activated receptor 2. *Proc Natl Acad Sci U S A.* **94**: 8884-8889.

Koshikawa N, Hasegawa S, Nagashima Y, Mitsuhashi K, Tsubota Y, Miyata S, Miyagi Y, Yasumitsu H, Miyazaki K, 1998, Expression of trypsin by epithelial cells of various tissues, leukocytes, and neurons in human and mouse. *Am J Pathol.* **153**: 937-944.

Kuno Y, Ina K, Nishiwaki T, Tsuzuki T, Shimada M, Imada A, Nishio Y, Nobata K, Suzuki T, Ando T, Hibi K, Nakao A, Yokoyama T, Yokoyama Y, Kusugami K, 2002, Possible involvement of neutrophil elastase in impaired mucosal repair in patients with ulcerative colitis. *J Gastroenterol.* **37** Suppl **14**: 22-32.

Kurten RC, Cadena DL, Gill GN, 1996, Enhanced degradation of EGF receptors by a sorting nexin, SNX1. *Science* **272**: 1008-1010.

Linden DR, Manning BP, Bunnett NW, Mawe GM, 2001, Agonists of proteinase-activated receptor 2 excite guinea pig ileal myenteric neurons. *Eur J Pharmacol.* **431**: 311-314.

Lourbakos A, Chinni C, Thompson P, Potempa J, Travis J, Mackie EJ, Pike RN, 1998, Cleavage and activation of proteinase-activated receptor-2 on human neutrophils by gingipain-R from Porphyromonas gingivalis. *FEBS Lett.* **435**: 45-48.

Lourbakos A, Potempa J, Travis J, D'Andrea MR, Andrade-Gordon P, Santulli R, Mackie EJ, Pike RN, 2001, Arginine-Specific Protease from Porphyromonas gingivalis Activates Protease-Activated Receptors on Human Oral Epithelial Cells and Induces Interleukin-6 Secretion. *Infect Immun.* **69**: 5121-5130.

Lungarella G, Gardi C, de Santi MM, Luzi P, 1985, Pulmonary vascular injury in pancreatitis: evidence for a major role played by pancreatic elastase. *Exp Mol Pathol.* **42**: 44-59.

Macfarlane SR, Seatter MJ, Kanke T, Hunter GD, Plevin R, 2001, Proteinase-activated receptors. *Pharmacol Rev.* **53**: 245-282.

Madamanchi NR, Li S, Patterson C, Runge MS, 2001, Thrombin regulates vascular smooth muscle cell growth and heat shock proteins via the JAK-STAT pathway. *J Biol Chem.* **276**: 18915-18924.

Marshall BJ, 1983, Unidentified curved bacilli on gastric epithelium in active chronic gastritis. *Lancet* **1**: 1273-1275.

Marshall BJ, Warren JR, 1984, Unidentified curved bacilli in the stomach of patients with gastritis and peptic ulceration. *Lancet* **1**: 1311-1315.

Mendall MA, Goggin PM, Molineaux N, Levy J, Toosy T, Strachan D, Camm AJ, Northfield TC, 1994, Relation of Helicobacter pylori infection and coronary heart disease. *Br Heart J.* **71**: 437-439.

Missy K, Plantavid M, Pacaud P, Viala C, Chap H, Payrastre B, 2001, Rho-kinase is involved in the sustained phosphorylation of myosin and the irreversible platelet aggregation induced by PAR1 activating peptide. *Thromb Haemost.* **85**: 514-520.

Molino M, Barnathan ES, Numerof R, Clark J, Dreyer M, Cumashi A, Hoxie JA, Schechter N, Woolkalis M, Brass LF, 1997, Interactions of mast cell tryptase with thrombin receptors and PAR-2. *J Biol Chem.* **272**: 4043-4049.

Mossner J, Bodeker H, Kimura W, Meyer F, Bohm S, Fischbach W, 1992, Isolated rat pancreatic acini as a model to study the potential role of lipase in the pathogenesis of acinar cell destruction. *Int J Pancreatol.* **12**: 285-296.

Mule F, Pizzuti R, Capparelli A, Vergnolle N, 2004, Evidence for the presence of functional protease activated receptor 4 (PAR4) in the rat colon. *Gut* **53**: 229-234.

Nakanishi-Matsui M, Zheng YW, Sulciner DJ, Weiss EJ, Ludeman MJ, Coughlin SR, 2000, PAR3 is a cofactor for PAR4 activation by thrombin. *Nature* **404**: 609-613.

Nishikawa H, Kawai K, Nishimura S, Tanaka S, Araki H, Al-Ani B, Hollenberg MD, Kuroda R, Kawabata A, 2002, Suppression by protease-activated receptor-2 activation of gastric acid secretion in rats. *Eur J Pharmacol.* **447**: 87-90.

Nyaruhucha CN, Kito M, Fukuoka SI, 1997, Identification and expression of the cDNA-encoding human mesotrypsin(ogen), an isoform of trypsin with inhibitor resistance. *J Biol Chem.* **272**: 10573-10578.

Nystedt S, Emilsson K, Wahlestedt C, Sundelin J, 1994, Molecular cloning of a potential proteinase activated receptor [see comments]. *Proc Natl Acad Sci U S A.* **91**: 9208-9212.

Nystedt S, Larsson AK, Aberg H, Sundelin J, 1995a, The mouse proteinase-activated receptor-2 cDNA and gene. Molecular cloning and functional expression. *J Biol Chem.* **270**: 5950-5955.

Nystedt S, Emilsson K, Larsson AK, Strombeck B, Sundelin J, 1995b, Molecular cloning and functional expression of the gene encoding the human proteinase-activated receptor 2. *Eur J Biochem.* **232**: 84-89.

O'Brien PJ, Prevost N, Molino M, Hollinger MK, Woolkalis MJ, Woulfe DS, Brass LF, 2000, Thrombin responses in human endothelial cells. Contributions from receptors other than PAR1 include the transactivation of PAR2 by thrombin-cleaved PAR1. *J Biol Chem.* **275**: 13502-13509.

Ossovskaya VS, Bunnett NW, 2004, Protease-activated receptors: contribution to physiology and disease. *Physiol Rev.* **84**: 579-621.

Pang G, Buret A, O'Loughlin E, Smith A, Batey R, Clancy R, 1996, Immunologic, functional, and morphological characterization of three new human small intestinal epithelial cell lines. *Gastroenterology* **111**: 8-18.

Pawlinski R, Pedersen B, Schabbauer G, Tencati M, Holscher T, Boisvert W, Andrade-Gordon P, Frank RD, Mackman N, 2004, Role of tissue factor and protease-activated receptors in a mouse model of endotoxemia. *Blood* **103**: 1342-1347.

Raia V, Maiuri L, de Ritis G, de Vizia B, Vacca L, Conte R, Auricchio S, Londei M, 2000, Evidence of chronic inflammation in morphologically normal small intestine of cystic fibrosis patients. *Pediatr Res.* **47**: 344-350.

Raithel M, Schneider HT, Hahn EG, 1999, Effect of substance P on histamine secretion from gut mucosa in inflammatory bowel disease. *Scand J Gastroenterol.* **34**: 496-503.

Raithel M, Winterkamp S, Pacurar A, Ulrich P, Hochberger J, Hahn EG, 2001, Release of mast cell tryptase from human colorectal mucosa in inflammatory bowel disease. *Scand J Gastroenterol.* **36**: 174-179.

Rasmussen UB, Vouret-Craviari V, Jallat S, Schlesinger Y, Pages G, Pavirani A, Lecocq JP, Pouyssegur J, Van Obberghen-Schilling E, 1991, cDNA cloning and expression of a hamster alpha-thrombin receptor coupled to Ca2+ mobilization. *FEBS Lett.* **288**: 123-128.

Reed DE, Barajas-Lopez C, Cottrell G, Velazquez-Rocha S, Dery O, Grady EF, Bunnett NW, Vanner SJ, 2003, Mast cell tryptase and proteinase-activated receptor 2 induce hyperexcitability of guinea-pig submucosal neurons. *J Physiol.* **547**: 531-542.

Riewald M, Petrovan RJ, Donner A, Mueller BM, Ruf W, 2002, Activation of endothelial cell protease activated receptor 1 by the protein C pathway. *Science* **296**: 1880-1882.

Rodriguez-Linares B, Watson SP, 1994, Phosphorylation of JAK2 in thrombin-stimulated human platelets. *FEBS Lett.* **352**: 335-338.

Roosterman D, Schmidlin F, Bunnett NW, 2003, Rab5a and rab11a mediate agonist-induced trafficking of protease-activated receptor 2. *Am J Physiol Cell Physiol.* **284**: C1319-1329.

Sambrano GR, Huang W, Faruqi T, Mahrus S, Craik C, Coughlin SR, 2000, Cathepsin G activates protease-activated receptor-4 in human platelets. *J Biol Chem.* **275**: 6819-6823.

Scase TJ, Heath MF, Evans RJ, 1997, Cloning of PAR3 cDNA from human platelets, and human erythroleukemic and human promonocytic cell lines. *Blood* **90**: 2113-2114.

Scheele G, Bartelt D, Bieger W, 1981, Characterization of human exocrine pancreatic proteins by two-dimensional isoelectric focusing/sodium dodecyl sulfate gel electrophoresis. *Gastroenterology* **80**: 461-473.

Schwartz LB, Lewis RA, Austen KF, 1981, Tryptase from human pulmonary mast cells. Purification and characterization. *J Biol Chem.* **256**: 11939-11943.

Sharma A, Tao X, Gopal A, Ligon B, Andrade-Gordon P, Steer ML, Perides G, 2005, Protection against acute pancreatitis by activation of protease-activated receptor-2. *Am J Physiol Gastrointest Liver Physiol.* **288**: G388-395.

Smyth RL, Croft NM, O'Hea U, Marshall TG, Ferguson A, 2000, Intestinal inflammation in cystic fibrosis. *Arch Dis Child* **82**: 394-399.

Stead RH, Tomioka M, Quinonez G, Simon GT, Felten SY, Bienenstock J, 1987, Intestinal mucosal mast cells in normal and nematode-infected rat intestines are in intimate contact with peptidergic nerves. *Proc Natl Acad Sci U S A.* **84**: 2975-2979.

Steinhoff M, Vergnolle N, Young SH, Tognetto M, Amadesi S, Ennes HS, Trevisani M, Hollenberg MD, Wallace JL, Caughey GH, Mitchell SE, Williams LM, Geppetti P, Mayer EA, Bunnett NW, 2000, Agonists of proteinase-activated receptor 2 induce inflammation by a neurogenic mechanism. *Nat Med.* **6**: 151-158.

Sun G, Stacey MA, Schmidt M, Mori L, Mattoli S, 2001, Interaction of mite allergens der p3 and der p9 with protease-activated receptor-2 expressed by lung epithelial cells. *J Immunol.* **167**: 1014-1021.

Szmola R, Kukor Z, Sahin-Toth M, 2003, Human mesotrypsin is a unique digestive protease specialized for the degradation of trypsin inhibitors. *J Biol Chem.* **278**: 48580-48589.

Takeuchi T, Shuman MA, Craik CS, 1999, Reverse biochemistry: use of macromolecular protease inhibitors to dissect complex biological processes and identify a membrane-type serine protease in epithelial cancer and normal tissue. *Proc Natl Acad Sci U S A.* **96**: 11054-11061.

Takeuchi T, Harris JL, Huang W, Yan KW, Coughlin SR, Craik CS, 2000, Cellular localization of membrane-type serine protease 1 and identification of protease-activated receptor-2 and single-chain urokinase-type plasminogen activator as substrates. *J Biol Chem.* **275**: 26333-26342.

Tancharoen S, Sarker KP, Imamura T, Biswas KK, Matsushita K, Tatsuyama S, Travis J, Potempa J, Torii M, Maruyama I, 2005, Neuropeptide release from dental pulp cells by RgpB via proteinase-activated receptor-2 signaling. *J Immunol.* **174**: 5796-5804.

Trejo J, Altschuler Y, Fu HW, Mostov KE, Coughlin SR, 2000, Protease-activated receptor-1 down-regulation: a mutant HeLa cell line suggests novel requirements for PAR1 phosphorylation and recruitment to clathrin-coated pits. *J Biol Chem.* **275**: 31255-31265.

Uehara A, Sugawara S, Muramoto K, Takada H, 2002, Activation of human oral epithelial cells by neutrophil proteinase 3 through protease-activated receptor-2. *J Immunol.* **169**: 4594-4603.

Uehara A, Muramoto K, Takada H, Sugawara S, 2003, Neutrophil serine proteinases activate human nonepithelial cells to produce inflammatory cytokines through protease-activated receptor 2. *J Immunol.* **170**: 5690-5696.

Uehara A, Sugawara Y, Sasano T, Takada H, Sugawara S, 2004, Proinflammatory cytokines induce proteinase 3 as membrane-bound and secretory forms in human oral epithelial cells and antibodies to proteinase 3 activate the cells through protease-activated receptor-2. *J Immunol.* **173**: 4179-4189.

Vergnolle N, 2000, Review article: proteinase-activated receptors - novel signals for gastrointestinal pathophysiology. *Aliment Pharmacol Ther.* **14**: 257-266.

Vergnolle N, Hollenberg MD, Sharkey KA, Wallace JL, 1999, Characterization of the inflammatory response to proteinase-activated receptor-2 (PAR2)-activating peptides in the rat paw. *Br J Pharmacol.* **127**: 1083-1090.

Vergnolle N, Macnaughton WK, Al-Ani B, Saifeddine M, Wallace JL, Hollenberg MD, 1998, Proteinase-activated receptor 2 (PAR2)-activating peptides: identification of a receptor distinct from PAR2 that regulates intestinal transport. *Proc Natl Acad Sci U S A.* **95**: 7766-7771.

Vergnolle N, Bunnett NW, Sharkey KA, Brussee V, Compton SJ, Grady EF, Cirino G, Gerard N, Basbaum AI, Andrade-Gordon P, Hollenberg MD, Wallace JL, 2001, Proteinase-activated receptor-2 and hyperalgesia: A novel pain pathway. *Nat Med.* **7**: 821-826.

Vergnolle N, Cellars L, Mencarelli A, Rizzo G, Swaminathan S, Beck P, Steinhoff M, Andrade-Gordon P, Bunnett NW, Hollenberg MD, Wallace JL, Cirino G, Fiorucci S, 2004, A role for proteinase-activated receptor-1 in inflammatory bowel diseases. *J Clin Invest.* **114**: 1444-1456.

Vu TK, Hung DT, Wheaton VI, Coughlin SR, 1991, Molecular cloning of a functional thrombin receptor reveals a novel proteolytic mechanism of receptor activation. *Cell* **64**: 1057-1068.

Wang J, Zheng H, Ou X, Fink LM, Hauer-Jensen M, 2002a, Deficiency of microvascular thrombomodulin and up-regulation of protease-activated receptor-1 in irradiated rat intestine: possible link between endothelial dysfunction and chronic radiation fibrosis. *Am J Pathol.* **160**: 2063-2072.

Wang J, Zheng H, Hollenberg MD, Wijesuriya SJ, Ou X, Hauer-Jensen M, 2003, Up-regulation and activation of proteinase-activated receptor 2 in early and delayed radiation injury in the rat intestine: influence of biological activators of proteinase-activated receptor 2. *Radiat Res.* **160**: 524-535.

Wang J, Zheng H, Ou X, Albertson CM, Fink LM, Herbert JM, Hauer-Jensen M, 2004, Hirudin ameliorates intestinal radiation toxicity in the rat: support for thrombin inhibition as strategy to minimize side-effects after radiation therapy and as countermeasure against radiation exposure. *J Thromb Haemost.* **2**: 2027-2035.

Wang Y, Zhou Y, Szabo K, Haft CR, Trejo J, 2002b, Down-regulation of protease-activated receptor-1 is regulated by sorting nexin 1. *Mol Biol Cell.* **13**: 1965-1976.

Whitcomb DC, Gorry MC, Preston RA, Furey W, Sossenheimer MJ, Ulrich CD, Martin SP, Gates LK, Jr., Amann ST, Toskes PP, Liddle R, McGrath K, Uomo G, Post JC, Ehrlich GD, 1996, Hereditary pancreatitis is caused by a mutation in the cationic trypsinogen gene. *Nat Genet.* **14**: 141-145.

Wiegand U, Corbach S, Minn A, Kang J, Muller-Hill B, 1993, Cloning of the cDNA encoding human brain trypsinogen and characterization of its product. *Gene* **136**: 167-175.

Wojcikiewicz RJ, 2004, Regulated ubiquitination of proteins in GPCR-initiated signaling pathways. *Trends Pharmacol Sci.* **25**: 35-41.

Xu WF, Andersen H, Whitmore TE, Presnell SR, Yee DP, Ching A, Gilbert T, Davie EW, Foster DC, 1998, Cloning and characterization of human protease-activated receptor 4. *Proc Natl Acad Sci U S A.* **95**: 6642-6646.

Zhu WJ, Yamanaka H, Obata K, Dai Y, Kobayashi K, Kozai T, Tokunaga A, Noguchi K, 2005, Expression of mRNA for four subtypes of the proteinase-activated receptor in rat dorsal root ganglia. *Brain Res.* **1041**: 205-211.

Chapter 2

Matrix Metalloproteinases in Gastric Cancer

Nikhil I. Khushalani[1] and Nithya Ramnath[2]
[1]*Department of Medicine, Veterans Affairs Medical Center, 3495 Bailey Ave, Buffalo, NY 14215*
[2]*Department of Medicine, Roswell Park Cancer Institute, Elm and Carlton Street, Buffalo, NY 14263*

1. INTRODUCTION

Despite its decreasing incidence, gastric cancer remains a major cause of morbidity and mortality worldwide. It is the second leading cause of cancer-related death with the incidence being highest in Japan, China, Eastern Europe and Latin America. In 2002, it was estimated that nearly 934,000 new cases were diagnosed with approximately 700,000 deaths from this disease (Parkin *et al* 2005). In the United States, approximately 22,000 new cases of gastric cancer will be diagnosed in the United States in 2005 with 11,500 deaths predicted (Jemal *et al* 2005).

Stomach cancer is often diagnosed at an advanced stage with delayed symptoms. Complete surgical resection remains the only curative modality of treatment. Despite curative attempts at surgery, the five-year survival remains poor at approximately 20%. Failure patterns include both local recurrence and systemic spread (including peritoneal metastases), particularly in those patients with serosal invasion by the primary tumor and in those with lymph node metastases. Hence attempts to improve outcomes in this disease have incorporated the use of adjuvant chemotherapy, radiation therapy or a combination thereof. This is regarded as the standard of care in the United States and the current Intergroup Adjuvant Therapy trial does not include an observation arm. The same treatment dogma does not hold true across the Atlantic or the Pacific where adjuvant therapy is considered investigational. In Japan, a systematic screening program has been adopted for gastric cancer, which may account for the declining mortality from this disease in that

U. Lendeckel and Nigel M. Hooper (eds.), Proteases in Gastrointestinal Tissue, 33-60.

country. Interestingly, stage for stage, Japanese patients appear to fare better than their counterparts in the United States (Noguchi *et al* 2000).

Another incompletely understood phenomenon has been observed over the past two decades regarding the epidemiology of stomach cancer. There has been a progressive decline in the incidence of tumors of the gastric body and distal stomach with a dramatic increase in the incidence of carcinomas of the gastro-esophageal junction and the gastric cardia.

Histologically, tumors of the stomach are divided into an intestinal variant and a diffuse type (Lauren's classification). The former tends to occur in older men and appears to follow a defined pattern of histological progression from metaplasia to dysplasia to carcinoma. The diffuse-type of gastric carcinoma has a higher propensity for younger age at presentation, with a genetic basis being suggested given a higher association with pernicious anemia and persons of blood group A. Germline mutations in the E-cadherin (CDH-1) gene have been found in hereditary diffuse gastric cancer and prophylactic gastrectomy needs to be considered in young patients from kindreds harboring this mutation. (Huntsman *et al* 2001)

In advanced gastric cancer, therapy is typically directed towards palliation. Combination chemotherapy is recommended for patients with a good performance status. A variety of regimens are available to choose from, with cisplatin, 5-fluoro-uracil, epirubicin, taxanes and irinotecan being the commonly used drugs. Activity of these drugs is modest, at best and there is an urgent need to identify novel agents. Improved understanding of the biology of neoplasia has allowed definition of cellular pathways that cause growth and replication of cancer cells. In keeping with this, translational research has moved the focus from traditional cytotoxic chemotherapy to biological compounds that specifically target the tumor or its micro-environment. There is evidence that molecular markers in gastric cancer may provide additional prognostic data in addition to clinical staging. Some markers studied to date include DNA copy number, microsatellite instability, thymidylate synthase, E-cadherin, beta-catenin, p53, COX-2, VEGFR, EGFR and matrix metalloproteinases (MMPs) (Scartozzi *et al* 2004). Development of drugs that target some of these receptors and proteases may lead to a higher therapeutic gain. Examples include epidermal growth factor receptor inhibitors, vascular endothelial growth factor inhibitors and matrix metalloproteinase inhibitors.

2. MATRIX METALLOPROTEINASES

Matrix metalloproteinases (MMPs) are a family of zinc dependent enzymes responsible for the proteolysis of components of the extracellular matrix (ECM). These are pro-enzymes that require activation by splitting off of a pro-peptide. More than twenty members of this family have so far been identified in humans. They are classified on the basis of their domain structure and substrate specificity into a number of groups: collagenases (MMP 1, 8 and 13), gelatinases (MMP-2 and 9), stromalysins (MMP 3 and 10), matrilysins (MMP 7 and 26), membrane type MMP's ([MT- MMPs]; MMPs 14, 15, 16, 17, 24 and 25) (Visse and Nagase 2003). The MT-MMPs are membrane-bound in contrast to the other MMPs that are secreted when activated. Normally MMPs are expressed only when and where needed such as during tissue remodeling during embryonic development and during wound healing. However, increased and/or aberrant expression of various MMPs can occur in physiological and pathological states such as inflammation, tissue healing and malignancy, including tumor cell invasion and metastasis (Woessner 1991).

2.1 Matrix metalloproteinases in cancer

MMPs are expressed in high levels in several cancers of epithelial origin and their level of expression often correlates to the aggressiveness phenotype (Lynch and Matrisian 2002). They contribute to the local growth and spread of malignant lesions (McCawley and Matrisian 2001). MMPs execute these functions by destroying the extracellular matrix, promoting tumor angiogenesis and by a variety of other actions including the activation and deactivation of growth factors and other active molecules. Both MMP-2 and MMP-9 have been implicated in the induction of the angiogenic switch in animal model systems, wherein the balance of pro-angiogenic factors such as bFGF (basic fibroblast growth factor) and VEGF (vascular endothelial growth factor) overcome the expression of angiogenic inhibitors such as angiostatin and thrombospondins (Rundhaug 2003). In addition to promoting metastasis, MMPs may also play a role in tumor initiation and progression (Egeblad and Werb 2002). These actions and the observation that MMPs are up regulated in many tumors have made them attractive targets for tumor drug development. The collagenases cleave interstitial collagen and also digest a number of ECM (extra-cellular matrix) related molecules. The gelatinases digest denatured collagen and gelatin. The stromalysins, besides digesting ECM components also activate a number of proMMPs, which in turn affect other MMPs. Matrilysins are involved in processing cell surface molecules such as fas-ligand and E-cadherin. Most MT-MMPs activate proMMP-2; they can also digest a number of ECM molecules. The unclassified MMPs of the ECM, also process a variety of non-matrix substrates and are involved in the cleavage of a number of growth factors, angiogenic factors as well as factors controlling cell migration (Table 1) (Visse and Nagase 2003).

After their initial discovery, MMPs were viewed as secretory products of neoplastic cells that degraded the basement membrane and ECM enabling local invasion and metastases. It is now well known that this process is far more complex involving angiogenesis, growth factor modulation, apoptosis, cell differentiation and immune surveillance (Coussens *et al* 2002). A schematic representation is depicted in Figure 1.

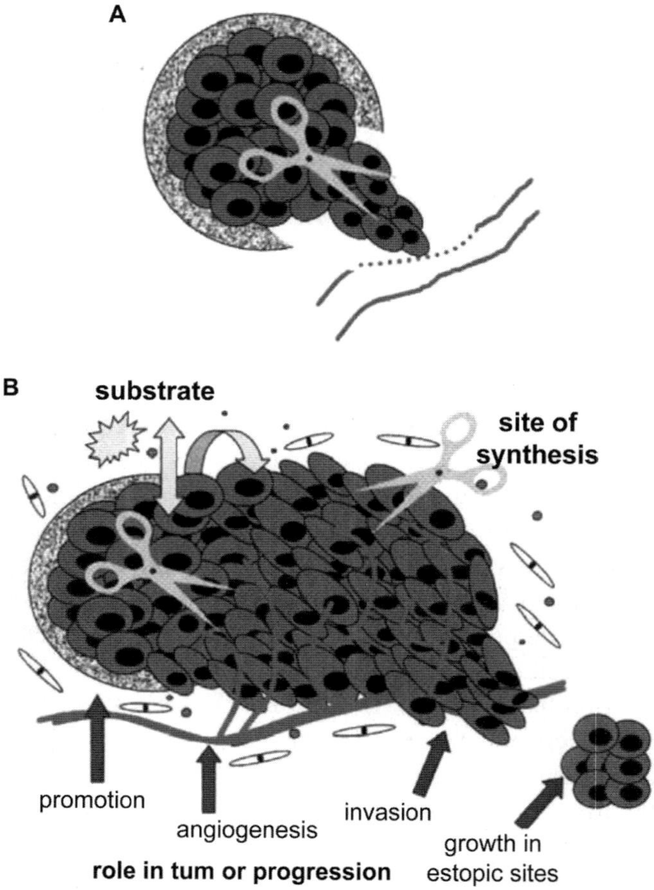

Figure 1: (a) Early view of MMP action in cancer. MMPs (represented by scissors) were viewed as secretory products of tumor cells, simply causing degradation of the BM and ECM. (b) Current multi-function view of MMP action in cancer. Tumor cells, stromal cells and infiltrating inflammatory cells secrete MMPs.

Reprinted with permission from Coussens LM, Fingleton B, Matrisian LM. 2002. Matrix metalloproteinase inhibitors and cancer: trials and tribulations. *Science* **295**:2387-92. Copyright 2002 AAAS

Table 1. Biological Activities Generated by MMP-Mediated Cleavage

Biological Effect	Responsible MMPs	Substrate Cleaved
Keratinocyte migration and reepithelialization	MMP-1	Type I collagen
Osteoclast activation	MMP-13	Type I collagen
Neurite outgrowth	MMP-2	Chondroitin sulphate proteoglycan
Adipocyte differentiation	MMP-7	Fibronectin
Cell migration	MMP-1,-2,-3	Fibronectin
Cell migration	MT1-MMP	CD44
Mammary epithelial cell apoptosis	MMP-3	Basement membrane
Mammary epithelial alveolar formation	MMP-3	Basement membrane
Epithelial-mesenchymal conversion (mammary epithelial cells)	MMP-3	E-cadherin
Mesenchymal cell differentiation with inflammatory phenotype	MMP-2	Not identified
Platelet aggregation	MMP-1	Not identified
Generation of angiostatin-like fragment	MMP-3,-7,-9, -12	Plasminogen
Generation of endostatin-like fragment	MMPs	Type XVIII collagen
Enhanced collagen affinity	MMP-2,-3,-7, -9,-13 (but not MMP-1)	BM-40 (SPARC/osteonectin)
Kidney tubulogenesis	MT1-MMP	Type I collagen
Release of bFGF	MMP-3,-13	Perlecan
Increased bioavailability of IGF1 and cell proliferation	MMP-1,-2,-3 MMPs MMP-11	IGFBP-3 IGFBP-5 IGFBP-1
Activation of VEGF	MMPs	CTGF
Epithelial cell migration	MMP-2, MT1-MMP	Laminin 5γ2 chain
Apoptosis (amnion epithelial cells)	Collagenase	Type I collagen
Proinflammatory	MMP-1,-3,-9	Processing IL-1β from the precursor
Tumor cell resistance	MMP-9	ICAM-1
Antiinflammatory	MMP-1,-2,-9	IL-1β degradation
Antiinflammatory	MMP-1,-2,-3,-13,-14	Monocyte chemo-attractant protein-3
Increased bioavailability of TGF-β	MMP-2,-3,-7	Decorin
Disrupted cell aggregation and increased cell invasion	MMP-3, MMP-7	E-cadherin
Reduced cell adhesion and spreading	MT1-MMP, MT2-MMP, MT3-MMP	Cell surface tissue transglutaminase
Fas receptor–mediated apoptosis	MMP-7	Fas ligand
Reduced IL-2 response	MMP-9	IL-2Rα

2.2 Regulation and activation of MMPs

MMPs are upregulated in many human cancers. Their expression in tumors has been shown to be a reaction to the presence of tumor cells. Contrary to earlier belief, MMPs are largely produced by the stromal cells and inflammatory cells infiltrating the tumor. The former secrete numerous cytokines such as TNF-α (tumor necrosis factor-alpha) and IL-1 (interleukin-1), growth factors and oncogenic proteins, which promote transcription of MMPs. Transforming growth factor-beta (TGF-β) may be a positive or negative regulator of MMP expression depending on the tumor cell type or the environment (Bissell and Radisky, 2001). The transcriptional activators of MMPs can be up regulated or down regulated by members of the signal transduction family such as the MAP kinases. Depending on the cell type, these members may stimulate or inhibit MMP expression. Members of the FOS and JUN family of oncogenes are contained in the transcription factor AP1, whose binding site at the promoter region of most MMP genes allows upregulation and increased expression of MMPs. MMP expression can also be affected by nucleotide polymorphisms in the promoter region of their genes, which in turn create or abolish transcription factor binding sites. Specific MMP-1 and -3 alleles have been associated with increased susceptibility to different cancers (D'Armiento *et al* 1995; Sternlicht *et al* 1999).

The main physiological inhibitors of MMPs are tissue inhibitors of metaric metalloproteinases (TIMPs), a family of low-molecular-weight proteins capable of specifically inhibiting the active forms of the MMPs by binding to the substrate binding site (Birkedal-Hansen *et al* 1993). There are four human TIMPs, all of which are secreted, low molecular-weight proteins that non-covalently bind to the active site of MMPs in a 1:1 ratio. It is likely that the imbalance between the MMPs and the TIMPs occurs early in tumorigenesis and increasing evidence suggests that this plays an important role in tumor invasion and metastasis (Liotta *et al* 1980; Nelson *et al* 2000).

MMPs are synthesized as inactive zymogens, in which an unpaired cysteine interacts with the catalytic Zn^{2+} of the active site rendering it inactive. They are activated by a complex mechanism in response to stimuli, which activates a proteolytic cascade resulting in the uncovering of the 'cysteine switch' on the surface within the pro-domain. Following this, additional sites are exposed for cleavage by other MMPs and the partially unfolded pro-domain now exposes other sites which may be further cleaved or allow ligand binding to substrates eventually culminating in protease activation (Bannikov *et al* 2002). Several of the MMPs (MT-MMP and MMP-3) have important roles as activators of other pro-MMPs (Knauper *et al* 1996), but they also require the co-operation of other classes of proteases such as the plasmin family to be activated. The activation of pro MMPs can occur in the extracellular (proMMP2 activation by MT1-MMP3) or intracellular space (MT-MM's). This becomes especially important when targeting MMPs in tumor cells.

3. ROLE OF MMPs IN GASTRIC CANCER

Studies performed in the past decade have attempted to improve our understanding of the molecular biology of hereditary and sporadic gastric cancer. Their relevance in a large cohort of unselected patients is undefined, though some may have prognostic significance. The availability of monoclonal antibodies has allowed characterization of the MMPs by immunohistochemistry (IHC) in formalin fixed paraffin blocks of patient specimens. Matrix metalloproteinases have been implicated in all stages of gastric carcinogenesis from susceptibility to metastasis. The following sections will summarize the status of our current knowledge of the MMPs, TIMPs and related proteases in gastric cancer.

3.1 Gelatinases in gastric cancer

Gelatinase A (MMP-2) and Gelatinase B (MMP-9) comprise this group of proteases. Following the activity of collagenases, further degradation of denatured interstitial collagen is undertaken by gelatinases. Both MMP-2 and MMP-9 have been implicated in tumor angiogenesis and growth (Itoh *et al* 1998; Kahari and Saarialho-Kere 1999; Kurizaki *et al* 1998). Along with MMP-7, these MMPs have been the most extensively studied in gastric cancer.

Pre-clinical studies in gastric carcinoma cell lines have revealed aberrant expression of MMPs with correlation to the invasive potential of the tumor cells (Koshikawa *et al* 1992; Schwartz *et al* 1994). Over-expression of gelatinases has been demonstrated in immunohistochemical studies performed on tissue samples of stomach cancer compared with surrounding normal gastric mucosa (D'Errico *et al* 1991; David *et al* 1994; Grigioni *et al* 1994; Parsons *et al* 1997a). Monig and colleagues examined 114 gastrectomy specimens in patients who underwent surgical resection with lymphadenectomy for primary gastric adenocarcinomas (Monig *et al* 2001). Surgery was deemed curative in 92% and approximately two-thirds of patients had nodal metastases. A semi-quantitative evaluation of MMP-2 immunohistochemical expression in formalin-fixed paraffin-embedded revealed a positive result in 82% of specimens with the intensity of staining correlating with the depth of the primary tumor, as well as with the nodal and distant metastatic status. In fact, all patients with N3 (22/22) or M+ (19/19) disease had positive MMP-2 expression. The authors concluded that MMP-2 expression was a predictor of disease progression in gastric cancer and suggested a possible prognostic role for this matrix metalloproteinase. While others studies have previously shown similar findings (Grigioni *et al* 1994), MMP-2 expression however, has not been consistently linked with clinical stage, tumor grade and prognosis. (Ko *et al* 1998; Allgayer *et al* 1998)

Immunohistochemistry does not distinguish between the precursor and active forms of MMPs, a disadvantage that is overcome by zymogen gel electrophoresis. Using this technique, the active form of gelatinase was demonstrated in gastric and colorectal tumor explants in a small study. Corresponding normal tissue in all but one case lacked this 66-kDa gelatinase suggesting that activated gelatinase may be unique to carcinogenesis (Yamagata *et al* 1991). In a series of experiments, Nomura *et al* have elegantly demonstrated that membrane-type matrix metalloproteinase (MT-MMP) which is required for activation of the zymogen of MMP-2 (proMMP-2) is expressed in human gastric carcinoma (Sato *et al* 1994; Nomura *et al* 1995; Nomura *et al* 1996). Using gelatin zymography they found a correlation between MT-MMP expression and gelatinase-A activation and further demonstrated that this activation occurs exclusively within carcinoma cells expressing MT-MMP, but not within normal gastric mucosa. In addition, the activation ratio of pro-MMP-2 was significantly higher in cases with lymphatic invasion and also correlated with advanced carcinoma. This suggests that activation of MMP-2 may be important in the progression and spread of gastric cancer. Evaluation of other proteases revealed increased production of MMP-1, MMP-3, MMP-9 and TIMP-1 by neoplastic cells (Nomura *et al* 1996).

An important observation was made by Miao *et al* regarding the susceptibility to gastric carcinoma and a functional polymorphism in the promoter region of the MMP-2 gene (Miao *et al* 2003). Previous studies had demonstrated that a *-1306C→T* polymorphism within the promoter of the MMP-2 gene decreased its activity and occurred with higher frequency in patients with lung cancer (Price *et al* 2001; Yu *et al* 2002). Testing this hypothesis in adenocarcinoma of the gastric cardia, 356 patients and 789 frequency-matched controls within an ethnic Chinese population were evaluated in a case-control study. Using high-performance liquid chromatography and direct DNA sequencing to determine MMP-2 genotypes, the authors demonstrated a greater than three-fold increase in the risk of development of gastric cardia adenocarcinoma in individuals harboring the *CC* genotype compared to those with the variant *CT* or *TT* genotypes. This risk was more pronounced in smokers and persons less than 60 years of age. It is unclear whether these results can be extended to tumors of the gastric body or of the distal stomach given the changing epidemiology of this disease.

It does purport a role for inherited susceptibility to some cancers based on protease genotyping.

Matrix metalloproteinase-9 (Gelatinase-B) is a 92-kDa enzyme that cleaves type IV collagen. In addition, it plays a role in the degradation of laminin, elastin and fibronectin (Zucker *et al* 2000). Given similarity in function, MMP-9 has often been studied in conjunction with MMP-2 in gastric cancer. In a study of 50 gastric cancer patients, Sier *et al* demonstrated significantly elevated tumor tissue levels of both gelatinases compared to tumor-free adjacent mucosa of the stomach (Sier *et al* 1996). Patients with high tumor levels of MMP-2 or MMP-9 had a significantly inferior survival, independent of histopathological prognostic variants. Another study examined MMP-1, MMP-3, TIMP-1 and TIMP-2 in addition to MMP-2 and MMP-9 in a group of 74 gastrectomy specimens by immunohistochemistry on formalin-fixed paraffin embedded tissue (Murray *et al* 1998). Nearly all cancers expressed MMP-2 (70/74 specimens; 94%) and more than two-thirds expressed MMP-1 (73%) and MMP-9 (70%). In contrast, MMP-3 expression was infrequent. The expression of MMP-1 and -9 correlated with the intestinal variant of stomach cancer but, unlike the Sier study, there was no correlation to overall survival in all the MMPs/ inhibitors evaluated. The normal stomach mucosa within the specimens did not demonstrate immunoreactivity for the proteases or their inhibitors suggesting a role for these enzymes in the process of tumorigenesis.

The variable results from studies examining MMPs individually clearly suggests that the process of cancer development is more complex and involves a dynamic interplay between the tumor cells, surrounding stroma and the host immune system (Heppner *et al* 1996; Nelson *et al* 2000; Bissell and Radisky 2001; Jacks and Weinberg 2002). Investigators in China evaluated MMP-9 in concert with its natural inhibitor TIMP-1 in 256 primary gastric carcinomas (Zhang *et al* 2003). In addition to independent correlation with stage, depth of invasion and nodal metastases, this study stratified patients into cohorts demonstrating a poorer prognosis for those patients whose tumors expressed MMP-9 but lacked TIMP-1. These tumors had a higher frequency of serosal invasion as well as nodal involvement. Others have evaluated the co-expression of MMPs and urokinase-type plasminogen activator (uPA), a member of the serine protease family that is active in degradation of the extra-cellular matrix (Migita *et al* 1999; Ji *et al* 2005). These serine proteases have been linked to tumor invasion and metastases in stomach cancer (Park *et al* 1997; Kaneko *et al* 2003). Single nucleotide polymorphisms in the promoter region of the MMP-9 gene have also been corroborated with the degree of tumor invasiveness, clinical stage and lymphatic involvement in gastric cancer (Matsumura *et al* 2005). These investigators reported that a *-1562C→T* polymorphism affects the prognosis and invasiveness phenotype of gastric cancer, though interestingly the frequency of this genotype was similar in control subjects.

The majority of studies discussed above looked at MMPs at the tissue level. Torii *et al* (1997) examined levels of MMP-9 in plasma and showed that these were higher in patients with gastric cancer than in normal subjects. There was a decline in concentration following surgical resection. Patients with early gastric cancer also exhibited higher mean values of and positivity rates for MMP-9 than healthy individuals. The preoperative plasma MMP-9 concentration correlated closely with the TNM stage. The authors concluded that plasma MMP-9 concentration could be used for detection of primary or recurrent gastric cancer, and for estimation of tumor extent (Torii *et al* 1997). Serum MMP-9 levels have also been associated with a prominent stromal reaction in this disease (Shen *et al* 2000).

As discussed earlier, diagnosis of stomach cancer is often delayed due to lack of specific symptoms. Even with early detection and resection, some gastric tumors have a propensity to recur. Hence identifying the molecular characteristics of these tumors may assist in therapeutic decisions (gastrectomy versus endoscopic mucosal resection), risk stratification and possibly, recommendations for adjuvant therapy in these individuals. Kabashima *et al* (1999) showed that lymph node positive intramucosal gastric carcinomas had a higher expression of MMP-9 compared to those that were node-negative. Other characteristics of these tumors included ulceration, larger size, poorly differentiated histology, and presence of lymphatic permeation. This suggests an early role for MMP-9 in tumor progression (Kabashima *et al* 2000).

Activity of MMP-2 and -9 has been shown to be associated with malignant ascites in a study by Sun and colleagues in 20/23 and 18/23 cases respectively (Sun *et al* 2003). There were six cases of gastric cancer with 5 demonstrating positive activity. They found no gelatinase activity within samples of non-malignant peritoneal fluid (cirrhotic and tuberculous; n=44). This observation supports further investigation into the development of matrix metalloproteinase inhibitors for intra-peritoneal use as this is a common site of failure in gastric cancer (Beattie and Smyth 1998; Parsons *et al* 1997b; Wada *et al* 2003).

3.2 Matrilysins and stromelysins in gastric cancer

The principle substrates for these enzymes include non-collagen matrix molecules, such as laminin, proteoglycans and fibronectin. In addition they play a role in the activation of other latent MMPs and thus indirectly effect collagen degradation. Matrilysins lack the carboxy-terminal hemopexin domain and include MMP-7 and MMP-26 (Parsons *et al* 1997a; Visse and Nagase 2003).

While the role of gelatinases A and B are well described in tumors including gastric cancer, there is emerging data on other MMPs. Pre-clinical studies in cell lines of prostate cancer and colon cancer suggested that MMP-7 was involved in progression of tumors (Powell *et al* 1993; Witty *et al* 1994). Honda *et al* used polymerase chain reaction based experiments to detect MMP-7 mRNA from 47 primary gastric tumors and paired adjacent normal gastric mucosa. Tumor tissue expressed higher levels in 41/47 (87%) cases. Greater depth of invasion and higher frequency of lympho-vascular permeation was noted in those cases that had a tumor/normal mRNA ration of greater than 2.1. Although these cases also had a higher rate of lymph node metastases, this was not statistically significant (Honda *et al* 1996). Similarly Yamashita *et al* showed that enhanced production of proMMP-7 (the inactive zymogen for MMP-7) correlated with invasion and metastasis (Yamashita *et al* 1998). Additionally the intestinal-variant of gastric carcinomas produced greater amounts of MMP-7 compared to the diffuse variety. The former more commonly metastasizes to the liver than to the peritoneum, which is a feature of the diffuse variety (Moriguchi *et al* 1991). This biologic feature appears similar to the pattern of metastases in colorectal cancer, a tumor where MMP-7 is often over-expressed (Itoh *et al* 1996; McDonnell *et al* 1991; Mori *et al* 1995). However, others have reported the contrary, in that higher levels of MMP-7 were noted in the diffuse versus intestinal variant of gastric cancer (Kitoh *et al* 2004). Ajisaki *et al* (2004) confirmed that strong positivity for MMP-7 (by immuno-histochemistry) within the primary lesion was associated with deep invasion of the gastric wall, nodal metastases, and infiltration of vessels or lymphatics. The five-year survival rate was nearly double in the weak expressers compared to those whose tumors were strongly positive (Ajisaka *et al* 2004). This difference in survival was even more pronounced when degree of nodal positivity (strong versus weak; 17% versus 68%) was considered. This work confirmed their earlier immunohistochemical observations concerning nodal involvement in gastric cancer (Ajisaka *et al* 2001). Liu *et al* also showed that increased expression of MMP-7 correlated with the invasive front particularly in tumors penetrating the muscularis propria and in clinical stages II-IV as against cancers confined to the submucosal layer or stage I gastric cancers respectively (Liu *et al* 2002a,b). Others have also confirmed the up-regulation of MMP-7 expression with serosal invasion suggesting the role this protease may play in tumor invasion (Adachi *et al* 1998; Chen *et al* 2004; Huachuan *et al* 2003; Zheng *et al* 2003).

Similar to studies of MMP2 and MMP-9, the matrilysin MMP-7 has been evaluated in early stage disease as well (Aihara *et al* 2005). Its expression and the nuclear accumulation of β-catenin were predictive of invasion and metastases in early, undifferentiated gastric carcinoma. The accumulation of β-catenin is believed to transactivate the MMP-7 promoter and contribute to neoplastic transformation (Crawford *et al* 1999). Detection of MMP-7 mRNA by reverse transcriptase-polymerase chain reaction (RT-PCR) in peritoneal fluid washings prior to surgical resection has been suggested as a means to identify patients who may benefit from intra-peritoneal therapy. This technique was used by Yonemura *et al* to correlate the MMP-7 RT-PCR assay (independently and in combination with standard cytology) to the risk of peritoneal dissemination in gastric cancer (Yonemura *et al* 2000, 2001).

Like matrilysins, the stromelysins also have broad substrate specificity. This group includes MMP-3, MMP-10 and MMP-11. MMP-3 also performs the important function of activating numerous proMMPs to generate a fully active enzyme, particularly MMP-1 (Suzuki *et al* 1990). Their role in gastric cancer is under investigation with relatively few studies reported to date. In Murray's study mentioned previously, the expression of MMP-3 was only noted in 27% of gastric cancer cases, far less than the frequency of MMP-2 and MMP-9 (Murray *et al* 1998) while an earlier study found no expression of stromelysin-1 (MMP-3) or stromelysin-2 (MMP-10) in ten gastric cancer samples examined (McDonnell *et al* 1991). Zhang *et al* (2004) evaluated an adenine nucleotide polymorphism (6A/5A) of the MMP-3 promoter in 417 patients with esophageal squamous cell carcinoma (ESCC) or gastric cardia adenocarcinoma. Smokers with at least one 5A allele had a higher risk of ESCC compared to 6A homozygotes; this polymorphism was also linked to the incidence of lymphatic metastases in ESCC, but no such correlation was found in gastric cancer (Zhang *et al* 2004).

3.3 Collagenases and membrane type-matrix metalloproteinases (MT-MMP) in gastric cancer

Since the first description of tadpole collagenase activity over four decades ago (Gross and Lapiere 1962), the history of the discovery and development of the matrix metalloproteinase family has been the subject of numerous review publications (Brinckerhoff and Matrisian 2002; Egeblad and Werb 2002; Parsons *et al* 1997a). MMP-1, MMP-8, MMP-13 and MMP-18 belong to the group of collagenases that are capable of digesting native collagens I, II and III at a specific site three-fourths from the N-terminus. Six MMPs (14, 15, 16, 17, 24 and 25) are MT-MMPs, a recently identified group of intrinsic plasma proteins. In addition to their ability to degrade the extracellular matrix, most of these enzymes serve as physiological activators of proMMP-2 (gelatinase-A) and have a role in angiogenesis.

Over-expression of MMP-1 has been linked to poor prognosis in several gastro-intestinal cancers and malignant melanoma (Ito *et al* 1999; Murray *et al* 1996; Nikkola *et al* 2002). Inoue *et al* (1999) reported a similar conclusion in gastric cancer where MMP-1 expression was detected in 75% cases and was associated with nodal and peritoneal metastases. An interaction between tumor cells and stromal cells (fibroblasts) may be responsible for regulation of MMP-1 protein expression (Sakurai *et al* 1997a; Sakurai *et al* 1997b). Histopathological correlation to the intestinal variant (as opposed to the diffuse form) in gastric carcinoma has also been demonstrated but there was no association between MMP-1 and survival (Migita *et al* 1999; Murray *et al* 1998). The role of collagenase-3 (MMP-13) in gastric cancer tumorigenesis is yet undefined, but recent work suggests it may involve an interplay with MMP-2 and MT1-MMP (Elnemr *et al* 2003).

Emerging data suggest that MT-MMPs function in physiologic and pathologic conditions, including tumor progression (Sato *et al* 2005; Sounni and Noel 2005). In gastric cancer, MT1-MMP co-localized with MMP-2 in tumor cells; microdissection revealed activated MMP-2 in invasive nests of tumor cells suggesting its induction in tumor associated stromal tissue followed by activation on the tumor cell surface (Nomura *et al* 1995). This landmark report was the first to demonstrate MT-MMP-assisted activation of the inactive zymogen form of MMP-2 in human gastric cancer. In a small study of 25 gastric cancer patients, a difference of MT1-MMP expression of up to 10-fold was noted between tumor and normal tissue (Caenazzo *et al* 1998). A larger study by Bando *et al* identified MT-MMP expression as an independent factor for poor prognosis in gastric cancer (Bando *et al* 1998).

3.4 TIMPs in gastric cancer

The tissue inhibitor of matrix metalloproteinase (TIMP) family comprises four members (TIMP-1 to TIMP-4) that are physiologic regulators of MMPs. These small proteins with molecular weights of approximately 21 kDa perform other biologic functions in addition to MMP inhibition. An imbalance between proteases and their naturally occurring inhibitors may affect the integrity of the ECM, a pre-requisite for neoplastic progression.

Tsuchiya *et al* (1993) injected human gastric cancer cells (derived from the cell line KKLS) into the chorioallantoic membrane vein of a fertilized chicken egg. Embryo livers were harvested and examined 7 days later. They found that TIMP levels were undetectable in the cells from metastatic colonies derived from chick embryonic liver. Furthermore, expression of a transfected TIMP-1 complementary DNA in this particular cell line caused the inhibition of metastasis. This suggested that TIMP-1 was crucial for steps involved in metastasis of gastric cancer. Watanabe *et al* (1996) confirmed the role of TIMP-1 in metastasis using an orthotopic transplantation mouse metastasis model demonstrating that expression of a transfected TIMP-1 gene in the cell line inhibited metastasis.

In clinical trials, the balance between MMPs and TIMPs is important in determining invasiveness and metastatic potential of gastric cancer (Joo *et al* 2000; Zhang *et al* 2003). In the latter study, an imbalance between MMP-9 (increased) and its inhibitor TIMP-1 (decreased) was associated with survival. Contrary to these results for TIMP-1, plasma and tissue levels of TIMP-1 have been correlated to tumor invasion and aggressiveness in gastric cancer (Mimori *et al* 1997; Yoshikawa *et al* 1999, 2001). These discrepancies may be related to additional functions of TIMPs that occur independent of MMP activity (Hornebeck *et al* 2005). Koyama *et al* studied the expression of MMPs and their inhibitors TIMP-2 and -4 in tumor and tumor infiltrating lymphocytes; they were able to show increased expression of MMP-2, -9, MT1-MMP and TIMP-2 and -4 in both tumor cells as well as in the tumor infiltrating lymphocytes, suggesting a host response to the tumors (Koyama 2004).

These inhibitory functions have led to the use of TIMPs as anti-cancer agents using gene transfer methodology. Unfortunately laboratory studies to date have demonstrated little success with low efficacy and poor specificity (Chau *et al* 2003).

3.5 Helicobacter pylori, matrix metalloproteinases and gastric cancer

The role of *Helicobacter pylori* in the pathogenesis of chronic atrophic gastritis and gastric cancer is well known (Nomura *et al* 1991; Parsonnet *et al* 1991) and this organism is classified as a class I carcinogen. Infection with *H. pylori* strains possessing the cagA pathogenicity island confer a higher risk (odds ratio = 1.9) of developing gastric cancer, particularly the intestinal variant of the distal stomach (Blaser *et al* 1995). In vitro, *H. pylori* stimulates the secretion of MMPs from gastric epithelial cells (Bebb *et al* 2003; Gooz *et al* 2001, 2003; Wroblewski *et al* 2003). Interestingly, infection with cagA + strains have been found to be associated with increased expression of MMP-7 in gastric epithelial cells compared to infection with cagA - strains (Crawford *et al* 2003). This differential induction may be one of several mechanisms that eventually lead to mucosal damage and augmentation of the risk of cancer development.

4. MATRIX METALLOPROTEINASE INHIBITORS

As evidenced by laboratory and clinical data, MMPs play a crucial role in cancer development and progression. Hence pharmacologic inhibition of the MMP cascade would be expected to dramatically alter the therapeutic armamentarium we have available at present. Unfortunately, the enthusiasm for matrix metalloproteinase inhibitors (MMPIs) has been somewhat diminished by their less than stellar success in the clinic to date. Numerous reasons have been put forth for this seeming paradox. The complexity of the interactions of the MMPs with other proteases, the multiplicity of their targets, the stage of the tumor, the selectivity of the agent used and the study design, including the validity of defined endpoints are some of the more critical issues that need to be addressed. Excellent reviews of these topics have been published (Chau *et al* 2003; Hidalgo and Eckhardt 2001; Hoekstra *et al* 2001; Ramnath and Creaven 2004).

Pharmacological inhibition as an approach to anti-cancer therapy has mainly targeted MMP activity in the extracellular matrix. However there are a series of steps (induction, transcription, translation, secretion, activation and degradation) within the MMP activation pathway that can serve as potential targets for intervention.

4.1 MMPIs in gastric cancer

Batimastat

This was the first MMPI in clinical trials in patients with cancer. It is a potent non-selective inhibitor of MMP-1, -2, -3, -7 and -9. Its major disadvantage is lack of oral bioavailability. Hence clinical evaluation was restricted to intra-peritoneal and intra-pleural use for malignant effusions. Although initial results were promising (Beattie and Smyth 1998; Wojtowicz-Praga *et al* 1996), further development of this drug has ceased.

Marimastat

Marimastat (BB-2516; TA-2516) was the first oral MMPI to undergo evaluation in clinical trials. It is an orally administered, low molecular weight peptido-mimetic agent with a hydroxamate group that is closely related to batimastat. Marimastat is a potent and reversible inhibitor of MMP-1, -2, -3, -7, -9, and -12.

Marimastat has been evaluated in pre-clinical models of gastric cancer. In a human xenograft model, this drug reduced tumor growth rate and increased survival (Watson *et al* 1999). In another human gastric cancer xenograft, TMK-1, this drug inhibited the peritoneal spread of tumor both independently as well as in combination with mitomycin-C (Kimata *et al* 2002). No human studies with this combination have been reported.

The initial phase I study in healthy volunteers established the maximum tolerated dose at 800mg single oral dose (Millar *et al* 1998). This drug was well tolerated with no accumulation in the plasma with continuous daily dosing for 6 days. Subsequently, several phase I-II studies were undertaken with varying doses and schedules; by itself and in combination with chemotherapy (Hoekstra *et al* 2001; Primrose *et al* 1999; Wojtowicz-Praga *et al* 1998). The dose limiting toxicity was severe inflammatory polyarthritis appearing in the first month and often persisting for 8 weeks or longer, even after discontinuation of treatment. This led to careful re-examination of dose, plasma concentrations and range of biologic activity. At doses that did not cause this disabling side effect (5-10 mg twice a day), plasma concentrations were well below the range for biologic activity. The higher doses that were required to block the MMPs could not be achieved because of adversity. Several Phase II studies in a variety of solid tumors were initiated examining surrogate markers as end-points rather than the traditional Phase II end-point of response rates. There was a dose dependent inhibition on the rate of tumor marker elevation, but no impact on survival. It was noted that patients who achieved a complete biological response (if the tumor marker did not rise above the pretreatment values during the first 4 weeks on treatment) had a longer survival (Nemunaitis *et al* 1998).

Tierney *et al* performed a pilot study of Marimastat in advanced, inoperable gastric and gastro-esophageal cancers. Thirty-five patients with advanced tumors were recruited. Initially Marimastat was given at a dose of 50mg twice daily but then reduced to 25 mg once daily after the first 6 patients when a parallel study using 100mg twice daily reported "inflammatory polyarthritis" in 5/6 patients. The drug demonstrated good oral bioavailability with higher plasma trough levels compared with healthy volunteers suggesting that patients with advanced malignancies might have alterations in hepatic metabolism of the drug. Despite the reduced dose, about one-third of the patients developed arthralgia/myalgia, being reversible in most. Additionally, in four patients using marimastat for more than 3 months, a subcutaneous skin thickening of the palmar surface of the hands resembling Dupuytren's disease developed. At endoscopy, 10 patients showed an increased fibrotic cover of the tumor, 8 had decreased hemorrhagic appearance, and in at least 2 cases there was evidence of increased stromal fibroblastic tissue (Tierney *et al* 1999).

Following this pilot study, British Biotech supported a large phase III randomized trial of marimastat versus placebo in patients with advanced gastric cancer, previously untreated or stable after initial treatment with 5-

fluorouracil (Bramhall *et al* 2002). This study recruited 369 patients, randomizing them to marimastat 10mg bid versus placebo. The median survival was 138 days for placebo and 160 days for marimastat ($p = 0.024$), with 2-year survival of 3% and 9% respectively. There was also a significant benefit in progression-free survival. Ten percent of patients on the marimastat arm withdrew from the study due to musculoskeletal pain. This condition characterized by inflammation of axial or appendicular joints, occurred around the 2nd or 3rd month of treatment and led to contractures of the hands in 5 patients. There was also an increase (>5%) in side effects such as anemia, jaundice, weight loss and ascites in the marimastat arm compared with placebo. Although the survival benefit can be considered modest, this trial was the first to demonstrate a therapeutic gain for a MMPI in clinical evaluation, particularly in the sub-set of patients who had received chemotherapy previously.

Studies evaluating the efficacy of marimastat in other tumor types including pancreas, lung, breast, prostate and brain have been completed or are ongoing.

CP-471,358

In vitro this drug is a potent inhibitor of MMP-2 and MMP-9 inhibitor. In a phase I study in 38 patients with advanced solid tumors, the dose limiting toxicity of orally administered CP-471,358 was grade III myalgia and arthralgia, similar to that seen with treatment with most matrix metalloproteinase inhibitors. This was seen with all dose levels and schedules except one (150mg bid). Although the joint symptoms observed were reversible on cessation of treatment, a drug-free interval of one week did not abrogate the recurrence of adversity. This represents a limitation for potential long-term use of this compound (Planting *et al* 2005).

Newer directions in MMPI development

As the molecular biology of gastric cancer continues to unfold, rational development of newer MMPIs may translate into better clinical outcomes. Several MMPs including the gelatinases and the MT-MMPs have been linked to angiogenesis (Handsley and Edwards 2005). MMP-2 and MMP-9 cause an imbalance in the angiogenic switch in favor of pro-angiogenesis factors such as VEGF and bFGF. Therefore specifically targeting these MMPs may be more appropriate in gastric cancer, though the compounds tested so far have been hampered by the notable musculoskeletal adversity. MMPs are known to inhibit shedding of membrane bound proteins, including tumor necrosis factor-α. Inhibition of MMPs and the closely related proteins ADAMs (a disintegrin and metalloproteinase domain) and ADAMTs (a disintegrin and metalloproteinase with thrombospondin motifs), which have ‘sheddase’ activity have been implicated with the musculoskeletal side effects noted with several agents of this class. In keeping with the concept of rational design, BMS -275291 was designed to avoid the inhibition of the sheddases (Naglich *et al* 2001). In a phase I study of this MMPI in advanced cancer, there was no dose limiting joint toxicity (Rizvi *et al* 2004). In another novel concept, Lockhart and colleagues used a wound angiogenesis assay rather than standard Phase I trial end-points (maximum tolerated dose) to evaluate BMS-275291 (Lockhart *et al* 2003). However further development of this compound is on hold following a negative Phase II/III study in advanced non-small cell lung cancer (Leighl, 2004).

4.2 Other approaches to inhibition of MMPs

The clear lack of major clinical success in the few MMPIs tested in trials of gastric cancer to date have underscored the importance of investigating novel agents to target the tumor and its micro-environment. The following have been carried out in pre-clinical models using gastric cancer cell lines. Whether this eventually lives up to the promise of therapeutic efficacy *in-vivo* remains to be seen.

4.2.1 Inhibition of transforming growth factor-beta (TGF-β)

TGF-β is thought to play an important role in invasive gastric cancer (Pasche 2001). One mechanism put forth involves an increase in urokinase-type plasminogen activator (uPA) and MMP-9 expression (Festuccia *et al* 2000).

Interferon-gamma: Using the human gastric cell line GCTM-1, Kuga *et al* (2003) showed that TGF-β induced enhanced MMP-9 and uPA expression; this was inhibited by interferon-gamma with decrease in the invasiveness of the carcinoma cells. Interferon-gamma could be a potential new therapeutic tool, particularly in gastric carcinomas with high levels of TGF-beta.

Tranilast: N-3,4-dimethoxycinamoyl anthranilic acid (tranilast) inhibited the metastasis of gastric cancer cells that were co-cultured with gastric fibroblasts; this was putatively mediated by decreasing MMP-2 and TGF-β production by the fibroblasts (Yashiro *et al* 2003).

Protein-bound polysaccharide (PSK): Zhang *et al* (2000) demonstrated inhibition of TGF-β and therefore of MMP-2 and -9 in a gastric and pancreatic cancer cell lines by a protein-bound polysaccharide, PSK that has been used as a biological response modifier. This resulted in decreased invasiveness but did not affect cell viability or proliferation in these tumor cell lines.

4.2.2 Prevention of lymphatic and peritoneal metastases

R-94138: As outlined in previous sections, several MMPs have been associated with lymphatic and peritoneal dissemination and thus poorer prognosis in gastric cancer. Peritoneal injection of R-94138, an MMPI, in orthotopic nude mice models decreased lymphatic permeation and lymph nodal invasion by the cancer cells. This could potentially translate into useful adjuvant therapy to prevent peritoneal dissemination (Matsuoka *et al* 2001). The same was confirmed by Igarashi *et al* (1999) when R-94138 was combined with chemotherapy.

4.2.3 Induction of TIMP-1 and TIMP-2

TIMP-1 and -2 are naturally occurring inhibitors of MMPS. Attempts have been made to increase the TIMPs; one such method in a pre-clinical model involved use of conjugated linoleic acid (CLA); it appeared that c9, t11-CLA inhibited type IV collagenases (MMP-2 and -9) and inhibited invasion by increasing the expression of TIMP-1 and TIMP-2 mRNA (Chen *et al* 2003).

4.2.4 Anti-sense oligonucleotides

Pre-clinical testing of anti-sense oligonucleotides specifically directed against MMP-7 inhibited invasion without affecting proliferation. This could be potentially developed for use against peritoneal dissemination of gastric cancer provided technical constraints are resolved.

4.2.5 Inhibition of MMP modulators

Green tea: Epigallocatechin gallate (EGCG), a green tea catechin has been shown to inhibit MMPs in human gastric cancer AGS cells potentially by inhibiting upstream modulators of AP-1, a transcription factor as well as suppression of mitogen activated protein kinase (Kim *et al* 2004).

5. CONCLUSIONS

Gastric cancer remains a major public health problem worldwide in the 21st century. Moreover the dramatic rise in the incidence of proximal stomach tumors and those of the gastro-esophageal junction is a disconcerting trend. Despite significant advances, the heterogeneity in histopathology and molecular biology of this disease constitutes an impediment to complete molecular delineation, similar to many other epithelial malignancies. The therapeutic plateau reached with traditional cytotoxic therapy makes this a fertile ground for the investigation of targeted therapy; much of this will be contingent upon pursuing the development of agents such as matrix metalloproteinase inhibitors or their close counterparts, and with the appropriate collaboration between academia and industry. The limited success of these compounds so far should not be a deterrent to further investigation; rather, the challenges of future research efforts would be in identifying the appropriate substrate at the correct time point in the process of gastric carcinogenesis, using these agents in combination with chemotherapy or other targeted drugs, evaluating their efficacy in the setting of minimal residual disease (eg. adjuvant therapy) and identifying surrogate markers of response to the inhibitors of matrix metalloproteinases.

REFERENCES

Adachi Y, Itoh F, Yamamoto H, Matsuno K, Arimura Y, Kusano M, Endoh T, Hinoda Y, Oohara M, Hosokawa M, Imai K, 1998, Matrix metalloproteinase matrilysin (MMP-7) participates in the progression of human gastric and esophageal cancers. *Int J Oncol.* **13:** 1031-1035.

Aihara R, Mochiki E, Nakabayashi T, Akazawa K, Asao T, Kuwano H, 2005, Clinical significance of mucin phenotype, beta-catenin and matrix metalloproteinase 7 in early undifferentiated gastric carcinoma. *Br J Surg.* **92:** 454-462.

Ajisaka H, Fushida S, Yonemura Y, Miwa K, 2001, Expression of insulin-like growth factor-2, c-MET, matrix metalloproteinase-7 and MUC-1 in primary lesions and lymph node metastatic lesions of gastric cancer. *Hepatogastroenterol.* **48:** 1788-1792.

Ajisaka H, Yonemura Y, Miwa K, 2004, Correlation of lymph node metastases and expression of matrix metalloproteinase-7 in patients with gastric cancer. *Hepatogastroenterol.* **51:** 900-905.

Allgayer H, Babic R, Beyer BC, Grutzner KU, Tarabichi A, Schildberg FW, Heiss MM, 1998, Prognostic relevance of MMP-2 (72-kD collagenase IV) in gastric cancer. *Oncology* **55:** 152-160.

Bando E, Yonemura Y, Endou Y, Sasaki T, Taniguchi K, Fujita H, Fushida S, Fujimura T, Nishimura G, Miwa K, Seiki M, 1998, Immunohistochemical study of MT-MMP tissue status in gastric carcinoma and correlation with survival analyzed by univariate and multivariate analysis. *Oncol Rep.* **5:** 1483-1488.

Bannikov GA, Karelina TV, Collier IE, Marmer BL, Goldberg GI, 2002, Substrate binding of gelatinase B induces its enzymatic activity in the presence of intact propeptide. *J Biol Chem.* **277:** 16022-16027.

Beattie GJ and Smyth JF, 1998, Phase I study of intraperitoneal metalloproteinase inhibitor BB94 in patients with malignant ascites. *Clin Cancer Res.* **4:** 1899-1902.

Bebb JR, Letley DP, Thomas RJ, Aviles F, Collins HM, Watson SA, Hand NM, Zaitoun A, Atherton JC, 2003, Helicobacter pylori upregulates matrilysin (MMP-7) in epithelial cells in vivo and in vitro in a Cag dependent manner. *Gut* **52:** 1408-1413.

Birkedal-Hansen H, Moore WG, Bodden MK, Windsor LJ, Birkedal-Hansen B, DeCarlo A, Engler JA, 1993, Matrix metalloproteinases: a review. *Crit Rev Oral Biol Med.* **4:** 197-250.

Bissell MJ and Radisky D, 2001, Putting tumours in context. *Nat Rev Cancer* **1:** 46-54.

Blaser MJ, Perez-Perez GI, Kleanthous H, Cover TL, Peek RM, Chyou PH, Stemmermann GN, Nomura A, 1995, Infection with Helicobacter pylori strains possessing cagA is associated with an increased risk of developing adenocarcinoma of the stomach. *Cancer Res.* **55:** 2111-2115.

Bramhall SR, Hallissey MT, Whiting J, Scholefield J, Tierney G, Stuart RC, Hawkins RE, McCulloch P, Maughan T, Brown PD, Baillet M, Fielding JW, 2002, Marimastat as maintenance therapy for patients with advanced gastric cancer: a randomised trial. *Br J Cancer* **86:** 1864-1870.

Brinckerhoff CE and Matrisian LM, 2002, Matrix metalloproteinases: a tail of a frog that became a prince. *Nat Rev Mol Cell Biol.* **3:** 207-214.

Caenazzo C, Onisto M, Sartor L, Scalerta R, Giraldo A, Nitti D, Garbisa S, 1998, Augmented membrane type 1 matrix metalloproteinase (MT1-MMP):MMP-2 messenger RNA ratio in gastric carcinomas with poor prognosis. *Clin Cancer Res.* **4:** 2179-2186.

Chau I, Rigg A, Cunningham D, 2003, Matrix metalloproteinase inhibitors--an emphasis on gastrointestinal malignancies. *Crit Rev Oncol Hematol.* **45:** 151-176.

Chen BQ, Yang YM, Gao YH, Liu JR, Xue YB, Wang XL, Zheng YM, Zhang JS, Liu RH, 2003, Inhibitory effects of c9, t11-conjugated linoleic acid on invasion of human gastric carcinoma cell line SGC-7901. *World J Gastroenterol.* **9:** 1909-1914.

Chen JQ, Zhan WH, He YL, Peng JS, Wang JP, Cai SR, Ma JP, 2004, Expression of heparanase gene, CD44v6, MMP-7 and nm23 protein and their relationship with the invasion and metastasis of gastric carcinomas. *World J Gastroenterol.* **10:** 776-782.

Coussens LM, Fingleton B, Matrisian LM, 2002, Matrix metalloproteinase inhibitors and cancer: trials and tribulations. *Science* **295:** 2387-2392.

Crawford HC, Fingleton BM, Rudolph-Owen LA, Goss KJ, Rubinfeld B, Polakis P, Matrisian LM, 1999, The metalloproteinase matrilysin is a target of beta-catenin transactivation in intestinal tumors. *Oncogene* **18:** 2883-2891.

Crawford HC, Krishna US, Israel DA, Matrisian LM, Washington MK, Peek RM Jr., 2003, Helicobacter pylori strain-selective induction of matrix metalloproteinase-7 in vitro and within gastric mucosa. *Gastroenterol.* **125:** 1125-1136.

D'Armiento J, DiColandrea T, Dalal SS, Okada Y, Huang MT, Conney AH, Chada K, 1995, Collagenase expression in transgenic mouse skin causes hyperkeratosis and acanthosis and increases susceptibility to tumorigenesis. *Mol Cell Biol.* **15:** 5732-5739.

D'Errico A, Garbisa S, Liotta LA, Castronovo V, Stetler-Stevenson WG, Grigioni WF, 1991, Augmentation of type IV collagenase, laminin receptor, and Ki67 proliferation antigen associated with human colon, gastric, and breast carcinoma progression. *Mod Pathol.* **4:** 239-246.

David L, Nesland JM, Holm R, Sobrinho-Simoes M, 1994, Expression of laminin, collagen IV, fibronectin, and type IV collagenase in gastric carcinoma. An immunohistochemical study of 87 patients. *Cancer* **73:** 518-527.

Egeblad M and Werb Z, 2002, New functions for the matrix metalloproteinases in cancer progression. *Nat Rev Cancer* **2:** 161-174.

Elnemr A, Yonemura Y, Bandou E, Kinoshita K, Kawamura T, Takahashi S, Tochiori S, Endou Y, Sasaki T, 2003, Expression of collagenase-3 (matrix metalloproteinase-13) in human gastric cancer. *Gastric Cancer* **6:** 30-38.

Festuccia C, Angelucci A, Gravina GL, Villanova I, Teti A, Albini A, Bologna M, 2000, Osteoblast-derived TGF-beta1 modulates matrix degrading protease expression and activity in prostate cancer cells. *Int J Cancer* **85:** 407-415.

Gooz M, Gooz P, Smolka AJ, 2001, Epithelial and bacterial metalloproteinases and their inhibitors in H. pylori infection of human gastric cells. *Am J Physiol Gastrointest Liver Physiol.* **281:** G823-G832.

Gooz M, Shaker M, Gooz P, Smolka AJ, 2003, Interleukin 1beta induces gastric epithelial cell matrix metalloproteinase secretion and activation during Helicobacter pylori infection. *Gut* **52:** 1250-1256.

Grigioni WF, D'Errico A, Fortunato C, Fiorentino M, Mancini AM, Stetler-Stevenson WG, Sobel ME, Liotta LA, Onisto M, Garbisa S, 1994, Prognosis of gastric carcinoma revealed by interactions between tumor cells and basement membrane. *Mod Pathol.* **7:** 220-225.

Gross J and Lapiere CM, 1962, Collagenolytic activity in amphibian tissues: a tissue culture assay. *Proc Natl Acad Sci U S A.* **48:** 1014-1022.

Handsley MM, Edwards DR, 2005, Metalloproteinases and their inhibitors in tumor angiogenesis. *Int J Cancer* **115:** 849-860.

Heppner KJ, Matrisian LM, Jensen RA, Rodgers WH, 1996, Expression of most matrix metalloproteinase family members in breast cancer represents a tumor-induced host response. *Am J Pathol.* **149:** 273-282.

Hidalgo M and Eckhardt SG, 2001, Development of matrix metalloproteinase inhibitors in cancer therapy. *J Natl Cancer Inst.* **93:** 178-193.

Hoekstra R, Eskens FA, Verweij J, 2001, Matrix metalloproteinase inhibitors: current developments and future perspectives. *Oncologist* **6:** 415-427.

Honda M, Mori M, Ueo H, Sugimachi K, Akiyoshi T, 1996, Matrix metalloproteinase-7 expression in gastric carcinoma. *Gut* **39:** 444-448.

Hornebeck W, Lambert E, Petitfrere E, Bernard P, 2005, Beneficial and detrimental influences of tissue inhibitor of metalloproteinase-1 (TIMP-1) in tumor progression. *Biochimie* **87:** 377-383.

Huachuan Z, Xiaohan L, Jinmin S, Qian C, Yan X, Yinchang Z, 2003, Expression of matrix metalloproteinase-7 involving in growth, invasion, metastasis and angiogenesis of gastric cancer. *Chin Med Sci J.* **18:** 80-86.

Huntsman DG, Carneiro F, Lewis FR, MacLeod PM, Hayashi A, Monaghan KG, Maung R, Seruca R, Jackson CE, Caldas C, 2001, Early gastric cancer in young, asymptomatic carriers of germ-line E-cadherin mutations. *N Engl J Med.* **344:** 1904-1909.

Igarashi N, Kubota T, Otani Y, Matsuzaki SW, Watanabe M, Teramoto T, Kumai K, Tamaki K, Tanzawa K, Kobayashi T, Kitajima M, 1999, Preventive effect of matrix metalloproteinase inhibitor, R-94138, in combination with mitomycin C or cisplatin on peritoneal dissemination of human gastric cancer cell line TMK-1 in nude mice. *Jpn J Cancer Res.* **90:** 116-121.

Inoue T, Yashiro M, Nishimura S, Maeda K, Sawada T, Ogawa Y, Sowa M, Chung KH, 1999, Matrix metalloproteinase-1 expression is a prognostic factor for patients with advanced gastric cancer. *Int J Mol Med.* **4:** 73-77.

Ito T, Ito M, Shiozawa J, Naito S, Kanematsu T, Sekine I, 1999, Expression of the MMP-1 in human pancreatic carcinoma: relationship with prognostic factor. *Mod Pathol.* **12:** 669-674.

Itoh F, Yamamoto H, Hinoda Y, Imai K, 1996, Enhanced secretion and activation of matrilysin during malignant conversion of human colorectal epithelium and its relationship with invasive potential of colon cancer cells. *Cancer* **77:** 1717-1721.

Itoh T, Tanioka M, Yoshida H, Yoshioka T, Nishimoto H, Itohara S, 1998, Reduced angiogenesis and tumor progression in gelatinase A-deficient mice. *Cancer Res.* **58:** 1048-1051.

Jacks T and Weinberg RA, 2002, Taking the study of cancer cell survival to a new dimension. *Cell* **111:** 923-925.

Jemal A, Murray T, Ward E, Samuels A, Tiwari RC, Ghafoor A, Feuer EJ, Thun MJ, 2005, Cancer statistics, 2005. *CA Cancer J Clin.* **55:** 10-30.

Ji F, Chen YL, Jin EY, Wang WL, Yang ZL, Li YM, 2005, Relationship between matrix metalloproteinase-2 mRNA expression and clinicopathological and urokinase-type plasminogen activator system parameters and prognosis in human gastric cancer. *World J Gastroenterol.* **11:** 3222-3226.

Joo YE, Seo KS, Kim HS, Rew JS, Park CS, Kim SJ, 2000, Expression of tissue inhibitors of metalloproteinases (TIMPs) in gastric cancer. *Dig Dis Sci.* **45:** 114-121.

Kabashima A, Maehara Y, Kakeji Y, Baba H, Koga T, Sugimachi K, 2000, Clinicopathological features and overexpression of matrix metalloproteinases in intramucosal gastric carcinoma with lymph node metastasis. *Clin Cancer Res.* **6:** 3581-3584.

Kahari VM and Saarialho-Kere U, 1999, Matrix metalloproteinases and their inhibitors in tumour growth and invasion. *Ann Med.* **31:** 34-45.

Kaneko T, Konno H, Baba M, Tanaka T, Nakamura S, 2003, Urokinase-type plasminogen activator expression correlates with tumor angiogenesis and poor outcome in gastric cancer. *Cancer Sci.* **94:** 43-49.

Kim HS, Kim MH, Jeong M, Hwang YS, Lim SH, Shin BA, Ahn BW, Jung YD, 2004, EGCG blocks tumor promoter-induced MMP-9 expression via suppression of MAPK and AP-1 activation in human gastric AGS cells. *Anticancer Res.* **24:** 747-753.

Kimata M, Otani Y, Kubota T, Igarashi N, Yokoyama T, Wada N, Yoshimizu N, Fujii M, Kameyama K, Okada Y, Kumai K, Kitajima M, 2002, Matrix metalloproteinase inhibitor, marimastat, decreases peritoneal spread of gastric carcinoma in nude mice. *Jpn J Cancer Res.* **93:** 834-841.

Kitoh T, Yanai H, Saitoh Y, Nakamura Y, Matsubara Y, Kitoh H, Yoshida T, Okita K, 2004, Increased expression of matrix metalloproteinase-7 in invasive early gastric cancer. *J Gastroenterol.* **39:** 434-440.

Knauper V, Will H, Lopez-Otin C, Smith B, Atkinson SJ, Stanton H, Hembry RM, Murphy G, 1996, Cellular mechanisms for human procollagenase-3 (MMP-13) activation. Evidence that MT1-MMP (MMP-14) and gelatinase a (MMP-2) are able to generate active enzyme. *J Biol Chem.* **271:** 17124-17131.

Ko BK, Cho HR, Choi DW, Nam CW, Park CJ, Kim GY, Kim SS, Woo YJ, Huh J, Kim MY, 1998, Reduced expression of tissue inhibitor of metalloproteinase in nodal metastasis of stomach cancer. *J Korean Med Sci.* **13:** 286-290.

Koshikawa N, Yasumitsu H, Umeda M, Miyazaki K, 1992, Multiple secretion of matrix serine proteinases by human gastric carcinoma cell lines. *Cancer Res.* **52:** 5046-5053.

Koyama S, 2004, Enhanced cell surface expression of matrix metalloproteinases and their inhibitors, and tumor-induced host response in progression of human gastric carcinoma. *Dig Dis Sci.* **49:** 1621-1630.

Kuga H, Morisaki T, Nakamura K, Onishi H, Noshiro H, Uchiyama A, Tanaka M, Katano M, 2003, Interferon-gamma suppresses transforming growth factor-beta-induced invasion of gastric carcinoma cells through cross-talk of Smad pathway in a three-dimensional culture model. *Oncogene* **22:** 7838-7847.

Kurizaki T, Toi M, Tominaga T, 1998, Relationship between matrix metalloproteinase expression and tumor angiogenesis in human breast carcinoma. *Oncol Rep.* **5:** 673-677.

Leighl NB, Shepherd F, Paz-Ares L, *et al,* 2004, Randomized phase II-III study of matrix metalloproteinase inhibitor (MMPI) BMS-275291 in combination with paclitaxel (P) and carboplatin (C) in advanced non-small cell lung cancer. *J Clin Oncol., 2004 ASCO Annual Meeting Proceedings (Post-Meeting Edition).* **22:** Abstract #7038.

Liotta LA, Tryggvason K, Garbisa S, Hart I, Foltz CM, Shafie S, 1980, Metastatic potential correlates with enzymatic degradation of basement membrane collagen. *Nature* **284:** 67-68.

Liu XP, Kawauchi S, Oga A, Tsushimi K, Tsushimi M, Furuya T, Sasaki K, 2002a, Prognostic significance of matrix metalloproteinase-7 (MMP-7) expression at the invasive front in gastric carcinoma. *Jpn J Cancer Res.* **93:** 291-295.

Liu XP, Oga A, Suehiro Y, Furuya T, Kawauchi S, Sasaki K, 2002b, Inverse relationship between matrilysin expression and proliferative activity of cells in advanced gastric carcinoma. *Hum Pathol.* **33:** 741-747.

Lockhart AC, Braun RD, Yu D, Ross JR, Dewhirst MW, Humphrey JS, Thompson S, Williams KM, Klitzman B, Yuan F, Grichnik JM, Proia AD, Conway DA, Hurwitz HI, 2003, Reduction of wound angiogenesis in patients treated with BMS-275291, a broad spectrum matrix metalloproteinase inhibitor. *Clin Cancer Res.* **9:** 586-593.

Lynch CC and Matrisian LM, 2002, Matrix metalloproteinases in tumor-host cell communication. *Differentiation* **70:** 561-573.

Matsumura S, Oue N, Nakayama H, Kitadai Y, Yoshida K, Yamaguchi Y, Imai K, Nakachi K, Matsusaki K, Chayama K, Yasui W, 2005, A single nucleotide polymorphism in the MMP-9 promoter affects tumor progression and invasive phenotype of gastric cancer. *J Cancer Res Clin Oncol.* **131:** 19-25.

Matsuoka T, Yashiro M, Sawada T, Ishikawa T, Ohira M, Hirakawa K, Chung YS, 2001, Effect of a matrix metalloproteinase inhibitor on a lymph node metastatic model of gastric cancer cells passaged by orthotopic implantation. *J Exp Clin Cancer Res.* **20:** 213-218.

McCawley LJ and Matrisian LM, 2001, Matrix metalloproteinases: they're not just for matrix anymore! *Curr Opin Cell Biol.* **13:** 534-540.

McDonnell S, Navre M, Coffey RJ Jr., Matrisian LM, 1991, Expression and localization of the matrix metalloproteinase pump-1 (MMP-7) in human gastric and colon carcinomas. *Mol Carcinog.* **4:** 527-533.

Miao X, Yu C, Tan W, Xiong P, Liang G, Lu W, Lin D, 2003, A functional polymorphism in the matrix metalloproteinase-2 gene promoter (-1306C/T) is associated with risk of development but not metastasis of gastric cardia adenocarcinoma. *Cancer Res.* **63:** 3987-3990.

Migita T, Sato E, Saito K, Mizoi T, Shiiba K, Matsuno S, Nagura H, Ohtani H, 1999, Differing expression of MMPs-1 and -9 and urokinase receptor between diffuse- and intestinal-type gastric carcinoma. *Int J Cancer.* **84:** 74-79.

Millar AW, Brown PD, Moore J, Galloway WA, Cornish AG, Lenehan TJ, Lynch KP, 1998, Results of single and repeat dose studies of the oral matrix metalloproteinase inhibitor marimastat in healthy male volunteers. *Br J Clin Pharmacol.* **45:** 21-26.

Mimori K, Mori M, Shiraishi T, Fujie T, Baba K, Haraguchi M, Abe R, Ueo H, Akiyoshi T, 1997, Clinical significance of tissue inhibitor of metalloproteinase expression in gastric carcinoma. *Br J Cancer* **76:** 531-536.

Monig SP, Baldus SE, Hennecken JK, Spiecker DB, Grass G, Schneider PM, Thiele J, Dienes HP, Holscher AH, 2001, Expression of MMP-2 is associated with progression and lymph node metastasis of gastric carcinoma. *Histopathology* **39:** 597-602.

Mori M, Barnard GF, Mimori K, Ueo H, Akiyoshi T, Sugimachi K, 1995, Overexpression of matrix metalloproteinase-7 mRNA in human colon carcinomas. *Cancer* **75:** 1516-1519.

Moriguchi S, Kamakura T, Odaka T, Nose Y, Maehara Y, Korenaga D, Sugimachi K, 1991, Clinical features of the differentiated and undifferentiated types of advanced gastric carcinoma: univariate and multivariate analyses. *J Surg Oncol.* **48:** 202-206.

Murray GI, Duncan ME, Arbuckle E, Melvin WT, Fothergill JE, 1998, Matrix metalloproteinases and their inhibitors in gastric cancer. *Gut* **43:** 791-797.

Murray GI, Duncan ME, O'Neil P, Melvin WT, Fothergill JE, 1996, Matrix metalloproteinase-1 is associated with poor prognosis in colorectal cancer. *Nat Med.* **2:** 461-462.

Naglich JG, Jure-Kunkel M, Gupta E, Fargnoli J, Henderson AJ, Lewin AC, Talbott R, Baxter A, Bird J, Savopoulos R, Wills R, Kramer RA, Trail PA, 2001, Inhibition of angiogenesis and metastasis in two murine models by the matrix metalloproteinase inhibitor, BMS-275291. *Cancer Res.* **61:** 8480-8485.

Nelson AR, Fingleton B, Rothenberg ML, Matrisian LM, 2000, Matrix metalloproteinases: biologic activity and clinical implications. *J Clin Oncol.* **18:** 1135-1149.

Nemunaitis J, Poole C, Primrose J, Rosemurgy A, Malfetano J, Brown P, Berrington A, Cornish A, Lynch K, Rasmussen H, Kerr D, Cox D, Millar A, 1998, Combined analysis of studies of the effects of the matrix metalloproteinase inhibitor marimastat on serum tumor markers in advanced cancer: selection of a biologically active and tolerable dose for longer-term studies. *Clin Cancer Res.* **4:** 1101-1109.

Nikkola J, Vihinen P, Vlaykova T, Hahka-Kemppinen M, Kahari VM, Pyrhonen S, 2002, High expression levels of collagenase-1 and stromelysin-1 correlate with shorter disease-free survival in human metastatic melanoma. *Int J Cancer* **97:** 432-438.

Noguchi Y, Yoshikawa T, Tsuburaya A, Motohashi H, Karpeh MS, Brennan MF, 2000, Is gastric carcinoma different between Japan and the United States? *Cancer* **89:** 2237-2246.

Nomura A, Stemmermann GN, Chyou PH, Kato I, Perez-Perez GI, Blaser MJ, 1991, Helicobacter pylori infection and gastric carcinoma among Japanese Americans in Hawaii. *N Engl J Med.* **325:** 1132-1136.

Nomura H, Fujimoto N, Seiki M, Mai M, Okada Y, 1996, Enhanced production of matrix metalloproteinases and activation of matrix metalloproteinase 2 (gelatinase A) in human gastric carcinomas. *Int J Cancer* **69:** 9-16.

Nomura H, Sato H, Seiki M, Mai M, Okada Y, 1995, Expression of membrane-type matrix metalloproteinase in human gastric carcinomas. *Cancer Res.* **55:** 3263-3266.

Park IK, Kim BJ, Goh YJ, Lyu MA, Park CG, Hwang ES, Kook YH, 1997, Co-expression of urokinase-type plasminogen activator and its receptor in human gastric-cancer cell lines correlates with their invasiveness and tumorigenicity. *Int J Cancer* **71:** 867-873.

Parkin DM, Bray F, Ferlay J, Pisani P, 2005, Global cancer statistics, 2002. *CA Cancer J Clin.* **55:** 74-108.

Parsonnet J, Friedman GD, Vandersteen DP, Chang Y, Vogelman JH, Orentreich N, Sibley RK, 1991, Helicobacter pylori infection and the risk of gastric carcinoma. *N Engl J Med.* **325:** 1127-1131.

Parsons SL, Watson SA, Brown PD, Collins HM, Steele RJ, 1997a, Matrix metalloproteinases. *Br J Surg.* **84:** 160-166.

Parsons SL, Watson SA, Steele RJ, 1997b. Phase I/II trial of batimastat, a matrix metalloproteinase inhibitor, in patients with malignant ascites. *Eur J Surg Oncol.* **23:** 526-531.

Pasche B, 2001, Role of transforming growth factor beta in cancer. *J Cell Physiol.* **186:** 153-168.

Planting A, van der Gaast A, Schoffski P, Bartkowski M, Verheij C, Noe D, Ferrante K, Verweij J, 2005, A phase I and pharmacologic study of the matrix metalloproteinase inhibitor CP-471,358 in patients with advanced solid tumors. *Cancer Chemother Pharmacol.* **55:** 136-142.

Powell WC, Knox JD, Navre M, Grogan TM, Kittelson J, Nagle RB, Bowden GT, 1993, Expression of the metalloproteinase matrilysin in DU-145 cells increases their invasive potential in severe combined immunodeficient mice. *Cancer Res.* **53:** 417-422.

Price SJ, Greaves DR, Watkins H, 2001, Identification of novel, functional genetic variants in the human matrix metalloproteinase-2 gene: role of Sp1 in allele-specific transcriptional regulation. *J Biol Chem.* **276:** 7549-7558.

Primrose JN, Bleiberg H, Daniel F, Van Belle S, Mansi JL, Seymour M, Johnson PW, Neoptolemos JP, Baillet M, Barker K, Berrington A, Brown PD, Millar AW, Lynch KP, 1999, Marimastat in recurrent colorectal cancer: exploratory evaluation of biological activity by measurement of carcinoembryonic antigen. *Br J Cancer* **79:** 509-514.

Ramnath N and Creaven PJ, 2004. Matrix metalloproteinase inhibitors. *Curr Oncol Rep.* **6:** 96-102.

Rizvi NA, Humphrey JS, Ness EA, Johnson MD, Gupta E, Williams K, Daly DJ, Sonnichsen D, Conway D, Marshall J, Hurwitz H, 2004, A phase I study of oral BMS-275291, a novel nonhydroxamate sheddase-sparing matrix metalloproteinase inhibitor, in patients with advanced or metastatic cancer. *Clin Cancer Res.* **10:** 1963-1970.

Rundhaug JE, 2003, Matrix metalloproteinases, angiogenesis, and cancer: commentary re: A C Lockhart *et al*, Reduction of wound angiogenesis in patients treated with BMS-275291, a broad spectrum matrix metalloproteinase inhibitor. *Clin Cancer Res.* **9:** 551-554.

Sakurai Y, Otani Y, Kameyama K, Hosoda Y, Okazaki I, Kubota T, Kumai K, Kitajima M, 1997a, Expression of interstitial collagenase (matrix metalloproteinase-1) in gastric cancers. *Jpn J Cancer Res.* **88:** 401-406.

Sakurai Y, Otani Y, Kameyama K, Igarashi N, Kubota T, Kumai K, Kitajima M, 1997b, The role of stromal cells in the expression of interstitial collagenase (matrix metalloproteinase-1) in the invasion of gastric cancer. *J Surg Oncol.* **66:** 168-172.

Sato H, Takino T, Miyamori H, 2005, Roles of membrane-type matrix metalloproteinase-1 in tumor invasion and metastasis. *Cancer Sci.* **96:** 212-217.

Sato H, Takino T, Okada Y, Cao J, Shinagawa A, Yamamoto E, Seiki M, 1994, A matrix metalloproteinase expressed on the surface of invasive tumour cells. *Nature* **370:** 61-65.

Scartozzi M, Galizia E, Freddari F, Berardi R, Cellerino R, Cascinu S, 2004, Molecular biology of sporadic gastric cancer: prognostic indicators and novel therapeutic approaches. *Cancer Treat Rev.* **30:** 451-459.

Schwartz GK, Wang H, Lampen N, Altorki N, Kelsen D, Albino AP, 1994, Defining the invasive phenotype of proximal gastric cancer cells. *Cancer* **73:** 22-27.

Shen KH, Chi CW, Lo SS, Kao HL, Lui WY, Wu CW, 2000, Serum matrix metalloproteinase-9 level associated with stromal reaction in patients with gastric cancer. *Anticancer Res.* **20:** 1307-1310.

Sier CF, Kubben FJ, Ganesh S, Heerding MM, Griffioen G, Hanemaaijer R, van Krieken JH, Lamers CB, Verspaget HW, 1996, Tissue levels of matrix metalloproteinases MMP-2 and MMP-9 are related to the overall survival of patients with gastric carcinoma. *Br J Cancer.* **74:** 413-417.

Sounni NE and Noel A, 2005, Membrane type-matrix metalloproteinases and tumor progression. *Biochimie* **87:** 329-342.

Sternlicht MD, Lochter A, Sympson CJ, Huey B, Rougier JP, Gray JW, Pinkel D, Bissell MJ, Werb Z, 1999, The stromal proteinase MMP3/stromelysin-1 promotes mammary carcinogenesis. *Cell* **98:** 137-146.

Sun XM, Dong WG, Yu BP, Luo HS, Yu JP, 2003, Detection of type IV collagenase activity in malignant ascites. *World J Gastroenterol.* **9:** 2592-2595.

Suzuki K, Enghild JJ, Morodomi T, Salvesen G, Nagase H, 1990, Mechanisms of activation of tissue procollagenase by matrix metalloproteinase 3 (stromelysin). *Biochemistry* **29:** 10261-10270.

Tierney GM, Griffin NR, Stuart RC, Kasem H, Lynch KP, Lury JT, Brown PD, Millar AW, Steele RJ, Parsons SL, 1999, A pilot study of the safety and effects of the matrix metalloproteinase inhibitor marimastat in gastric cancer. *Eur J Cancer* **35:** 563-568.

Torii A, Kodera Y, Uesaka K, Hirai T, Yasui K, Morimoto T, Yamamura Y, Kato T, Hayakawa T, Fujimoto N, Kito T, 1997, Plasma concentration of matrix metalloproteinase 9 in gastric cancer. *Br J Surg.* **84:** 133-136.

Tsuchiya Y, Sato H, Endo Y, Okada Y, Mai M, Sasaki T, Seiki M, 1993, Tissue inhibitor of metalloproteinase 1 is a negative regulator of the metastatic ability of a human gastric cancer cell line, KKLS, in the chick embryo. *Cancer Res.* **53:** 1397-1402.

Visse R and Nagase H, 2003, Matrix metalloproteinases and tissue inhibitors of metalloproteinases: structure, function, and biochemistry. *Circ Res.* **92:** 827-839.

Wada N, Otani Y, Kubota T, Kimata M, Minagawa A, Yoshimizu N, Kameyama K, Saikawa Y, Yoshida M, Furukawa T, Fujii M, Kumai K, Okada Y, Kitajima M, 2003, Reduced angiogenesis in peritoneal dissemination of gastric cancer through gelatinase inhibition. *Clin Exp Metastasis* **20:** 431-435.

Watanabe M, Takahashi Y, Ohta T, Mai M, Sasaki T, Seiki M, 1996, Inhibition of metastasis in human gastric cancer cells transfected with tissue inhibitor of metalloproteinase 1 gene in nude mice. *Cancer* **77:** 1676-1680.

Watson SA, Morris TM, Collins HM, Bawden LJ, Hawkins K, Bone EA, 1999, Inhibition of tumour growth by marimastat in a human xenograft model of gastric cancer: relationship with levels of circulating CEA. *Br J Cancer* **81:** 19-23.

Witty JP, McDonnell S, Newell KJ, Cannon P, Navre M, Tressler RJ, Matrisian LM, 1994, Modulation of matrilysin levels in colon carcinoma cell lines affects tumorigenicity in vivo. *Cancer Res.* **54:** 4805-4812.

Woessner JF Jr., 1991, Matrix metalloproteinases and their inhibitors in connective tissue remodeling. *FASEB J.* **5:** 2145-2154.

Wojtowicz-Praga S, Low J, Marshall J, Ness E, Dickson R, Barter J, Sale M, McCann P, Moore J, Cole A, Hawkins MJ, 1996, Phase I trial of a novel matrix metalloproteinase inhibitor batimastat (BB-94) in patients with advanced cancer. *Invest New Drugs* **14:** 193-202.

Wojtowicz-Praga S, Torri J, Johnson M, Steen V, Marshall J, Ness E, Dickson R, Sale M, Rasmussen HS, Chiodo TA, Hawkins MJ, 1998, Phase I trial of Marimastat, a novel matrix metalloproteinase inhibitor, administered orally to patients with advanced lung cancer. *J Clin Oncol.* **16:** 2150-2156.

Wroblewski LE, Noble PJ, Pagliocca A, Pritchard DM, Hart CA, Campbell F, Dodson AR, Dockray GJ, Varro A, 2003, Stimulation of MMP-7 (matrilysin) by Helicobacter pylori in human gastric epithelial cells: role in epithelial cell migration. *J Cell Sci.* **116:** 3017-3026.

Yamagata S, Yoshii Y, Suh JG, Tanaka R, Shimizu S, 1991, Occurrence of an active form of gelatinase in human gastric and colorectal carcinoma tissues. *Cancer Lett.* **59:** 51-55.

Yamashita K, Azumano I, Mai M, Okada Y, 1998, Expression and tissue localization of matrix metalloproteinase 7 (matrilysin) in human gastric carcinomas. Implications for vessel invasion and metastasis. *Int J Cancer* **79:** 187-194.

Yashiro M, Murahashi K, Matsuoka T, Nakazawa K, Tanaka H, Osaka H, Koyama T, Ohira M, Chung KH, 2003, Tranilast (N-3,4-dimethoxycinamoyl anthranilic acid): a novel inhibitor of invasion-stimulating interaction between gastric cancer cells and orthotopic fibroblasts. *Anticancer Res.* **23:** 3899-3904.

Yonemura Y, Endou Y, Fujita H, Fushida S, Bandou E, Taniguchi K, Miwa K, Sugiyama K, Sasaki T, 2000, Role of MMP-7 in the formation of peritoneal dissemination in gastric cancer. *Gastric Cancer* **3:** 63-70.

Yonemura Y, Fujimura T, Ninomiya I, Kim BS, Bandou E, Sawa T, Kinoshita K, Endo Y, Sugiyama K, Sasaki T, 2001, Prediction of peritoneal micrometastasis by peritoneal lavaged cytology and reverse transcriptase-polymerase chain reaction for matrix metalloproteinase-7 mRNA. *Clin Cancer Res.* **7:** 1647-1653.

Yoshikawa T, Saitoh M, Tsuburaya A, Kobayashi O, Sairenji M, Motohashi H, Yanoma S, Noguchi Y, 1999, Tissue inhibitor of matrix metalloproteinase-1 in the plasma of patients with gastric carcinoma. A possible marker for serosal invasion and metastasis. *Cancer* **86:** 1929-1935.

Yoshikawa T, Tsuburaya A, Kobayashi O, Sairenji M, Motohashi H, Yanoma S, Noguchi Y, 2001, Intratumoral concentrations of tissue inhibitor of matrix metalloproteinase 1 in patients with gastric carcinoma a new biomartker for invasion and its impact on survival. *Cancer* **91:** 1739-1744.

Yu C, Pan K, Xing D, Liang G, Tan W, Zhang L, Lin D, 2002, Correlation between a single nucleotide polymorphism in the matrix metalloproteinase-2 promoter and risk of lung cancer. *Cancer Res.* **62:** 6430-6433.

Zhang H, Morisaki T, Matsunaga H, Sato N, Uchiyama A, Hashizume K, Nagumo F, Tadano J, Katano M, 2000, Protein-bound polysaccharide PSK inhibits tumor invasiveness by down-regulation of TGF-beta1 and MMPs. *Clin Exp Metastasis* **18:** 343-352.

Zhang J, Jin X, Fang S, Li Y, Wang R, Guo W, Wang N, Wang Y, Wen D, Wei L, Kuang G, Dong Z, 2004, The functional SNP in the matrix metalloproteinase-3 promoter modifies susceptibility and lymphatic metastasis in esophageal squamous cell carcinoma but not in gastric cardiac adenocarcinoma. *Carcinogenesis* **25:** 2519-2524.

Zhang S, Li L, Lin JY, Lin H, 2003, Imbalance between expression of matrix metalloproteinase-9 and tissue inhibitor of metalloproteinase-1 in invasiveness and metastasis of human gastric carcinoma. *World J Gastroenterol* **9:** 899-904.

Zheng HC, Sun JM, Li XH, Yang XF, Zhang YC, Xin Y, 2003, Role of PTEN and MMP-7 expression in growth, invasion, metastasis and angiogenesis of gastric carcinoma. *Pathol Int.* **53:** 659-666.

Zucker S, Cao J, Chen WT, 2000, Critical appraisal of the use of matrix metalloproteinase inhibitors in cancer treatment. *Oncogene* **19:** 6642-6650.

Chapter 3

Proteases in Helicobacter pylori-Mediated Diseases

Thomas Wex, Michael Zack, and Peter Malfertheiner
Department of Gastroenterology, Hepatology and Infectious Diseases, Otto-von-Guericke University, Leipziger Str. 44, D-39120 Magdeburg, Germany

1. INTRODUCTION

1.1 General remarks

A recent medline search (May 2005) linking protease or peptidase-related publications with gastroduodenal disorders retrieved about 4.500 entries. This number as well as the usage of distinct cell models, various methodologies and the different designs of clinical studies limit the possibility to present a comprehensive and critical review of proteases and their functional implications in the upper gastrointestinal tract. Therefore, we only included H. pylori-associated diseases leaving out the autoimmune-mediated disorders (sprue and autoimmune gastritis), the role of non-steroidal anti-inflammatory drugs (NSAID) as well the abnormal gastric reflux as cause for the gastroesophageal reflux disease (GERD).

Taken into consideration that the majority of the potential readers will rather come from the field of proteases than from gastroenterology, we decided to use the gastroduodenal diseases as scaffold for this chapter. Within this chapter, we discuss (I) basic pathophysiological mechanisms and (II) review relevant data from the field of proteases. Due to the enormous number of publications, we could only consider a fraction of original literature. The lack of any particular article or findings concerning certain proteases is not related to the quality of publication. The linkage between the basic pathophysiological mechanisms and the role of proteases discussed should enable others to put their specific protease into the context to gastric physiology and related diseases.

U. Lendeckel and Nigel M. Hooper (eds.), Proteases in Gastrointestinal Tissue, 61-87.

1.2 Studies, models, methods and statistics

Regardless whether projects are functionally or clinically-orientated, each study has its limits. Therefore, results of single studies are rather limited to the specific experimental conditions, methods or models. Whether specific findings do indeed reflect general phenomena needs to be confirmed by several studies using different approaches and methods. With respect to the topic of this chapter several common and specific aspects need to be critically considered. For the initiation of a new project it is urgent to consider the advantages and disadvantages of the study design and methods to obtain an acceptable compromise for answering the question raised.

First, one if not the most important issue is the material used for analysis. Cell lines mostly used for investigating the regulatory and functional aspects are easy to handle. They represent a single cell type and *in vitro* analyses usually provide consistent results. However, all of these models (e.g. gastric cancer cells AGS, MKN or NCI-87) do not correspond to their normal counterparts such as gastric epithelium. The latter represent terminally differentiate cells, which do not proliferate. On the other hand, the usage of *ex vivo* material (e.g. biopsies, surgical specimens) has other limitations. Tissue samples are generally complex and contain different cell types, for instance tumor cells, immune cells, fibroblasts, endothelial and nerve cells. The highly variable degree of this cellular composition among patients with identical diagnosis (e.g. gastric adenocarcinoma) requires the usage of different methods (e.g. ELISA, immunohistochemistry) and appropriate *in vitro* models to identify the cell type that is responsible for changes in the expression pattern of specific genes.

Second, another critical factor is the usage of analytic methods. Due to complex regulation of most genes, which includes transcriptional and post-transcriptional regulation as well as proteolytic processing of polypeptides, one should investigate both the transcript as well as the protein level. Due to the miniaturization of methods and higher sensitivity (e.g. real-time RT-PCR), limited material is increasingly less an issue. If material, in particular for clinical studies, is indeed limited, the protein expression should be preferentially analyzed, because its represents the functional level. While ELISA and RIA lead primarily to numeric data allowing direct quantitative comparisons, Western blot and immunohistochemistry generate semi-quantitative data at best. These data should be solely analyzed by nonparametric statistics, which lead usually to higher numbers of experiments. On the other hand, microscopy-based methods allow the identification of cells and subcellular localization of proteins permitting functional conclusions with respect to cellular and subcellular compartments.

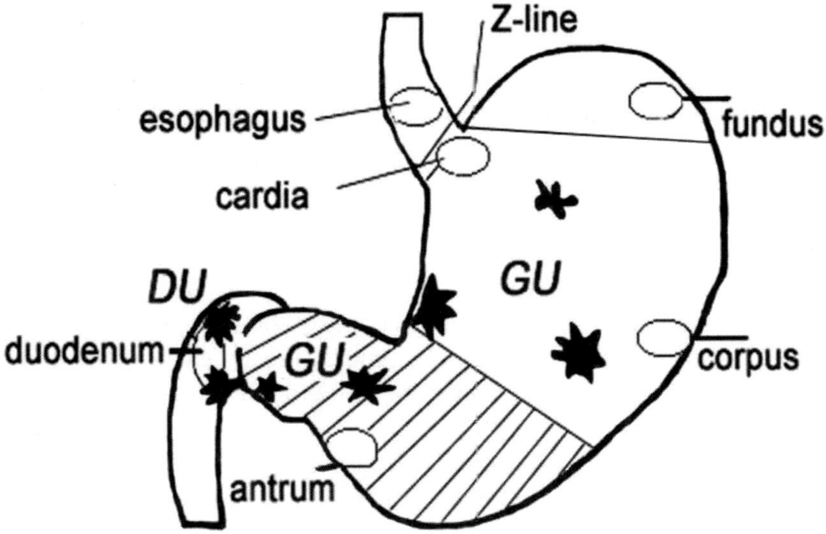

Figure 1: Schematic illustration of the stomach. Open circles represent the localizations of biopsies (duodenal bulb, antrum, corpus, cardia and distal esophagus) mostly taken during endoscopy in clinical studies. Furthermore, the antrum predominantly infected by H.pylori in Caucasian population is identified by lines. Please note that the *H.pylori*-induced gastritis can also affect the whole stomach up to the distal esophagus. Typical localizations of either duodenal or gastric ulcers are indicated by black stars. Gastric ulcers are associated with adenocarcinoma at higher rates than antral ulcers, but gastric cancer does develop at all locations in the stomach.

Third, based on cellular composition, the stomach can be basically divided into different segments, the cardia, the fundus, the corpus and the antrum (Figure 1). The gastric mucosa comprises five types of specialized cells, the surface and neck mucous producing cells, the acid-secreting parietal cells, the enzyme-producing chief cells, endocrine cells and stem cells, which are differentially localized and consequently determine the distinct functionality of the different regions. Therefore, *ex vivo* analyses of gastric tissue should always include a standardized protocol for gastroduodenoscopy and a histological evaluation of tissue specimens to prevent a mixture of biopsies from these anatomical regions.

Fourth, if gene expression analyses are performed with respect to pathological processes (e.g. inflammation, tumors), it is quite important to consider that these processes are always associated with wide cellular changes such as infiltration of immune cells, tumor-associated stroma, dedifferentiation of cell types or metaplastic changes. For instance, the appearance of specialized intestinal metaplasia, known as Barrett's metaplasia, in the distal esophagus is naturally linked with the expression of intestine-specific genes such as transcription factors (CDX-1, CDX-2) or hydrolytic enzymes (CD26: dipeptidyl peptidase IV, sucrose isomaltase). Gastric inflammation, termed as gastritis, is constantly accompanied by increased cytokine production, which are produced by the infiltrating immune cells. Here, a critical view is necessary for the differentiation, whether the change of gene expression is really a new feature of a preexisting cell type (e.g. gastric epithelium), or it just reflects the change of cellular composition in the tissue sample analyzed.

Fifth, in order to draw general conclusions appropriate statistical analyses are indispensable. With respect to this issue, clinically-orientated studies mostly present higher standards than functionally-focused projects, which are often limited to the comparison of one parameter and the usage of Student's T-test. Furthermore, clinical studies mostly include the complex interactions of a disease and apply more often multivariate analysis that leads to identification of less but more universally valid findings. In order to prevent major pitfalls, all data should be thoroughly analyzed with respect to their intrinsic property and distribution pattern. For instance, non-parametric data (e.g. scoring-based data sets from immunohistochemistry) or not normally distributed data form quantitative RT-PCR (e.g. if samples with missing expression are included) have to be solely analyzed with nonparametric tests. Last but not least, appropriate controls are a key issue of all statistical analyses. Since the gene expression pattern is dependent on numerous parameters (age, gender, medication), groups should be matched for maximal numbers of these factors.

2. PROTEASES IN GASTRIC PHYSIOLOGY

After the oral cavity, responsible for the mechanical breakup of the diet, the stomach represents the second compartment of the alimentary tract. Here, the first step of protein degradation takes place. Typically, 50-100 g of protein are consumed each day. Since the proteins are too large to be absorbed by the intestine, they must be hydrolyzed to yield their constituent amino acids, which can be absorbed. The proteolytic enzymes responsible for degrading proteins are produced by three different organs: the stomach (pepsinogens), the pancreas (chymotrypsin) and the small intestine (e.g. aminopeptidases), from those we only discuss the pepsinogens.

Pepsinogens are zymogens of pepsins. The aspartic gastric proteases of the vertebrates belong to the peptidase family A1 [MEROPS database: http://merops.sanger.ac.uk/]. To date, five groups, namely pepsinogens A, B, C, F and prochymosin are known (Kageyama 2002). All of them are expressed as inactive precursors and converted to their active forms at pH below 5.0 by autoactivation that involves intramolecular and intermolecular reactions (Richter *et al* 1998). For humans, pepsin A and pepsin C/gastricsin are the two major gastric proteases, while pepsins B and F have been characterized from other species (Narita *et al* 2002). The chymosin gene represents a pseudogene in humans (Ord *et al* 1990). In the last decade, the analysis of serum pepsinogen A and C levels has been established as biomarkers for the gastric mucosa permitting the identification of subjects with severe atrophic gastritis (discussed in section 4.1).

The release of gastric acid and pepsinogens is highly regulated and involves several gastric hormones. Together with central acting hormones like acetylcholine, adrenaline and somatostatin, locally acting gastric peptides such gastrin-17 / gastrin-34 or ghrelin regulate gastric physiology (Rosicka *et al* 2002). The complex network is greatly affected by the H.pylori-infection (Kaneko *et al* 2002), and these changes are one important component in the subsequent development of diseases as illustrated in Figure 2. With respect to the expression of proteases, it is noteworthy that the biosynthesis of active forms of most hormones includes extensive proteolytic processing by subtilisin-like proconvertases (PC-1, PC-2) as well as lysosomal cathepsins and exopeptidases (Rehfeld *et al* 2003). While the expression of gastric hormones in context with gastroduodenal diseases has been studied quite extensively (Vaananen *et al* 2003), the role of proteases involved in the biosynthesis of these hormones has been investigated on a limited scale so far. In addition to the specific expression of pepsinogens in the stomach, the gastroduodenal mucosa expresses a variety of other proteases and several protease inhibitors.

3. HELICOBACTER PYLORI

3.1 Pathophysiology of Helicobacter pylori-mediated diseases

Twenty years after the discovery of Helicobacter pylori (H.pylori) by Marshall and Warren (Marshall *et al* 1984), we know that the infection of the stomach by the gram-negative microaerophil bacterium is the most common cause for chronic gastritis, peptic ulcers and gastric malignancies (adenocarcinoma and mucosa-associated lymphoid tissue lymphoma) (Dunn *et al* 1997, Moayyedi *et al* 2004). Interestingly, the infection by H.pylori can lead to quite divergent pathologies. Two of them are duodenal ulcer and gastric adenocarcinoma, which clinically represent two alternative H.pylori-induced diseases. The main factor deciding the pathways of H.pylori-associated diseases is the acid-secreting capacity of the stomach, which depends on the topography of the H.pylori infection (Suerbaum *et al* 2002).

H.pylori-induced antral predominant gastritis results in hypergastrinemia, which stimulates acid secretion and increases the risk for duodenal ulceration. In contrast, H.pylori-induced pan- or corpus-predominant gastritis suppresses acid production leading to hypochlorhydria that enhances risk for gastric ulcer and adenocarcinoma (Figure 2). The interaction between bacterium and gastric mucosa results in various molecular changes of epithelial cells including cytoskeletal rearrangement, intracellular phosphorylation, the expression of pro-inflammatory cytokines as well as the induction of a Th1-immune response (Blaser *et al* 2004). The cytokine pattern and chronic gastritis affects various cell types that are important for the acid-homeostasis, including somatostatin-producing D cells, gastrin-secreting G cells and acid-producing parietal cells. These changes in the expression pattern of cytokines and hormones can be associated with histomorphological modifications of the gastric architecture. Both the development of atrophic gastritis and the presence of intestinal metaplasia represent premalignant conditions for the gastric carcinogenesis (Correa 1995). However, it is notable that despite the fact that literally all H.pylori-infected individuals develop a chronic gastritis, severe complications occur only in a subset of H.pylori-infected subjects (Figure 2). About 5-15% of all H.pylori-infected individuals develop an ulcer disease during their life, whereas only 1% will eventually develop gastric cancer (Suerbaum *et al* 2002). Very recently, a gastric cancer mouse model suggested an involvement of bone marrow-derived stem cells for the development of H.pylori-induced gastric adenocarcinoma (Houghton *et al* 2004), however its importance for the human disease still needs to be shown.

To identify subjects with higher risk for the development of severe gastroduodenal diseases and to evaluate "biological markers" for this stratification is an actual challenge in the field of gastroenterology.

3.2 Proteases of Helicobacter pylori

Since H.pylori-induced diseases, in particular duodenal and gastric ulcer, are associated with extensive tissue damage, bacterial proteases were assumed to play an important role in this process. Several studies addressed this issue and investigated the functional implications of these proteases in context to H.pylori infection.

After the first characterization of the H.pylori genome in 1997 (Tomb *et al* 1997), the genomes of several other H.pylori strains were characterized (Ge *et al* 1999). Based on data of 11 H.pylori strains, the genome size of this bacterium was shown to range from 1.6 to 1.73 Mb. The genomes of H.pylori strains encode between 1.500 to 1.600 different putative proteins (open reading frames). From those about 2/3 have been functionally characterized or at least based on their sequence a putative function has been predicted

(Ge *et al* 1999). Among them are at least 20 protease-encoding genes (Tomb *et al* 1997). Since none of the corresponding gene products have been associated with clinical features so far, there is only limited knowledge concerning their potential pathogenetic importance. Based on their homology to genes of better characterized bacteria like E.coli or Salmonella spec., the ClpXP protease could be potentially involved in the heat shock response (Kim *et al* 2003). Furthermore, the serine protease HtrA (HP1019) was characterized as component of the secretome, which comprises all secreted proteins of this bacterium (Bumann *et al* 2002). Interestingly, HtrA belongs to the 150 most abundant proteins in H.pylori and represents an antigen recognized by the majority of sera obtained by H.pylori-infected patients (Haas *et al* 2002). Whether this protease is directly involved in the pathogenesis of H.pylori-infection has not been investigated. However, taken into account the presence of the endogenous serine protease inhibitor SLPI in gastric mucosa and its downregulation in H.pylori-associated diseases (Wex *et al* 2004a), a "crosstalk" between the HtrA protease and host factors like SLPI seems to be possible. The role of HtrA for the bacterium has not been studied, but there are contradictory results from mutational analysis. While Salama and co-workers identified the HtrA protease as an essential gene for the survival of H.pylori (Salama *et al* 2004), others were able to establish HtrA-deficient strains (S. Backert Otto-von-Guericke University Magdeburg, personal communication). Furthermore, a secreted collagenase (HP0169) as virulence factor for the gastric colonization of H.pylori was described (Kavermann *et al* 2003). In addition to its own proteases and in analogy to other bacteria, H.pylori is also capable to capture host proteases on its membrane and to activate them (Lahteenmaki *et al* 2001). Plasminogen, as precursor of the serine protease plasmin, was shown to bind to the cell surface of the H.pylori strain CCUG17874, where it was activated to cell-bound plasmin by tissue-type plasminogen activator (Pantzar *et al* 1998). Meanwhile, the two plasminogen-binding proteins (HP0508 and HP0863) of H.pylori have been characterized and identified in a variety of strains suggesting that the capture of plasminogen and its subsequent activation at the bacterial surface might be a general phenomenon for this bacterium (Jonsson *et al* 2004). The surface acquisition of protease activity may enhance the virulence of H.pylori. However, it is notable that these findings were obtained from *in vitro* studies ignoring the different compartments of plasminogen (peripheral circulation) and H.pylori (gastric lumen, mucosa). Taken into account recent data concerning the possible interaction between H.pylori and intramucosal compartments by the disruption of the epithelial junction by CagA, the plasminogen binding is potentially possible, but its proposed role in pathophysiology still needs to be proven.

Although, the knowledge concerning H.pylori-derived proteases is still incomplete, their role for the pathology of H.pylori-associated diseases should not been neglected and future studies will shed light into this field.

4. HOST PROTEASES AND INHIBITORS

4.1 H.pylori-induced gastritis

Gastritis, by definition, is a histopathological entity characterized by the chronic and active inflammation of the gastric mucosa, which is mainly caused by the H.pylori infection (60-70%), NSAID-associated or bile-induced chemical reactive gastritis (20–30 %) and to smaller extent by autoimmune processes (Stolte *et al* 2001). The inflammatory infiltrate is composed of T-cells, B-lymphocytes and plasma cells. The number of these infiltrating cells defines the chronicity of gastritis. The infiltration of the lamina propria and gastric epithelium by polymorph nuclear leukocytes (mostly neutrophil granulocytes) reflects the activity of the inflammation (Dixon *et al* 1996). Almost all autoimmune and a small portion of H.pylori-induced gastric inflammation lead to the development of atrophic gastritis. This type of gastritis is characterized by the subsequent loss of antral and corpus glands including the destruction of parietal and chief cells, which secret gastric acid and pepsinogens, respectively (Faller *et al* 2005). The two major pepsinogens (A and C) are differentially expressed. Pepsinogen A is secreted only by the chief cells of the corpus mucosa, and therefore its serum level decreases with increasing grade of corpus atrophy (Asaka *et al* 1992). In contrast, the expression of pepsinogen C is less restricted; corpus chief cells, antral glands and the Brunner glands of the proximal duodenum secrete this protease in large quantities (Plebani 1993). The ratio of pepsinogen A and C serum concentrations in healthy individuals is between 5-6 to 1. Depending on the topology of gastritis (antrum- or corpus-predominant) and its severity this ratio is reduced (Aoki *et al* 1997, Broutet *et al* 2003). In combination with serum gastrin-17, a peptide hormone of the alimentary tract, and the presence of anti-H.pylori antibodies, the determination of the pepsinogen ratio offers a noninvasive method for characterizing different forms of gastritis in serum for defining increased risks for severe complications like ulcer disease or gastric cancer (Vaananen *et al* 2003).

As illustrated in figure 2, the infection by H.pylori leads in all subjects to a chronic gastritis. In a minority of patients the chronic gastritis progresses into an atrophic gastritis that can eventually lead to gastric cancer.

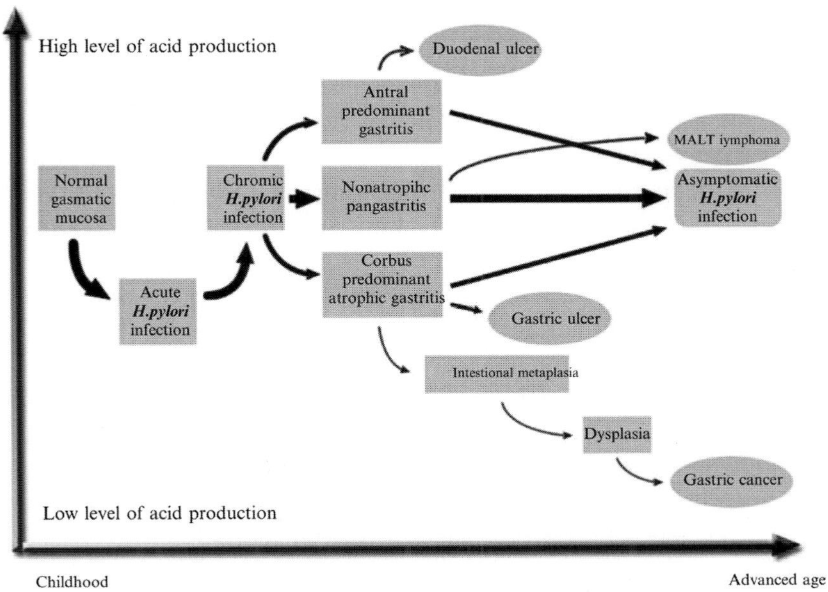

Figure 2: Natural history of H.pylori-mediated gastroduodenal diseases. H.pylori infection is usually acquired in childhood. Acute H.pylori infection causes transient hypochlorhydria and is rarely diagnosed. Chronic gastritis will develop in virtually all persistently colonized subjects, but 80 to 90 percent will never have any symptoms. The further clinical course is highly variable and depends on bacterial and host factors. Patients with higher acid output are likely to have antral-predominant gastritis, which predisposes them to duodenal ulcers. Patients with lower acid output are more likely to have gastritis in the body of the stomach, which predisposes them to gastric ulcer and can initiate a sequence of events that, in rare cases, leads to gastric carcinoma. Another infrequent complication of H.pylori infection is the formation of mucosa-associated lymphoid tissue (MALT) in gastric mucosa, from which malignant lymphoma can arise (adapted from Suerbaum et al 2002).

Since the research on tumor tissue (as an endpoint of pathological changes) is highly accepted, first studies were aimed at the comparison of protease activities in tissue homogenates from normal and cancer tissues. Using peptide-based substrates, elevated proteolytic activities for cathepsins B, L, H and D as well as collagenase were identified in gastric cancer tissue (Vasishta *et al* 1985, Watanabe *et al* 1987). Further characterization of these cancer-associated protease activities revealed several aspects. First, the higher activities were due to an upregulation of gene expression that was mostly accompanied by elevated transcript levels. Second, the higher proteolytic activities in tumor-derived tissue correlated with a diminished expression of the corresponding inhibitor leading to an imbalance of the protease / inhibitor equilibrium. Third, novel cancer-specific protease forms, regulated by alternative splicing and/or alternative promoters, were identified that contribute to the higher proteolytic activities. For instance, a cathepsin L-like activity was isolated from gastric cancer tissue that differed in its biochemical properties such as apparent molecular weight and isoelectric point (Chung 1990). Alternative splice variants in gastric or other cancers are known from cathepsins B, L and E (Cao *et al* 1994, Arora *et al* 2002, Seth *et al* 2003, Tatnell *et al* 2003). The expression of tumor-specific cathepsin B forms lead to the aberrant intracellular trafficking of cathepsin B that is observed in some human cancers. Splice variants of cathepsin B have been associated with membrane- and mitochondria-associated cathepsin B activity (Mehtani *et al* 1998, Sinha *et al* 2001, Muntener *et al* 2004). The functional relevance of this different subcellular distribution in tumor cells has not been fully elucidated. However, taken together with the findings of other studies, it is highly likely that the altered distribution of cathepsin B is an important cause for the upregulation of this protease in gastric cancer. Khan *et al* identified a negative correlation between the cathepsin B expression of gastric cancer cells and tumor-associated laminin that is a major component of the basement membrane (Khan *et al* 1998). Increased cathepsin B expression by tumor cells, associated with decreased tumor-derived laminin, could represent one mechanism for local tumor progression and metastasis.

Based on recent data, a functional role of cathepsins, in particular cathepsin B, for regulating the intrinsic pathway of programmed cell death (Debatin 2004) in gastric epithelium and related tumors has been proposed. First, it was shown that at least one isoform of cathepsin B exists that is translocated into the mitochondrial compartment (Muntener *et al* 2004). Second, lysosomal thiol-dependent cathepsins are known to cleave the bcl-2 family member "bid" implying a regulatory role of these proteases for the initiation of apoptosis (Stoka *et al* 2001; Cirman *et al* 2004).

After the discovery of an association between certain proteases with gastric cancer, studies investigating earlier stages of gastric tumorgenesis were initiated. Farinati *et al* determined a significant upregulation of cathepsins B, L and urokinase-type plasminogen activator (uPA) and its inhibitor type-1 (PAI-1) in tissue homogenates of gastric biopsies from patients with chronic atrophic gastritis and existing metaplasia (Farinati *et al* 1996). In addition, a gradual increase of cathepsin B and uPA expression was identified comparing patients with and without dysplastic changes. Notably, the changes of cathepsin B and L levels occurred at later stage in the gastritis–carcinoma sequence. The gene expression analysis at the transcript level of patients without atrophy and intestinal metaplasia did not show an upregulation of cathepsins B, L and K (Buhling *et al* 2004). Similar findings were reported for the tissue kallikrein. While the presence of an active chronic H.pylori infection did not lead to changes of tissue kallikrein levels (Naidoo *et al* 1997), both ulcer disease and gastric cancer exhibited a significant increase of kallikrein expression (Sawant *et al* 2001).

The central role of the plasminogen activators for the fibrinolytic system and its known alterations in H.pylori-mediated diseases has lead to studies focusing on the role of the serine proteases uPA and tissue-type plasminogen activator (tPA). While uPA expression was found to be increased in H.pylori-mediated gastritis, tPA levels were significantly decreased (Gotz *et al* 1996).

Important histological criteria of the chronic active gastritis are the presence of neutrophil granulocytes and lymphocytic infiltrates. In context to this infiltration, proteases specifically expressed in these cells were found to be upregulated in gastritis. For instance, the activities of neutrophil-associated serine proteases like cathepsin G, proteinase-3 and elastase were found to be elevated in an animal model as well as in human H.pylori-induced gastritis (Yoshida *et al* 2002, Nilius *et al* 2000). The higher proteolytic activity of these proteases is considered to be involved in the degradation of extracellular matrix and tissue damage seen in gastritis and subsequent diseases. Functionally, it is notable that the increased cellular expression of these serine proteases is associated with strong reduction of the secretory leukocyte protease inhibitor (SLPI) expression in the gastric mucosa of H.pylori-mediated diseases (Wex *et al* 2004a, b). Taken into consideration the multiple properties of SLPI including anti-inflammatory and antimicrobial effects, the reduction of this mucosa-protective factor might contribute to the inflammation and impaired repair mechanisms. Recent reports provided evidence that SLPI might not only interfere with the degradation of extracellular matrix components, but indirectly also regulates the activation of transcription factors of the NFκB family by inhibiting the degradation of the inhibitor IκB and IRAK. Decreased SLPI levels in gastric mucosa will therefore further boost the NFκB-mediated inflammation (Taggart *et al* 2002). The SLPI knock-out model clearly demonstrated that in the absence of SLPI, proepithelin (PEPI), an epithelial growth factor, is increasingly converted to epithelin (EPI). PEPI and EPI exert opposing activities. EPI inhibits the growth of epithelial cells but induce them to secrete the neutrophil attractant IL-8, while PEPI blocks neutrophil activation by tumor necrosis factor, preventing release of oxidants and proteases. The authors concluded that the equilibrium between SLPI and elastase determines the ratio of PEPI and EPI, which affects repair processes of gastric mucosa and represents a link between innate immunity and wound healing (Zhu *et al* 2002).

Histological characterization of inflamed tissue sections or mucosa-associated lymphoid tissue lymphoma (MALT) revealed a higher proportion of intraepithelial cytotoxic lymphocytes than in normal gastric mucosa, which is almost devoid of lymphocytes (Oberhuber *et al* 1998; de Bruin *et al* 1994). The expression of granzyme B, a serine protease of cytotoxic T cells (Oberhuber *et al* 1998, Suzuki *et al* 2003), as well as cathepsin W, a thiol-dependent cathepsin of NK cells and CTL (Wex *et al* 2001) were induced in chronic gastritis. However, this increase was basically associated with higher numbers of infiltrating cytotoxic cells into the inflamed mucosa and not caused by the gastric epithelium (Buhling *et al* 2004).

Furthermore, the thiol-dependent carboxypeptidase cathepsin X was identified to be upregulated in H.pylori-gastritis (Kruger *et al* 2005). However, here two independent cellular events are involved. At first, infiltrating macrophages constitutively expressing cathepsin X are one source of increased mucosal cathepsin X levels. Second, the antral surface epithelium expresses cathepsin X *de novo* that represents a real new cellular characteristic of normal gastric epithelium (Kruger *et al* 2005). The observation that gastric cancer cells contain higher cathepsin X levels and H.pylori can also induce cathepsin X in gastric cancer cell lines strongly suggest a functional role of this protease in H.pylori-mediated diseases (Kruger *et al* 2005). The findings concerning the upregulation of cathepsin X illustrate the complexity of gastric pathophysiology and the need for performing comprehensive analysis including the analysis of *ex vivo* material and *in vitro* studies.

Matrix metalloproteases (MMP) and membrane-type matrix metalloproteases (MT-MMP) comprise more than 20 different proteases (mostly family M10) that differ in the expression profile, substrate specificity, subcellular localization and functional implications. Based on the important role of certain members of this protease family in cancer, including gastric cancer, these proteases have been studied to a large extent in chronic gastritis and premalignant lesions in the stomach. MMP-9- and MMP-2-derived activities were strongly upregulated in H.pylori-infected gastric mucosa, whereas the expression of the tissue inhibitors of MMPs TIMP-1 and TIMP-2 was unchanged. This upregulation, in particular of MMP-9, could be assigned to the increased number of macrophages infiltrating the inflamed mucosa (Bergin *et al* 2004). The upregulation of MMP-9 during H.pylori-induced gastritis could be completely reversed to normal levels after the successful eradication of the bacterium proving the direct linkage between the H.pylori-induced MMP-9 expression and chronic gastritis (Danese *et al* 2004). Other studies confirmed these findings and identified MMP-7 (Wroblewski *et al* 2003; Koyama 2004), ADAM-10 and -17 (Yoshimura *et al* 2002), MMP-1 (Menges *et al* 2000) and MT1-MMP (Koyama 2004) as target genes in H.pylori infection. The association between the upregulation of MMP- 7 and bacterial factors revealed a unique role of the CagA for the induction of MMP-7 (Crawford *et al* 2003). The induction of MMP-7 was strongly dependent on the presence of the cagA gene, while the expression of VacA, another important bacterial pathogenic factor, was irrelevant (Bebb *et al* 2003).

4.2 H.pylori-induced gastric and duodenal ulcer disease

Since the development of gastric and duodenal ulcer disease is a direct consequence of a preexisting H.pylori infection, dysregulations of the equilibrium between proteases and their corresponding inhibitors are in part similar between the chronic-active gastritis and ulcer diseases. As illustrated in Figure 2, both gastric and duodenal ulcer disease are distinct entities of the H.pylori infection mostly determined by alterations of gastric pH and the location of the infection. Naturally, similar molecular changes including changes of protease expression were described for these pathologies. Like in asymptomatic chronic active gastritis, active duodenal ulcer disease was associated with lower tPA levels (Ben-Hamida *et al* 1998) and higher uPA levels (Herszenyi *et al* 1997). The subsequent alterations of the fibrinolytic system are important factors for the impaired healing of ulcers and the associated increased risk of severe gastroduodenal bleeding events. Furthermore, an upregulation of tryptase was identified both in duodenal and gastric ulcer (Plebani *et al* 1992) and higher levels of chymase were described in H.pylori-mediated gastritis (Matsuo *et al* 2003). However, both findings can be attributed to the higher number of mast cells infiltrating the inflamed tissue and do not reflect a new feature of the gastric epithelium (Hall *et al* 2003).

As discussed earlier, pepsinogens are the main aspartic proteases of the stomach and their functional implications for peptic and duodenal ulcer were established already 20 years ago. In general, both forms of ulcer are associated with higher pepsin activities or levels (Pearson *et al* 1986). However, it is notable that changes of mucosal and systemic pepsinogen levels and the corresponding pepsin activities do not always correlate (Vianello *et al* 1994). Therefore, investigations aimed at the determination of proteolytic activities in gastroduodenal diseases should be performed rather by taking mucosal biopsies than using serum samples. The upregulation of pepsinogens in ulcer disease is strongly linked to normal or higher acid secretion in this subgroup of H.pylori-infected patients. Once atrophic gastritis develops in the stomach, both acid and pepsinogen release is strongly impaired (see section 4.1). In addition to pepsinogens, the aspartic cathepsins D and E (Samloff *et al* 1989) as well as the thiol-dependent cathepsins B and L were found to be increased in biopsies from patients with active ulcer disease (Herszenyi *et al* 1997). Furthermore, several MMPs such as MMP-1, -2, -7 and 10 are known to be upregulated in ulcer and the surrounding tissue (Saarialho-Kere *et al* 1996; Menges *et al* 2000; Yokoyama *et al* 2000). Similarly to their role in gastric cancer, MMPs seem to be important for the degradation of extracellular matrix components and the epithelial remodeling occurring in the gastroduodenal ulceration. Animal models of gastric ulcer disease clearly showed that the induction of MMPs and TIMPs is not restricted to the epithelial cell layer only, but also includes stromal cells (Calabro *et al* 2004).

4.3 Gastric cancer

Gastric cancer comprises several types of tumors, the adenocarcinoma with either intestinal or diffuse type and the mucosa-associated lymphoid tissue lymphoma (MALT-lymphoma) (Crew *et al* 2004). Although, the role of H.pylori is still being debated for proximal gastric cancer (located at the esophageal gastric junction), there is a general agreement that H.pylori accounts for approximately 70 % of gastric tumors (Marshall *et al* 2005). With respect to the tumorgenesis of adenocarcinoma it is notable that in most cases the development of the tumor is preceded by the appearance of intestinal metaplasia in the stomach (Nardone *et al* 2004). The transdifferentiation of normal gastric intestinal-type mucosa is associated with the induction and subsequent constitutive expression of genes usually expressed in intestine. Among these "upregulated" genes are several proteases like neprilysin (CD10), aminopeptidase N (CD13), dipeptidylpepdidase IV (CD26) (Carl-McGrath *et al* 2004). The presence of these proteases in areas of intestinal metaplasia or their induction compared to normal gastric mucosa is in fact "normal". The pathological condition is not the upregulation of these genes, but the existence of intestinal-type tissue in the gastric mucosa. The linkage of CD10 to distinct cell types has been exploited for the characterization of MALT-lymphoma (Ohshima *et al* 2001), the differentiation between intestinal and specialized metaplasia (Sarbia *et al* 2004) and the discrimination of gastric adenocarcinoma (Tajima *et al* 2001).

One key feature of cancer cells is their resistance to apoptosis leading to prolonged survival of cell clones and facilitate the enrichment of somatic mutations. The regulation of apoptosis involves the proteasome as largest and most powerful proteolytic compartment. The degradation of the poly-ubiquitinated IκB, the inhibitor of the relA-dimers, is a prerequisite for the induction anti-apoptotic genes as XIAP (Ng *et al* 2002). The inhibition of NFκB signaling (Wang *et al* 1999) or the usage of proteasome inhibitors resulted in a normalization of apoptose rates and could be a future strategy for the chemotherapy of gastric cancer (Fan *et al* 2001). Furthermore, an upregulation of distinct proteasome subunits was identified in gastric cancer (Jang *et al* 2004) that could contribute to the higher activity of the protasome-mediated degradation seen in gastric cancer (Bossola *et al* 2001, Yokozaki *et al* 2001).

Lysosomal cathepsins have been investigated in context to gastric cancer for 20 years. After the identification of increased cathepsin-derived activities in tumor tissue compared to normal gastric mucosa (Vasishita *et al* 1985,

Watanabe *et al* 1987), these findings were subsequently correlated to clinical characteristics of the patients. In a recent study, cytosolic cathepsin D levels were negatively correlated to the survival of patients suffering from gastric adenocarcinoma (Del Casar *et al* 2004). In this study, only patients with primarily resectable cancer were included. Both the expression of cathepsin D and the patients' age correlated negatively with the survival rate. However, the age was the only independent prognostic factor, limiting the importance of the upregulated cathepsin D expression. In addition to higher cathepsin D levels, a different subcellular distribution pattern of this protease was demonstrated in gastric cancer. While cathepsin D appears in normal tissue as granular staining, gastric tumors show an abnormal cytoplasmic localization. Interestingly, this staining pattern was associated with stronger submucosal infiltration (Kashida *et al* 2001). Up to now, most studies have confirmed the upregulation of cathepsin D in gastric cancer and have proven that not only the expression of cathepsin D by the tumor itself is important, but the stromal compartment plays an important role as well (Allgayer *et al* 1998, Ikeguchi *et al* 2001).

In addition to cathepsin D, the thiol-dependent cathepsins B and L are also found to be upregulated in gastric cancer (Hirano *et al* 1993, Plebani *et al* 1995). Similar to cathepsin D, a higher expression of cathepsin B and L correlated with the invasive potential of the tumor cells (Dohchin *et al* 2000). As discussed earlier, several tumor-specific cathepsin B isoforms were identified (Gong *et al* 1993, Berquin *et al* 1995). Functionally, the increased cathepsin-derived activity in gastric cancer might be important for the degradation of extracellular matrix as well as in the regulation of neoangiogenesis (Jedeszko *et al* 2004, Sloane *et al* 2005). The regulation of cathepsin B expression in tumor tissue is not well understood. In part, genetic rearrangements might be the primary cause for the upregulation of cathepsin B. In esophageal cancer about 13% of patients had an amplification of the locus 8p22-23 that includes the cathepsin B gene (Hughes *et al* 1998). In most cases, the altered expression results from elevated transcription, use of alternative promoters and alternative splicing (Yan *et al* 2003). As shown for cathepsin D, the increased expression of cathepsin B and L is not only limited to the tumor tissue. The surrounding stromal compartment including macrophages, infiltrating lymphocytes and fibroblasts exhibit also higher cathepsin B expression and were functionally involved in the intra- and pericellular degradation of DQ-collagen IV (Sameni *et al* 2003).

Even most publications provide concordant results with respect to the induction of cathepsins in gastric cancer, there are studies (e.g. for cathepsin D, Russo *et al* 2000) in which the upregulation could not be demonstrated. The underlying reasons for these differences might be diverse and potential causes were extensively discussed in the first section of this chapter. A recent paper dealing with the upregulation of cathepsin B in gastric cancer examplarily shows the problems in the assessment of expression changes in tumor tissue (Ebert *et al* 2005). While the authors were able to confirm the generally accepted correlation between higher cathepsin B levels and advanced tumor stage/tumor progression, the isolation of pure tumor cells by magnetic beads technique showed an upregulation of cathepsin B in only 6 out of 10 cases. Based on this finding, it can be concluded that the overexpression of cathepsin B is not a mandatory feature of all gastric cancer, but if present, there is a lot of evidence that the higher expression of this protease is unfavorable for the patient.

Although the role of protease inhibitors for regulating the activity of proteases is well recognized, only a limited number of these inhibitors has been evaluated with respect to gastroduodenal diseases. Stefin B, a cysteine protease inhibitor, was found to be decreased in gastric cancer (Russo *et al* 2000). Furthermore, TIMP-2 and PAI-1 levels were analyzed in patients with gastric cancer and found to be associated in part with clinical features (Allgayer *et al* 1998).

The most attention concerning gastric cancer has been attracted by the matrix metalloproteases and their inhibitors. Since 1994, over 400 reviews have summarized the current knowledge in this field. Taken into account the presence of a specific chapter dealing with these proteases in this book, we only want to list the most prominent MMPs and TIMPs studied in gastric cancer, which are almost identical to those identified in chronic gastritis and ulcer disease. The upregulation of MMP-1, -2, -7, - 9, -13 and MT1-MMP in gastric cancer has been confirmed by several groups, different methods and distinct ethnicities and can be therefore considered to be a general feature of gastric adenocarcinoma. From the functional point of view, it is important to mention that the upregulation of these proteases is often associated with unchanged levels of the corresponding inhibitors (TIMPs) resulting in an increased proteolytic activity (Zhang *et al* 2003). This imbalance affects a variety of cellular processes like angiogenesis, motility, cell cycle regulation, growth factor and receptor interactions and eventually supports the development and spreading of the initial tumor clone (Yasui *et al* 2005). In addition to the epigenetic dysregulation of MMPs in gastric cancer, the investigation of gene polymorphisms in MMP genes has been constantly growing over the last years. For instance, promoter polymorphisms in the MMP-1 and -9 genes have been identified and correlated to an increased risk for an invasive phenotype (Matsumura *et al* 2004, 2005). However, these analyses have just been started for the field of gastric cancer, and further studies are needed to strengthen the initial findings.

4.4 *In vitro* models of H.pylori-infection

In order to investigate the interaction between H.pylori and gastric mucosa and to identify cellular pathways, *in vitro* models using gastric tumor cell lines were established (Takagi *et al* 2000). The usage of these cell models confirmed the known protease interactions from clinical studies as well as identified new candidates from the proteolytic field. The coculture of H.pylori with gastric tumor cell lines demonstrated an upregulation of MMP-9, uPA (Kitadai *et al* 2003) and identified protease-activated receptors as important components of mucosal host defense (Toyoda *et al* 2003, Kaunitz *et al* 2004). These receptors are specifically activated by either thrombin (PAR-1, 3, 4) or trypsin/tryptase (PAR-2) and mediate a variety of gastric functions like the motility of the smooth muscle cell layers within the esophageal and gastric mucosa (Vergnolle 2000, Kawabata 2003).

In addition to the induction of gastritis, H.pylori-infection broadly affects epithelial cells directly. One major phenomenon is the induction of apoptosis (Xia *et al* 2001). The coculture of the bacterium with different cell lines revealed a predominant induction of the intrinsic (mitochondrial) pathway including the action of caspases 3, 6, 7, 8 and 9 (Potthoff *et al* 2002, Maeda *et al* 2002, Shibayama *et al* 2001) that was also confirmed by clinical studies using *ex vivo* material (Hoshi *et al* 1998). Interestingly, rather conflicting data have been obtained for the caspase-1, the interleukin-1 converting enzyme. A recent work on monocytic THP-1 cells identified the intracellular signals (TLR-4, Rac1/Pak1 pathway) for the activation of caspase-1 (Basak *et al* 2005), however an induction of caspase-1 has not been demonstrated in *ex vivo* analyses (Potthoff *et al* 2002, Tomita *et al* 2001). Considering the important regulatory role of IL-1B polymorphisms for the fate of H.pylori-infected patients (El-Omar *et al* 2000), caspase-1 as the final activating enzyme of this cytokine might be an interesting candidate to investigate in more detail.

The central role of the proteasome for the regulation of the cell cycle and the increased gastric epithelial cell turnover in subjects with gastritis were the rational base for investigating the effect of H.pylori on this proteolytic compartment. Using gastric tumor cell lines, it was demonstrated that p27, a cyclin-dependent kinase inhibitor, is decreased in the presence of H.pylori by proteasome-mediate degradation (Eguchi *et al* 2003, 2004). Lower p27 levels are thought to promote gastric tumorgenesis by inhibiting apoptotic pathways and might therefore, represent one piece of the numerous molecular changes induced by H.pylori during the development of precancerous lesion and subsequent adenocarcinoma.

In order to study the mechanisms leading to MMP upregulation in gastritis and gastric cancer, the co-cultivation of H.pylori and gastric cancer cell lines has been widely used. In general, the *in vitro* studies confirmed the findings obtained from tissue specimens and added information concerning the signal pathways involved. For instance, interleukin-1beta was a key mediator for the induction of MMP-1 and -3 in the gastric cancer cell line AGS (Gooz *et al* 2003), whereas MMP-9 induction was regulated via the NFκB pathway in these cells (Mori *et al* 2003). Using the ADAM-17 deficient mice, it was shown that this protease is essential for the H.pylori-dependent activation of epithelial growth factor receptor (EGFR) and downstream pathways including ERK1/2 and MMP-7 production (Yan *et al* 2005).

5. CONCLUSIONS

Proteases are important regulators for the gastric physiology and they are strongly involved in the pathogenesis of various gastroduodenal diseases. The upregulation of certain proteases, in particular, certain lysosomal cathepsins and matrix-metalloproteases in the H.pylori-mediated diseases has been successfully correlated with clinical and pathological characteristics of the patients. Although, a lot of data has been published and in part independently confirmed by several groups, only the analysis of the serum ratio between pepsinogen A and C in combination with the levels of gastrin-17 has been established as "biomarker" into the routine clinical work-up so far. Using this approach, also known as GASTROPANEL™ (BIOHIT, Helsinki, Finland), H.pylori-infected subjects suffering from atrophic gastritis can be specifically identified.

For other proteases, the limited number of prospective long-term studies in gastroduodenal diseases, compared to colon, lung or breast cancer, as well as the lack of consistent methodologies are the main problems that need to be resolved before potential markers such as cathepsin D can be implemented into the clinical practice. Furthermore, the role of protease inhibitors, with the exception of TIMPs, has been mostly neglected in the gastric compartment. Future work in this field as well as large prospective studies will lead to a better functional understanding of proteases and their inhibitors in gastric physiology and their potential use as "biomarker" for the identification of subgroups of patients who might have higher risk for distinct gastroduodenal diseases.

ACKNOWLEDGEMENTS

This work was supported in parts by the "Deutsche Forschungsgemeinschaft", Germany (We2170/3-1) and the NBL-3 program of the "Bundesministerium für Forschung und Technik" (01ZZ0407/PFG1).

We thank Ursula Stolz, Nadine Siebert and Simone Philipsen for their excellent work.

REFERENCES

Allgayer H, Basic R, Grutzner KU, Beyer BC, Tarabichi A, Schildberg FW, Heiss MM, 1998, Tumor-associated proteases and inhibitors in gastric cancer: analysis of prognostic impact and individual risk protease patterns. *Clin Exp Metastasis.* **16:** 62-73.

Aoki K, Misumi J, Kimura T, Zhao W, Xie T, 1997, Evaluation of cutoff levels for screening of gastric cancer using serum pepsinogens and distributions of levels of serum pepsinogen I, II and of PG I/PG II ratios in a gastric cancer case-control study. *J Epidemiol.* **7:** 143-151.

Arora S, Chauhan SS, 2002, Identification and characterization of a novel human cathepsin L splice variant. *Gene.* **293:** 123-131.

Asaka M, Kimura T, Kudo M, Takeda H, Mitani S, Miyazaki T, Miki K, Graham DY, 1992, Relationship of Helicobacter pylori to serum pepsinogens in an asymptomatic Japanese population. *Gastroenterology.* **102:** 760-766.

Basak C, Pathak SK, Bhattacharyya A, Mandal D, Pathak S, Kundu M, 2005, NF-kappaB- and C/EBPbeta-driven interleukin-1beta gene expression and PAK1-mediated caspase-1 activation play essential roles in interleukin-1beta release from Helicobacter pylori lipopolysaccharide-stimulated macrophages. *J Biol Chem.* **280:** 4279-4288.

Bebb JR, Letley DP, Thomas RJ, Aviles F, Collins HM, Watson SA, Hand NM, Zaitoun A, Atherton JC, 2003, Helicobacter pylori upregulates matrilysin (MMP-7) in epithelial cells in vivo and in vitro in a Cag dependent manner. *Gut.* **52:** 1408-1413.

Ben-Hamida A, Adesanya AA, Man WK, Spencer J, 1998, Histamine and tissue fibrinolytic activity in duodenal ulcer disease. *Dig Dis Sci.* **43:** 126-132.

Bergin PJ, Anders E, Sicheng W, Erik J, Jennie A, Hans L, Pierre M, Qiang PH, Marianne QJ, 2004, Increased production of matrix metalloproteinases in Helicobacter pylori-associated human gastritis. *Helicobacter.* **9:** 201-210.

Berquin IM, Cao L, Fong D, Sloane BF, 1995, Identification of two new exons and multiple transcription start points in the 5'-untranslated region of the human cathepsin-B-encoding gene. *Gene.* **159:** 143-149.

Blaser MJ, Atherton JC, 2004, Helicobacter pylori persistence: biology and disease. *J Clin Invest.* **113:** 321-333.

Bossola M, Muscaritoli M, Costelli P, Bellantone R, Pacelli F, Busquets S, Argiles J, Lopez-Soriano FJ, Civello IM, Baccino FM, Rossi Fanelli F, Doglietto GB, 2001, Increased muscle ubiquitin mRNA levels in gastric cancer patients. *Am J Physiol Regul Integr Comp Physiol.* **280:** R1518-1523.

Broutet N, Plebani M, Sakarovitch C, Sipponen P, Megraud F, 2003, Eurohepygast Study Group, Pepsinogen A, pepsinogen C, and gastrin as markers of atrophic chronic gastritis in European dyspeptics. *Br J Cancer.* **88:** 1239-1247.

de Bruin PC, Kummer JA, van der Valk P, van Heerde P, Kluin PM, Willemze R, Ossenkoppele GJ, Radaszkiewicz T, Meijer CJ, 1994, Granzyme B-expressing peripheral T-cell lymphomas: neoplastic equivalents of activated cytotoxic T cells with preference for mucosa-associated lymphoid tissue localization. *Blood.* **84:** 3785-3791.

Buhling F, Peitz U, Kruger S, Kuster D, Vieth M, Gebert I, Roessner A, Weber E, Malfertheiner P, Wex T, 2004, Cathepsins K, L, B, X and W are differentially expressed in normal and chronically inflamed gastric mucosa. *Biol Chem.* **385:** 439-445.

Bumann D, Aksu S, Wendland M, Janek K, Zimny-Arndt U, Sabarth N, Meyer TF, Jungblut PR, 2002, Proteome analysis of secreted proteins of the gastric pathogen Helicobacter pylori. *Infect Immun.* **70:** 3396-3403.

Calabro A, Grappone C, Pellegrini G, Evangelista S, Tramontana M, Schuppan D, Herbst H, Milani S, 2004, Spatial and temporal pattern of expression of interstitial collagenase, stromelysin/transin, gelatinase A, and TIMP-1 during experimental gastric ulcer healing. *Digestion.* **70:** 127-138.

Cao L, Taggart RT, Berquin IM, Moin K, Fong D, Sloane BF, 1994, Human gastric adenocarcinoma cathepsin B: isolation and sequencing of full-length cDNAs and polymorphisms of the gene. *Gene.* **139:** 163-169.

Carl-McGrath S, Lendeckel U, Ebert M, Wolter AB, Roessner A, Rocken C, 2004, The ectopeptidases CD10, CD13, CD26, and CD143 are upregulated in gastric cancer. *Int J Oncol.* **25:** 1223-1232.

Chung SM, 1990, Variant cathepsin L activity from gastric cancer tissue. *Jpn J Cancer Res.* **81:** 813-819.

Cirman T, Oresic K, Mazovec GD, Turk V, Reed JC, Myers RM, Salvesen GS, Turk B, 2004, Selective disruption of lysosomes in HeLa cells triggers apoptosis mediated by cleavage of Bid by multiple papain-like lysosomal cathepsins. *J Biol Chem.* **279:** 3578-3587.

Correa P, 1995, Helicobacter pylori and gastric carcinogenesis. *Am J Surg Pathol.* **19(Suppl 1):** S37-43.

Crawford HC, Krishna US, Israel DA, Matrisian LM, Washington MK, Peek RM Jr, 2003, Helicobacter pylori strain-selective induction of matrix metalloproteinase-7 in vitro and within gastric mucosa. *Gastroenterology.* **125:** 1125-1136.

Crew KD, Neugut AI, 2004 Epidemiology of upper gastrointestinal malignancies. *Semin Oncol.* **31:** 450-464.

D'Amico TA, Harpole DH Jr, 2000, Molecular biology of esophageal cancer. *Chest Surg Clin N Am.* **10:** 451-469.

Danese S, Papa A, Gasbarrini A, Ricci R, Maggiano N, 2004, Helicobacter pylori eradication down-regulates matrix metalloproteinase-9 expression in chronic gastritis and gastric ulcer. *Gastroenterology.* **126:** 369-371.

Debatin KM, 2004, Apoptosis pathways in cancer and cancer therapy. *Cancer Immunol Immunother.* **53:** 153-159.

Del Casar MJ, Vizoso FJ, Abdel-Laa O, Sanz L, Martin A, Daniela Corte M, Bongera M, Garcia Muniz JL, Fueyo A, 2004, Prognostic value of cytosolyc cathepsin D content in resectable gastric cancer. *J Surg Oncol.* **86:** 16-21.

Dixon MF, Genta RM, Yardley JH, Correa P, 1996, Classification and grading of gastritis. The updated Sydney System. International Workshop on the Histopathology of Gastritis, Houston 1994. *Am J Surg Pathol.* **20:** 1161-1181.

Dohchin A, Suzuki JI, Seki H, Masutani M, Shiroto H, Kawakami Y, 2000, Immunostained cathepsins B and L correlate with depth of invasion and different metastatic pathways in early stage gastric carcinoma. *Cancer.* **89:** 482-487.

Dunn BE, Cohen H, Blaser MJ, 1997, Helicobacter pylori. *Clin Microbiol Rev.* **10:** 720-741.

Ebert MP, Kruger S, Fogeron ML, Lamer S, Chen J, Pross M, Schulz HU, Lage H, Heim S, Roessner A, Malfertheiner P, Rocken C, 2005, Overexpression of cathepsin B in gastric cancer identified by proteome analysis. *Proteomics.* **5:** 1693-1704.

Eguchi H, Carpentier S, Kim SS, Moss SF, 2004, P27kip1 regulates the apoptotic response of gastric epithelial cells to Helicobacter pylori. *Gut.* **53:** 797-804.

Eguchi H, Herschenhous N, Kuzushita N, Moss SF, 2003, Helicobacter pylori increases proteasome-mediated degradation of p27(kip1) in gastric epithelial cells. *Cancer Res.* **63:** 4739-4746.

El-Omar EM, Carrington M, Chow WH, McColl KE, Bream JH, Young HA, Herrera J, Lissowska J, Yuan CC, Rothman N, Lanyon G, Martin M, Fraumeni JF Jr, Rabkin CS, 2000, Interleukin-1 polymorphisms associated with increased risk of gastric cancer. *Nature.* **404:** 398-402.

Faller G, Kirchner T, 2005,Immunological and morphogenic basis of gastric mucosa atrophy and metaplasia. *Virchows Arch.* **446:** 1-9

Fan XM, Wong BC, Wang WP, Zhou XM, Cho CH, Yuen ST, Leung SY, Lin MC, Kung HF, Lam SK, 2001, Inhibition of proteasome function induced apoptosis in gastric cancer. *Int J Cancer.* **93:** 481-488.

Farinati F, Herszenyi L, Plebani M, Carraro P, De Paoli M, Cardin R, Roveroni G, Rugge M, Nitti D, Grigioni WF, D'Errico A, Naccarato R, 1996, Increased levels of cathepsin B and L, urokinase-type plasminogen activator and its inhibitor type-1 as an early event in gastric carcinogenesis. *Carcinogenesis.* **17:** 2581-2587.

Ge Z, Taylor DE, 1999,Contributions of genome sequencing to understanding the biology of Helicobacter pylori. *Annu Rev Microbiol.* **53:** 353-587.

Gong Q, Chan SJ, Bajkowski AS, Steiner DF, Frankfater A, 1993, Characterization of the cathepsin B gene and multiple mRNAs in human tissues: evidence for alternative splicing of cathepsin B pre-mRNA. *DNA Cell Biol.* **12:** 299-309.

Gooz M, Shaker M, Gooz P, Smolka AJ, 2003, Interleukin 1beta induces gastric epithelial cell matrix metalloproteinase secretion and activation during Helicobacter pylori infection. *Gut.* **52:** 1250-1256.

Gotz JM, Vergouwe Y, Verspaget HW, Biemond I, Sier CF, Lamers CB, Veenendaal RA, 1996, Gastric mucosal plasminogen activators in Helicobacter pylori infection. *Dig Dis Sci.* **41:** 1577-1582.

Haas G, Karaali G, Ebermayer K, Metzger WG, Lamer S, Zimny-Arndt U, Diescher S, Goebel UB, Vogt K, Roznowski AB, Wiedenmann BJ, Meyer TF, Aebischer T, Jungblut PR, 2002, Immunoproteomics of Helicobacter pylori infection and relation to gastric disease. *Proteomics.* **2:** 313-324.

Hall W, Buckley M, Crotty P, O'Morain CA, 2003, Gastric mucosal mast cells are increased in Helicobacter pylori-negative functional dyspepsia. *Clin Gastroenterol Hepatol.* **1:** 363-369.

Herszenyi L, Plebani M, Carraro P, De Paoli M, Cardin R, Di Mario F, Kusstatscher S, Naccarato R, Farinati F, 1997, Impaired fibrinolysis and increased protease levels in gastric and duodenal mucosa of patients with active duodenal ulcer. *Am J Gastroenterol.* **92:** 843-847.

Hirano T, Yoshioka H, 1993, Serum cathepsin B levels, urinary excretion of cathepsin B and tissue cathepsin B content in the patients with gastric cancer. *Nippon Geka Hokan.* **62:** 217-221.

Hoshi T, Sasano H, Kato K, Yabuki N, Ohara S, Konno R, Asaki S, Toyota T, Tateno H, Nagura H, 1998, Immunohistochemistry of Caspase3/CPP32 in human stomach and its correlation with cell proliferation and apoptosis. *Anticancer Res.* **18:** 4347-4353.

Houghton J, Stoicov C, Nomura S, Rogers AB, Carlson J, Li H, Cai X, Fox JG, Goldenring JR, Wang TC, 2004, Gastric cancer originating from bone marrow-derived cells. *Science.* **306**: 1568-1571.

Hughes SJ, Glover TW, Zhu XX, Kuick R, Thoraval D, Orringer MB, Beer DG, Hanash S, 1998, A novel amplicon at 8p22-23 results in overexpression of cathepsin B in esophageal adenocarcinoma. *Proc Natl Acad Sci U S A.* **95:** 12410-12415.

Ikeguchi M, Fukuda K, Oka S, Yamaguchi K, Hisamitsu K, Tsujitani S, Sakatani T, Ueda T, Kaibara N, 2001, Clinicopathological significance of cathepsin D expression in gastric adenocarcinoma. *Oncology.* **61:** 71-78.

Jang JS, Cho HY, Lee YJ, Ha WS, Kim HW, 2004, The differential proteome profile of stomach cancer: identification of the biomarker candidates. *Oncol Res.* **14:** 491-499.

Jedeszko C, Sloane BF, 2004, Cysteine cathepsins in human cancer. *Biol Chem.* **385:** 1017-1027.

Jonsson K, Guo BP, Monstein HJ, Mekalanos JJ, Kronvall G, 2004, Molecular cloning and characterization of two Helicobacter pylori genes coding for plasminogen-binding proteins. *Proc Natl Acad Sci U S A.* **101:** 1852-1857.

Kageyama T, 2002, Pepsinogens, progastricsins, and prochymosins: structure, function, evolution, and development. *Cell Mol Life Sci.* **59:** 288-306.

Kaneko H, Konagaya T, Kusugami K, 2002, Helicobacter pylori and gut hormones. *J Gastroenterol.* **37:** 77-86.

Kashida H, Kawamata H, Ichikawa K, Morita K, Imura J, Fujimori T, 2001, Intracytoplasmic localization of cathepsin D reflects the invasive potential of gastric carcinoma. *J Gastroenterol.* **36:** 809-815.

Kaunitz JD, Akiba Y, 2004, Gastroduodenal mucosal defense: role of endogenous mediators. *Curr Opin Gastroenterol.* **20:** 526-532.

Kavermann H, Burns BP, Angermuller K, Odenbreit S, Fischer W, Melchers K, Haas R, 2003, Identification and characterization of Helicobacter pylori genes essential for gastric colonization. *J Exp Med.* **197:** 813-822.

Kawabata A, 2003, Gastrointestinal functions of proteinase-activated receptors. *Life Sci.* **74:** 247-254.

Kawachi H, Takizawa T, Eishi Y, Shimizu S, Kumagai J, Funata N, Koike M, 2003, Absence of either gastric or intestinal phenotype in microscopic differentiated gastric carcinomas. *J Pathol.* **199:** 436-446.

Khan A, Krishna M, Baker SP, Malhothra R, Banner BF, 1998, Cathepsin B expression and its correlation with tumor-associated laminin and tumor progression in gastric cancer. *Arch Pathol Lab Med.* **122:** 172-177.

Kim DY, Kim KK, 2003, Crystal structure of ClpX molecular chaperone from Helicobacter pylori. *J Biol Chem.* **278:** 50664-50670.

Kitadai Y, Sasaki A, Ito M, Tanaka S, Oue N, Yasui W, Aihara M, Imagawa K, Haruma K, Chayama K, 2003, Helicobacter pylori infection influences expression of genes related to angiogenesis and invasion in human gastric carcinoma cells. *Biochem Biophys Res Commun.* **311:** 809-814.

Koyama S, 2004, Significance of cell-surface expression of matrix metalloproteinases and their inhibitors on gastric epithelium and infiltrating mucosal lymphocytes in progression of Helicobacter pylori-associated gastritis. *Scand J Gastroenterol.* **39:** 1046-1053.

Krueger S, Kalinski T, Hundertmark T, Wex T, Kuester D, Peitz U, Ebert M, Nägler DK, Kellner U, Malfertheiner P, Naumann M, Röcken C, Roessner A, 2005, Upregulation of Cathepsin X in Helicobacter pylori Gastritis and Gastric Cancer. *J Pathol.* **in press.**

Lahteenmaki K, Kuusela P, Korhonen TK, 2001, Bacterial plasminogen activators and receptors. *FEMS Microbiol Rev.* **25:** 531-552.

Maeda S, Yoshida H, Mitsuno Y, Hirata Y, Ogura K, Shiratori Y, Omata M, 2002, Analysis of apoptotic and antiapoptotic signalling pathways induced by Helicobacter pylori. *Mol Pathol.* **55:** 286-293.

Marshall BJ, Warren JR, 1984, Unidentified curved bacilli in the stomach of patients with gastritis and peptic ulceration. *Lancet.* **1:** 1311-1315.

Marshall BJ, Windsor HM, 2005, The relation of Helicobacter pylori to gastric adenocarcinoma and lymphoma: pathophysiology, epidemiology, screening, clinical presentation, treatment, and prevention. *Med Clin North Am.* **89:** 313-344.

Matsumura S, Oue N, Kitadai Y, Chayama K, Yoshida K, Yamaguchi Y, Toge T, Imai K, Nakachi K, Yasui W, 2004, A single nucleotide polymorphism in the MMP-1 promoter is correlated with histological differentiation of gastric cancer. *J Cancer Res Clin Oncol.* **130:** 259-265.

Matsumura S, Oue N, Nakayama H, Kitadai Y, Yoshida K, Yamaguchi Y, Imai K, Nakachi K, Matsusaki K, Chayama K, Yasui W, 2005, A single nucleotide polymorphism in the MMP-9 promoter affects tumor progression and invasive phenotype of gastric cancer. *J Cancer Res Clin Oncol.* **131:** 19-25.

Matsuo T, Ikura Y, Ohsawa M, Ogami M, Kayo S, Yoshimi N, Hai E, Naruko T, Ohishi M, Higuchi K, Arakawa T, Ueda M, 2003, Mast cell chymase expression in Helicobacter pylori-associated gastritis. *Histopathology.* **43:** 538-549.

Mehtani S, Gong Q, Panella J, Subbiah S, Peffley DM, Frankfater A, 1998, In vivo expression of an alternatively spliced human tumor message that encodes a truncated form of cathepsin B. Subcellular distribution of the truncated enzyme in COS cells. *J Biol Chem.* **273:** 13236-13244.

Menges M, Chan CC, Zeitz M, Stallmach A, 2000, Higher concentration of matrix-metalloproteinase 1 (interstitial collagenase) in H. pylori-compared to NSAID-induced gastric ulcers. *Z Gastroenterol.* **38:** 887-891.

Moayyedi P, Hunt RH, 2004, Helicobacter pylori public health implications. *Helicobacter.* **9(Suppl 1):** 67-72.

Mori N, Sato H, Hayashibara T, Senba M, Geleziunas R, Wada A, Hirayama T, Yamamoto N, 2003, Helicobacter pylori induces matrix metalloproteinase-9 through activation of nuclear factor kappaB. *Gastroenterology.* **124:** 983-992.

Muntener K, Zwicky R, Csucs G, Rohrer J, Baici A, 2004, Exon skipping of cathepsin B: mitochondrial targeting of a lysosomal peptidase provokes cell death. *J Biol Chem.* **279:** 41012-41017.

Naidoo S, Ramsaroop R, Bhoola R, Bhoola KD, 1997, The evaluation of tissue kallikrein in Helicobacter pylori-associated gastric ulcer disease. *Immunopharmacology.* **36:** 263-269.

Nardone G, Rocco A, Malfertheiner P, 2004, Review article: helicobacter pylori and molecular events in precancerous gastric lesions. *Aliment Pharmacol Ther.* **20:** 261-270.

Narita Y, Oda S, Moriyama A, Kageyama T, 2002, Primary structure, unique enzymatic properties, and molecular evolution of pepsinogen B and pepsin B. *Arch Biochem Biophys.* **404:** 177-185.

Ng CP, Bonavida B, 2002, X-linked inhibitor of apoptosis (XIAP) blocks Apo2 ligand/tumor necrosis factor-related apoptosis-inducing ligand-mediated apoptosis of prostate cancer cells in the presence of mitochondrial activation: sensitization by overexpression of second mitochondria-derived activator of caspase/direct IAP-binding protein with low pl (Smac/DIABLO). *Mol Cancer Ther.* **1:** 1051-1058.

Nilius M, Vahldieck T, Repper I, Sokolowski A, Janowitz P, Malfertheiner P, 2000, Protease-protease inhibitor balance in the gastric mucosa. Influence of Helicobacter pylori infection. *Adv Exp Med Biol.* **477:** 445-454.

Oberhuber G, Bodingbauer M, Mosberger I, Stolte M, Vogelsang H, 1998, High proportion of granzyme B-positive (activated) intraepithelial and lamina propria lymphocytes in lymphocytic gastritis. *Am J Surg Pathol.* **22:** 450-458

Ohshima K, Kawasaki C, Muta H, Muta K, Deyev V, Haraoka S, Suzumiya J, Podack ER, Kikuchi M, 2001, CD10 and Bcl10 expression in diffuse large B-cell lymphoma: CD10 is a marker of improved prognosis. *Histopathology.* **39:** 156-162.

Ord T, Kolmer M, Villems R, Saarma M, 1990, Structure of the human genomic region homologous to the bovine prochymosin-encoding gene. *Gene.* **91:** 241-246.

Pantzar M, Ljungh A, Wadstrom T, 1998, Plasminogen binding and activation at the surface of Helicobacter pylori CCUG 17874. *Infect Immun.* **66:** 4976-4980.

Pearson JP, Ward R, Allen A, Roberts NB, Taylor WH, 1986, Mucus degradation by pepsin: comparison of mucolytic activity of human pepsin 1 and pepsin 3: implications in peptic ulceration. *Gut.* **27:** 243-8.

Plebani M, 1993, Pepsinogens in health and disease. *Crit Rev Clin Lab Sci.* **30:** 273-328.

Plebani M, Di Mario F, Battistel M, Basso D, Mantovani G, Giacomini A, Burlina A, 1992, Measurement of tryptase in endoscopic gastroduodenal biopsies: distribution and relationship with ulcer disease. *Clin Chim Acta.* **206:** 107-114.

Plebani M, Herszenyi L, Cardin R, Roveroni G, Carraro P, Paoli MD, Rugge M, Grigioni WF, Nitti D, Naccarato R, 1995, Cysteine and serine proteases in gastric cancer. *Cancer.* **76:** 367-375.

Potthoff A, Ledig S, Martin J, Jandl O, Cornberg M, Obst B, Beil W, Manns MP, Wagner S, 2002, Significance of the caspase family in Helicobacter pylori induced gastric epithelial apoptosis. *Helicobacter.* **7:** 367-377.

Rehfeld JF, Goetze JP, 2003, The posttranslational phase of gene expression: new possibilities in molecular diagnosis. *Curr Mol Med.* **3:** 25-38.

Richter C, Tanaka T, Yada RY, 1998, Mechanism of activation of the gastric aspartic proteinases: pepsinogen, progastricsin and prochymosin. *Biochem J.* **335:** 481-490.

Rosicka M, Krsek M, Jarkovska Z, Marek J, Schreiber V, 2002, Ghrelin – a new endogenous growth hormone secretagogue. *Physiol Res.* **51:** 435-441.

Russo A, Bazan V, Migliavacca M, Zanna I, Tubiolo C, Tumminello FM, Dardanoni G, Cajozzo M, Bazan P, Modica G, Latteri M, Tomasino RM, Colucci G, Gebbia N, Leto G, 2000, Prognostic significance of DNA ploidy, S-phase fraction, and tissue levels of aspartic, cysteine, and serine proteases in operable gastric carcinoma. *Clin Cancer Res.* **6:** 178-184.

Saarialho-Kere UK, Vaalamo M, Puolakkainen P, Airola K, Parks WC, Karjalainen-Lindsberg ML, 1996, Enhanced expression of matrilysin, collagenase, and stromelysin-1 in gastrointestinal ulcers. *Am J Pathol.* **148:** 519-526.

Salama NR, Shepherd B, Falkow S, 2004, Global transposon mutagenesis and essential gene analysis of Helicobacter pylori. *J Bacteriol.* **186:** 7926-7935.

Sameni M, Dosescu J, Moin K, Sloane BF, 2003, Functional imaging of proteolysis: stromal and inflammatory cells increase tumor proteolysis. *Mol Imaging.* **2:** 159-175.

Samloff IM, 1989, Peptic ulcer: the many proteinases of aggression. *Gastroenterology.* **96(Suppl 2):** 586-595.

Sarbia M, Donner A, Franke C, Gabbert HE, 2004, Distinction between intestinal metaplasia in the cardia and in Barrett's esophagus: the role of histology and immunohistochemistry. *Hum Pathol.* **35:** 371-376.

Sawant S, Snyman C, Bhoola K, 2001, Comparison of tissue kallikrein and kinin receptor expression in gastric ulcers and neoplasms. *Int Immunopharmacol.* **1:** 2063-2080.

Seth P, Mahajan VS, Chauhan SS, 2003, Transcription of human cathepsin L mRNA species hCATL B from a novel alternative promoter in the first intron of its gene. *Gene.* **321:** 83-91.

Shibayama K, Doi Y, Shibata N, Yagi T, Nada T, Iinuma Y, Arakawa Y, 2001, Apoptotic signaling pathway activated by Helicobacter pylori infection and increase of apoptosis-inducing activity under serum-starved conditions, *Infect Immun.* **69:** 3181-3189.

Sinha AA, Jamuar MP, Wilson MJ, Rozhin J, Sloane BF, 2001, Plasma membrane association of cathepsin B in human prostate cancer: biochemical and immunogold electron microscopic analysis. *Prostate.* **49:** 172-184.

Sloane BF, Yan S, Podgorski I, Linebaugh BE, Cher ML, Mai J, Cavallo-Medved D, Sameni M, Dosescu J, Moin K, 2005, Cathepsin B and tumor proteolysis: contribution of the tumor microenvironment. *Semin Cancer Biol.* **15:** 149-157.

Stoka V, Turk B, Schendel SL, Kim TH, Cirman T, Snipas SJ, Ellerby LM, Bredesen D, Freeze H, Abrahamson M, Bromme D, Krajewski S, Reed JC, Yin XM, Turk V, Salvesen GS, 2001, Lysosomal protease pathways to apoptosis. Cleavage of bid, not pro-caspases, is the most likely route. *J Biol Chem.* **276:** 3149-3157.

Stolte M, Meining A, 2001, The updated Sydney system: classification and grading of gastritis as the basis of diagnosis and treatment. *Can J Gastroenterol.* **15:** 591-598.

Suerbaum S, Michetti P, 2002, Helicobacter pylori infection. *N Engl J Med.* **347:** 1175-1186.

Suzuki T, Ito M, Hayasaki N, Ishihara A, Ando T, Ina K, Kusugami K, 2003, Cytotoxic molecules expressed by intraepithelial lymphocytes may be involved in the pathogenesis of acute gastric mucosal lesions. *J Gastroenterol.* **38:** 216-221.

Taggart CC, Greene CM, McElvaney NG, O'Neill S, 2002, Secretory leucoprotease inhibitor prevents lipopolysaccharide-induced IkappaBalpha degradation without affecting phosphorylation or ubiquitination. *J Biol Chem.* 277: 33648-33653.

Tajima Y, Shimoda T, Nakanishi Y, Yokoyama N, Tanaka T, Shimizu K, Saito T, Kawamura M, Kusano M, Kumagai K, 2001, Gastric and intestinal phenotypic marker expression in gastric carcinomas and its prognostic significance: immunohistochemical analysis of 136 lesions. *Oncology.* **61:** 212-220.

Takagi A, Watanabe S, Igarashi M, Koike J, Hasumi K, Deguchi R, Koga Y, Miwa T, 2000, The effect of Helicobacter pylori on cell proliferation and apoptosis in gastric epithelial cell lines. *Aliment Pharmacol Ther.* **14(Suppl 1):** 188-192.

Tatnell PJ, Cook M, Kay J, 2003, An alternatively spliced variant of cathepsin E in human gastric adenocarcinoma cells. *Biochim Biophys Acta.* **1625:** 203-206.

Tomb JF, White O, Kerlavage AR, Clayton RA, Sutton GG, Fleischmann RD, Ketchum KA, Klenk HP, Gill S, Dougherty BA, Nelson K, Quackenbush J, Zhou L, Kirkness EF, Peterson S, Loftus B, Richardson D, Dodson R, Khalak HG, Glodek A, McKenney K, Fitzegerald LM, Lee N, Adams MD, Hickey EK, Berg DE, Gocayne JD, Utterback TR, Peterson JD, Kelley JM, Cotton MD, Weidman JM, Fujii C, Bowman C, Watthey L, Wallin E, Hayes WS, Borodovsky M, Karp PD, Smith HO, Fraser CM, Venter JC, 1997, The complete genome sequence of the gastric pathogen Helicobacter pylori. *Nature.* **388:** 539-547.

Tomita T, Jackson AM, Hida N, Hayat M, Dixon MF, Shimoyama T, Axon AT, Robinson PA, Crabtree JE, 2001, Expression of Interleukin-18, a Th1 cytokine, in human gastric mucosa is increased in Helicobacter pylori infection. *J Infect Dis.* **183:** 620-627.

Toyoda N, Gabazza EC, Inoue H, Araki K, Nakashima S, Oka S, Taguchi Y, Nakamura M, Suzuki Y, Taguchi O, Imoto I, Suzuki K, Adachi Y, 2003, Expression and cytoprotective effect of protease-activated receptor-1 in gastric epithelial cells. *Scand J Gastroenterol.* **38:** 253-259.

Vaananen H, Vauhkonen M, Helske T, Kaariainen I, Rasmussen M, Tunturi-Hihnala H, Koskenpato J, Sotka M, Turunen M, Sandstrom R, Ristikankare M, Jussila A, Sipponen P, 2003, Non-endoscopic diagnosis of atrophic gastritis with a blood test. Correlation between gastric histology and serum levels of gastrin-17 and pepsinogen I: a multicentre study. *Eur J Gastroenterol Hepatol.* **15:** 885-891.

Vasishta A, Baker PR, Hopwood D, Holley PM, Cuschieri A, 1985, Proteinase-like peptidase activities in malignant and non-malignant gastric tissue. *Br J Surg.* **72:** 386-388.

Vergnolle N, 2000, Review article: proteinase-activated receptors - novel signals for gastrointestinal pathophysiology. *Aliment Pharmacol Ther.* **14:** 257-266.

Vianello F, Di Mario F, Plebani M, Germana B, Dal Santo P, Leandro G, Dotto P, Grassi SA, Battaglia G, Naccarato R, 1994, Pepsin concentration in gastroduodenal biopsy homogenates in chronic ulcer disease. *Dig Dis Sci.* **39:** 301-308.

Wang CY, Cusack JC Jr, Liu R, Baldwin AS Jr, 1999, Control of inducible chemoresistance: enhanced anti-tumor therapy through increased apoptosis by inhibition of NF-kappaB. *Nat Med.* **5:** 412-417.

Watanabe M, Higashi T, Hashimoto M, Tomoda I, Tominaga S, Hashimoto N, Morimoto S, Yamauchi Y, Nakatsukasa H, Kobayashi M, 1987, Elevation of tissue cathepsin B and L activities in gastric cancer. *Hepatogastroenterology.* **34:** 120-122.

Wex T, Buhling F, Wex H, Gunther D, Malfertheiner P, Weber E, Bromme D, 2001, Human cathepsin W, a cysteine protease predominantly expressed in NK cells, is mainly localized in the endoplasmic reticulum. *J Immunol.* **167:** 2172-2178.

Wex T, Sokic-Milutinovic A, Todorovic V, Bjelovic M, Milosavljevic T, Pesko P, Malfertheiner P, 2004, Down-regulation of secretory leukocyte protease inhibitor expression in gastric mucosa is a general phenomenon in Helicobacter pylori-related gastroduodenal diseases. *Dig Dis.* **22:** 390-395.

Wex T, Treiber G, Nilius M, Vieth M, Roessner A, Malfertheiner P, 2004, Helicobacter pylori-mediated gastritis induces local downregulation of secretory leukocyte protease inhibitor in the antrum. *Infect Immun.* **72:** 2383-2385.

Wroblewski LE, Noble PJ, Pagliocca A, Pritchard DM, Hart CA, Campbell F, Dodson AR, Dockray GJ, Varro A, 2003, Stimulation of MMP-7 (matrilysin) by Helicobacter pylori in human gastric epithelial cells: role in epithelial cell migration. *J Cell Sci.* **116:** 3017-3026.

Xia HH, Talley NJ, 2001, Apoptosis in gastric epithelium induced by helicobacter pylori infection: implications in gastric carcinogenesis. *Am J Gastroenterol.* **96:** 16-26.

Yan F, Krishna U, Peek Jr. RM, Kamel M, Frey M, Riggins K, Dempsey PJ, Polk DB, 2005. ADAM17 is required for Helicobacter Pylori-dependent EGFR and Erbb-3 Transactivation in Gastric Epithelial Cells. *Gastroenterology.* **128 (Suppl 2)**: A-117.

Yan S, Sloane BF, 2003, Molecular regulation of human cathepsin B: implication in pathologies. *Biol Chem.* **384:** 845-854.

Yasui W, Oue N, Aung PP, Matsumura S, Shutoh M, Nakayama H, 2005, Molecular-pathological prognostic factors of gastric cancer: a review. *Gastric Cancer.* **8:** 86-94.

Yokoyama T, Otani Y, Kurihara N, Sakurai Y, Kameyama K, Suzuki H, Igarashi N, Kimata M, Wada N, Kubota T, Kumai K, Kitajima M, 2000, Matrix metalloproteinase expression in cultured human gastric wall fibroblasts - interactions with Helicobacter pylori isolated from patients with ulcers. *Aliment Pharmacol Ther.* **14(Suppl 1):** 193-198.

Yokozaki H, Yasui W, Tahara E, 2001, Genetic and epigenetic changes in stomach cancer. *Int Rev Cytol.* **204:** 49-95.

Yoshida N, Sugimoto N, Ochiai J, Nakamura Y, Ichikawa H, Naito Y, Yoshikawa T, 2002, Role of elastase and active oxygen species in gastric mucosal injury induced by aspirin administration in Helicobacter pylori-infected Mongolian gerbils. *Aliment Pharmacol Ther.* **16(Suppl 2):** 191-197.

Yoshimura T, Tomita T, Dixon MF, Axon AT, Robinson PA, Crabtree JE, 2002, ADAMs (a disintegrin and metalloproteinase) messenger RNA expression in Helicobacter pylori-infected, normal, and neoplastic gastric mucosa. *J Infect Dis.* **185:** 332-340.

Zhang S, Li L, Lin JY, Lin H, 2003, Imbalance between expression of matrix metalloproteinase-9 and tissue inhibitor of metalloproteinase-1 in invasiveness and metastasis of human gastric carcinoma. *World J Gastroenterol.* **9:** 899-904.

Zhu J, Nathan C, Jin W, Sim D, Ashcroft GS, Wahl SM, Lacomis L, Erdjument-Bromage H, Tempst P, Wright CD, Ding A, 2002, Conversion of proepithelin to epithelins: roles of SLPI and elastase in host defense and wound repair. *Cell.* **111:** 867-878.

Chapter 4

Proteases in Pancreatic Disease

Avinash Sewpaul[1], Jeremy J. French[2], and Richard M. Charnley[1,2]
[1]*Department of Surgery, University of Newcastle upon Tyne;* [2]*HPB Surgical Unit, Freeman Hospital, Newcastle upon Tyne, United Kingdom*

1. OVERVIEW

In recent years, there have been substantial advances in our understanding of diseases of the exocrine pancreas as a consequence of the recent scientific progress in the underlying genetic, cellular, and molecular pathophysiology. This evidence-based review and critique of the traditional pathogenic theories, clearly shows that proteases and their inhibitors play a crucial role in these diseases.

2. PROTEOLYTIC ENZYMES AND ACUTE PANCREATITIS

2.1 Introduction

More than a century after its comprehensive description by Reginald Fitz (Fitz 1889) acute pancreatitis remains a common disorder with potentially devastating consequences. The incidence has been reported to be as high as 38 per 100,000 population per year and seems to be increasing (Corfield *et al* 1985). The aetiology of acute pancreatitis is varied and the outcome for an individual patient can be difficult to predict from the outset. Around 25% of patients will develop severe or life-threatening complications which require high dependency nursing or intensive care support (de Beaux *et al* 1995). Even though over the past 30 years the overall mortality has fallen from 25-30% to 6-10%, it has now remained at that level for a decade or more

U. Lendeckel and Nigel M. Hooper (eds.), Proteases in Gastrointestinal Tissue, 89-121.

(Neoptolemos *et al* 1995), and if complications develop may increase to 35% or higher (Banerjee 1999).

Although the exact molecular mechanisms involved in the pathogenesis of acute pancreatitis are not fully understood, the earliest events are thought to involve perturbations of normal acinar cell biology. Thus, an understanding of those events is dependent upon our knowledge of normal acinar cell biology.

Acute pancreatitis can be viewed as a disease which evolves in 3 phases:

1. An initiating phase,
2. A phase that involves acinar cell events including cell injury,
3. And an extra-acinar cell phase in which the response to acinar cell injury includes pancreatic as well as systemic complications.

The initiating phase of pancreatitis involves one or more processes (more commonly referred to as 'aetiologies'). These include biliary tract stone disease, alcohol, pancreatic trauma or ischaemia, exposure to certain drugs, hypercalcaemia, hypertriglyceridaemia, and obstructive lesions of the pancreatic duct. It is thought that an early and crucial event in the pathogenesis of all forms of acute pancreatitis is an interference with digestive enzyme secretion from pancreatic acinar cell (Steer 1999). The second phase would seem to involve a series of changes within pancreatic acinar cells culminating in the intra-acinar cell activation of digestive enzyme zymogens and acinar cell injury. In the third phase a number of extra-acinar cell events take place. These are to a great extent dependent on the local as well as systemic generation of inflammatory mediators such as cytokines, chemokines and others. Not only does acinar cell damage lead to a local inflammatory response but it is thought these inflammatory mediators also spill over into the general circulation. The severity of an episode of acute pancreatitis appears to be determined by the magnitude of the resultant systemic inflammatory response.

2.2 Acinar cell biology

The pancreatic acinar cell is a factory for protein synthesis. Proteins are assembled in the rough endoplasmic reticulum (RER), and transported to the golgi complex where post-translational modifications occur. More than 90% of the protein synthesised by acinar cells consists of digestive enzymes which are destined to be transported out of the cell. Those proteins, which exist primarily as inactive pro-enzymes or zymogens, are packaged in condensing vacuoles at the *trans* side of the golgi and carried towards the luminal plasma membrane. The condensing plasma vacuoles evolve into zymogen granules as the electron density of their content increases. At the plasma membrane, those zymogen granules fuse with the surface membrane and then release their contents into the acinar space. Acinar cells also synthesise enzymes which are not secreted. These enzymes are intracellularly transported to lysosomes where they act to digest intracellular substrates. As they traverse the golgi complex these lysosomal hydrolases are phosphorylated at the 6-position of mannose residues. This process ensures that they are bound to receptors in the golgi complex which recognise the mannose-6-phosphate label and then transported to the lysosomal compartment and thus away from the secretory pathway.

2.3 Acinar cell pathophysiology and the role of cysteine proteases in acute pancreatitis

Recent studies suggest that an abnormality in the intracellular transport and secretion of enzyme protein plays an important role in the evolution of acute pancreatitis (Niederau and Luthen 1999; Luthen *et al* 1998). This is accompanied by an increase of the intracellular concentration of Ca^{2+}, which is released from the RER. This increase of intracellular Ca^{2+} is followed shortly thereafter by cell dehydration and a blockade of protein secretion. All these changes result in activation of trypsinogen within the acinar cell (Luthen *et al* 1998). Hence, it is thought that the autodigestive process is likely to originate inside acinar cells and trypsinogen activation is considered to be a key step in the evolution of acute pancreatitis. Once trypsin has been activated however, its inhibition does not alter the course of pancreatitis because other proteases, which are activated by trypsin, finally cause the subsequent cell damage (Luthen *et al* 1993). The activation of pancreatic enzymes before their secretion from the acinar cell is one the most commonly reported theories for the pathogenesis of acute pancreatitis.

Under normal conditions, natural safeguards protect the pancreas from autodigestion by pancreatic proteases and include (Steer 1999; Reber 1991):

1. Enzyme synthesis, storage, and secretion as pro-enzymes or zymogens, which are segregated from the cytoplasm after their synthesized by various organelles and cell membranes. Activation of these pro-enzymes normally occurs in the duodenum, where enteropeptidase secreted by the duodenal mucosa activates trypsinogen to trypsin, which then activates the inactive pro-enzymes to their active state.
2. It is thought that strict segregation of the zymogens from the lysosomal hydrolases may be important to avoid the premature activation of the zymogens within the acinar cells .
3. The presence of pancreatic trypsin inhibitor and circulating antiproteases (including α_1-antitrypsin) which prevent activation of inactive

pancreatic pro-enzymes within pancreatic tissue or ducts. Larger amounts of liberated trypsin, however, can overwhelm these defence mechanisms resulting in enzyme activation.

There seems to be mounting evidence that the activation of trypsin in the acinar cell is a crucial initiating step (Whitcomb 1999; Lerch *et al* 2000; Saluja *et al* 1989; Hofbauer *et al* 1998; Saluja *et al* 1989). Cathepsin B has been shown to play a critical role in the activation of zymogens (Steer 1999; Lerch *et al* 2000; Saluja *et al* 1989; Niederau *et al* and Grendell 1988). Experimental models of acute pancreatitis showed coalescence of zymogen granules with lysosome vacuoles (a phenomenon termed 'co-localization' or 'crinophagy'), allowing for possible premature activation of trypsinogen by the lysosomal enzyme cathepsin B (Saluja *et al* 1989; Klonowski-Stumpe *et al* 1998). The organelles containing digestive zymogens and lysosomal hydrolases become increasingly fragile and liberate activated digestive enzymes into the cytoplasm, thereby initiating the activation cascade of proteolytic enzymes (Steer 1999).

A second theory postulates that trypsinogen activation occurs in the normal pathway under low pH conditions and becomes pathological only with a secretory blockade. Under normal conditions a fraction of the human trypsinogen, auto-activates to trypsin. This process is regulated by at least two different lines of defence. The first one is SPINK1 (serine protease inhibitor, Kazal type 1) (Witt *et al* 2001). When levels of trypsin activity are low, SPINK1 inhibits trypsin and prevents further auto-activation of trypsin and other pro-enzymes within the pancreas. During excessive trypsinogen activation however, the SPINK1 inhibitory capacity is overwhelmed and trypsin activity continues to increase. The second line of defence is represented by trypsin itself. To prevent uncontrolled enzyme activation, trypsin and trypsin-like enzymes, by means of a feedback mechanism, hydrolyze the chain connecting the two globular domains of the trypsin at R122H. This results in permanent inactivation of trypsin and prevents subsequent activation of other pro-enzymes. Mutations of the cationic trypsinogen gene responsible for a human form of hereditary pancreatitis have recently been discovered, reinforcing the link between these early events and the disease (Whitcomb *et al* 1996; Creighton *et al* 1999) Taken together, all these observations suggest that one of the earliest events during acute pancreatitis consists of inappropriate and premature activation of trypsinogen into active trypsin within the pancreas

To test this hypothesis, Halangk *et al.* (Halangk *et al* 2001) developed cathepsin B-deficient mice. After induction of pancreatitis, the pancreatic trypsin activity in these mice is more than 80% lower than in wild-type mice and pancreatic injury is 50% lower. It was also shown that the prevention of trypsinogen activation by genetic deletion of cathepsin B was incomplete.

This suggests that cathepsin B is not the only pathway involved in premature intra-acinar activation of trypsinogen; trypsinogen activation by other lysosomal enzymes has to be considered as an alternative. In the cathepsin B-deficient mice, although the reduction of trypsinogen activation correlates with a decrease of acinar cell necrosis, the systemic inflammatory response as well as the pancreatic leukocyte infiltration were not affected, indicating that these events are not cathepsin B-dependent.

2.4 Involvement of proteases in extra-acinar cell events in acute pancreatitis

Once triggered, the acinar cell initiates an unpredictable cascade of events that can lead to a spectrum of clinical scenarios ranging from mild, local interstitial inflammation, to severe necrosis, with spread into the peripancreatic spaces and the release of toxic factors into the systemic circulation or peritoneal space. The necrosis and vascular damage in acute pancreatitis is caused by pancreatic autodigestion by various proteolytic and lipolytic enzymes that are released within the organ. The noxious potential of various digestive enzymes on pancreatic acinar cells is strikingly different (Niederau *et al* 1995) On a molecular basis elastase, lipase, chymotrypsin, and phospholipase A_2 are more potent in damaging acinar cells when compared to trypsin (Niederau *et al* 1995). Although activation of trypsinogen initiates the cascade (Figure 1), this enzyme is the one least harmful to the pancreas in terms of direct damage; its main effect being the activation of other enzymes.

Systemically, the release of trypsin activates complement and the kallikrein-kinin system (Uehara *et al* 1989) Elevated systemic concentrations of products of the kallikrein-kinin system cause vasodilatation and may contribute to haemodynamic abnormalities (disseminated intravascular coagulation, shock, or renal failure) ultimately leading to multiple organ failure syndrome (Uehara *et al* 1989) The lipolytic enzyme phospholipase A_2 is activated by trypsin. In the presence of bile acids, phospholipase A_2 destroys cell membranes, causing pancreatic parenchymal necrosis. Various toxic cell membrane lysophospholipids and phospholipase A_2 reaching the circulation may be responsible for acute respiratory distress syndrome (Mirkovic 2000) to its well known effects on elastin within vessel walls, elastase appears to have a broad spectrum of action on many proteins, the variety of which is greater than generally assumed (Niederau *et al* 1995). Furthermore, Johnson *et al.* demonstrated that elastase can activate Toll-like receptor 4 (TLR4) inducing a systemic inflammatory response syndrome (SIRS) like reaction in mice (Johnson *et al* 2004). The injection of lipopolysaccharide (LPS) free pancreatic elastase solution into the peritoneal cavity of mice caused the release of heparin sulphate. Fifty per cent of the wild type of mice died whereas no TLR4 mutant mice died. In addition, studies demonstrated that elastase can stimulate resident macrophages within the lungs as well as the liver to produce large amounts of tumour necrosis factor (TNF) and Fas ligand (FasL) (Jaffray *et al* 2000; Yang *et al* 2004; Gallagher *et al* 2004). Lipase, unlike the other enzymes previously discussed, is synthesised in the acinar cell in its active form but does require the presence of bile acids for biological activity.

During acute pancreatitis an initially localised inflammatory process has the propensity to amplify to a generalised systemic inflammatory response. The severity of an episode of acute pancreatitis appears to be determined by the magnitude of such a systemic inflammatory response (Norman 1998). Inflammatory cytokines such as interleukin (IL)-1, tumour necrosis factor-α, IL-6, IL-8, and platelet activating factor (PAF) are considered to be the principal mediators in the transformation of acute pancreatitis from a local inflammatory process into a multiorgan dysfunction condition. The characterisation of the renin-angiotensin system (RAS) in the pancreas has been reported in experimental models as well as humans (Chappell *et al* 1991, 1992; Tahmasebi *et al* 1991). Further evidence for the existence of such a system came form the demonstration of angiotensin II receptors and expression of key renin-angitensin system component genes in pancreatic tissue (Leung *et al* 1997, 1998, 1999, 2000). The role of angiotensin II in acute pancreatitis is still not well known. Studies have shown that RAS may be involved in the generation of reactive oxygen species (ROS) (Griendling *et al* 1994) and apoptotic cell death (Yamada *et al* 1996).

Experimental studies show that pancreatic injury is mediated not only by pro-inflammatory mediators but also by the activation of inflammatory cells such as neutrophils, macrophages, and lymphocytes (Yamaguchi *et al* 1993; Xie *et al* 2001). Activation of endothelial cells permits the transendothelial migration of neutrophils, monocytes, and lymphocytes and mediators released by these cells such as neutrophil elastase. These factors may even be more damaging than pancreatic enzymes themselves (Frossard *et al* 1999). In a recent study, trypsinated serum was shown to induce the upregulation of both membrane-bound ICAM-1 on endothelial cells and soluble ICAM-1 (Hartwig *et al* 2004). These changes contribute to the early steps of leukocyte migration in acute pancreatitis. The role of soluble ICAM-1 remains to be investigated but levels of the molecule have been shown to correlate with the severity of the disease (Kaufman *et al* 1999a; Kaufman *et al* 1999b; Mandi *et al* 2000). In addition to hyper-cytokinemia resulting from the inflammatory process in the pancreas and peripancreatic tissues, there is evidence that cytokines are released by hyperactive macrophages when acute pancreatitis is complicated by infection. These cytokines activate neutrophils that have already infiltrated organs, such as lung, liver, and organs of the digestive tract

(Ogawa 1998). Decreased organ oxygen delivery (Sunamura *et al* 1998) and generation of oxygen derived free radicals also contribute to the injury (Gukovskaya *et al* 1996).

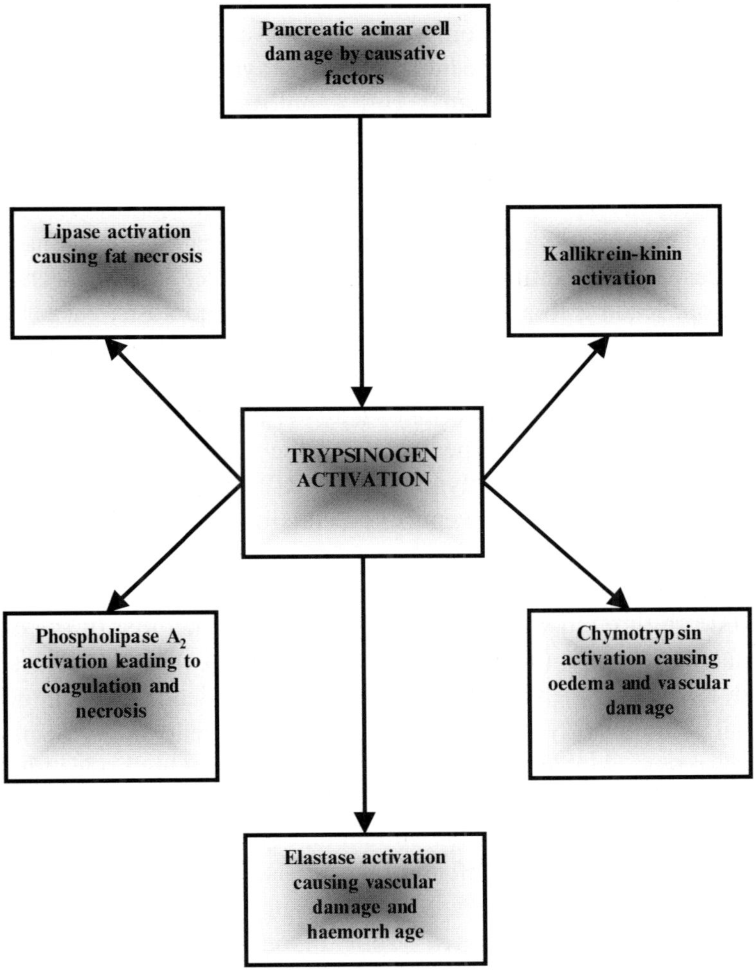

Figure 1: Trypsinogen activation-a key step in the evolution of acute pancreatitis.

2.5 Proteases and Cell death in acute pancreatitis

Clinical and experimental acute pancreatitis is characterised by cell death, the mechanisms of which remains unclear. Experimental models of acute pancreatitis have shown that severe acute pancreatitis (e.g., that induced by pancreatic duct ligation in the opossum, by choline-deficient and ethionine-supplemented diet in the mouse, or by caerulein hyperstimulation in the mouse) is associated primarily with necrosis but little apoptosis, whereas mild acute pancreatitis (e.g., that induced by pancreatic duct ligation or by caerulein hyperstimulation in the rat) is associated primarily with apoptotic cell death and little necrosis (Gukovskaya *et al* 1996; Kaiser *et al* 1999). The mechanisms of acinar cell apoptosis and necrosis in acute pancreatitis remain poorly understood.

A recent report (Gukovskaya *et al* 2002) has shown the role of the intrinsic pathway in acinar cell apoptosis. The results show that cholecystokinin (CCK) stimulates death signalling pathways in rat pancreatic acinar cells, including caspase activation, cytochrome c release, and mitochondrial depolarization, leading to apoptosis. In addition to apoptosis, caspases also regulate other processes in the pancreatic acinar cell that play key roles in pancreatitis; in particular, caspases negatively regulate necrosis and intra-acinar cell activation of trypsin (Gukovskaya *et al* 2002). PARP is a major target of effector caspases especially caspase-3 [52]. Caspase-mediated cleavage of polyADP-ribose polymerase (PARP) results in its inactivation. Thus, effector caspases may prevent ATP depletion and necrosis by cleaving PARP during apoptosis (Adams 2003).

As mentioned earlier, elastase may play a crucial role in hepatocyte injury and death through activation of Fas, which is a member of the tumour necrosis factor receptor (TNFR) family of receptors. FasL activates Fas-associated death domain (FADD) and unmasks its death effector domain (DED) that subsequently activates the caspase cascade and downstream effector caspases, including caspase-3, that ultimately leads to DNA cleavage and cell apoptosis (Yang *et al* 2004; Gallagher *et al* 2004; Hori *et al* 2000). The resolution of the inflammatory response is mediated by induction of apoptosis in the inflammatory cells. It has been reported that caspase-3 activation and apoptosis are delayed in neutrophils and peripheral blood mononuclear cells isolated from blood of patients with acute pancreatitis (O'Neill *et al* 2000; Salomone *et al* 2002). A delay in apoptosis in inflammatory cells correlated with the severity of pancreatitis (O'Neill *et al* 2000). The delay in apoptosis could be related to high levels of nuclear factor kappa B (NF-κB) activation in inflammatory cells in pancreatitis. Indeed, higher levels of NF-κB activity were observed in blood mononuclear cells from patients with severe pancreatitis (Satoh *et al* 2003).

Whereas caspases mediate only apoptotic type of cell death, cathepsins and calpain may cause both apoptosis and necrosis. Both genetic and pharmacologic blockade of cathepsin B inhibited necrosis in cerulein pancreatitis by about 50% (Halangk *et al* 2000; Van Acker *et al* 2002). These results suggest a mediatory role of cathepsin B in pancreatic necrosis. Cathepsin B deficiency did not affect apoptotic rate in caerulein-induced pancreatitis (Halangk *et al* 2000). The calcium-dependent protease, calpain, can also mediate apoptotic death (Kohli *et al* 1999). In particular, calpain is involved into hepatocyte cell death after ischemia/reperfusion injury (Wang 2000). In neutrophils calpain causes Bax activation and is indispensable for downstream activation of caspase-3 (Altznauer *et al* 2004).

The mechanisms of pancreatic fibrosis are not fully elucidated. Apoptosis has been suggested to be involved in the progression of pancreatic fibrosis. It has been reported that the renin-angiotensin system (RAS) plays a crucial role in the formation of fibrosis in acinar cells (Wang *et al* 2004). Wang *et al.* randomly divided Male Sprague-Dawley rats (200-300 g) into a normal group, a control group, and a losartan-treatment group. Pancreatic fibrosis was induced by infusion of 2% trinitrobenzene sulfonic acid into the pancreatic duct. Rats were treated with losartan (10 mg/kg) by gavage daily in the losartan-treatment group and an identical volume of sterile distilled water was administered to the control group. The administration of losartan resulted in inhibition of acinar cell apoptosis and down-regulation of Bax, Bak, and Bcl-2 mRNA expression. The Bax/Bcl-2 ratio was lower in losartan-treated rats than in control rats. The authors concluded that losartan prevents apoptosis of pancreatic acinar cell by blocking AT1R during the development of pancreatic fibrosis. This action may be associated with its regulation of apoptosis-associated genes, such as Bax, Bak, and Bcl-2 mRNA. The results of the study suggest that angiotensin II probably mediates pancreatic acinar cell apoptosis during the course of pancreatic fibrosis.

2.6 The role of Matrix Metalloproteinases in acute pancreatitis

Alterations of the balance of expression between matrix metalloproteases (MMPs) and their tissue inhibitors (TIMPs) in inflammatory diseases has been described, e.g. in active rheumatoid arthritis (Mc Cachren 1991) and Hashimoto's thyroiditis (Campo *et al* 1992). The exact role of MMPs in acute pancreatitis remains to be established.

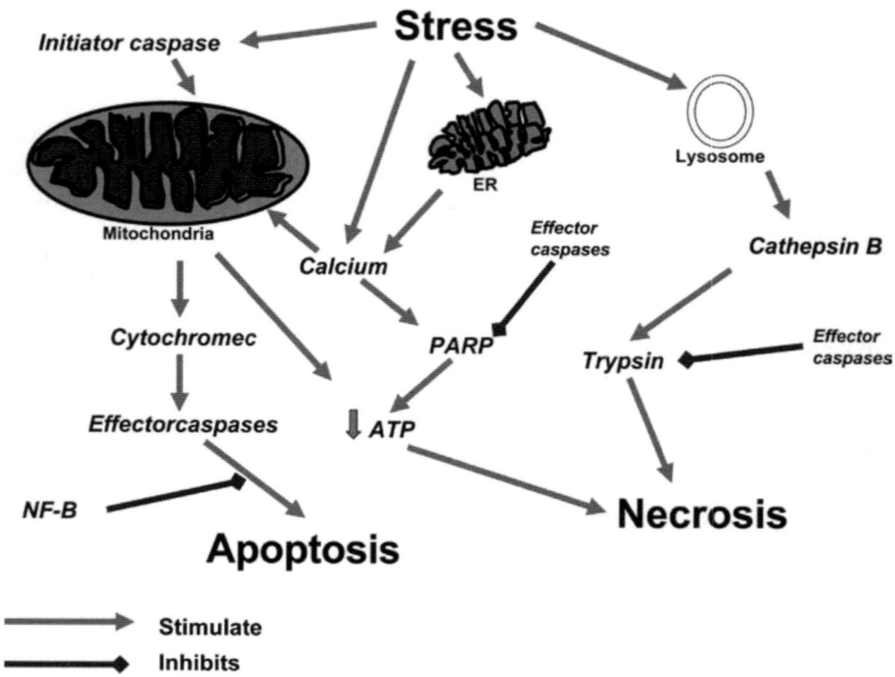

Figure 2: Cell death pathways in acute pancreatitis.

The majority of deaths from acute pancreatitis occur within the first 7 days and are usually associated with acute pulmonary failure (Johnson and Abu-Hilal 2004). Extracellular matrix degradation from MMP-2 and MMP-9 may result in capillary leak and play a causative role in the lung injury (Muhs *et al* 2001). Depletion of circulating polymorphonuclear neutrophils (PMNs) protects against the development of pancreatitis-induced lung injury, suggesting that PMNs occupy a critical position in the pathway leading to lung injury (Guice *et al* 1989). *In vivo* activation of MMP-2 and MMP-9 is thought to be dependent on at least two sources of proteases: neutrophil derived serine proteases and plasmin (Peppin and Weiss 1986). Neutrophils may play a central role in pulmonary injury through activation of MMPs, as well as release of PMN proteases and reactive oxygen species. A study Muhs *et al.* (Muhs *et al* 2001) provides insight into the role of MMP-2 and -9 in the evolution of local and distant organ injury following acute pancreatitis. The investigators propose a model of pulmonary injury following severe pancreatitis that involves chemotactic mediators activating PMNs and attracting them to the lung vasculature. The activated PMNs secrete pro-MMP-9 and neutrophil-derived serine proteases. These proteases activate pro-MMP-2, which is constitutively expressed in parenchyma cells. The active MMP-2 acts to degrade the basement membrane, allowing the activated PMNs to migrate into the interstitium. The resulting lung injury is a significant cause of morbidity and mortality in patients with acute pancreatitis.

The model of caerulein-induced pancreatitis in rats (Muller-Pilasch *et al* 1997) has offered new insight into the role of MMPs and their inhibitors in the development of pancreatic fibrosis. Surprisingly, increased MMP expression during days 2–4 after induction of pancreatitis could only be demonstrated for MMP-2 and MMP-3. Transcript levels of MMP-1 and MMP-9 did not change throughout the regeneration period.Twelve hours after the induction of pancreatitis, a marked increase of gelatinolytic and caseinolytic activity was observed at approximately 92 kD (MMP-9) and 45 kD (active MMP-3), respectively, which decreased 2 (MMP-9) or 3 (MMP-3) days after the end of cerulein infusion. Simultaneously, an increase of gelatinolytic activity of active MMP-2 (62 kD) was noted on day 2 reaching peak values on day 3 after the induction of pancreatitis, accompanied by a parallel a decrease of the 72-kD inactive form of MMP-2. Proteolytic activities detected by substrate zymographs and transcription levels of MMP-2 and TIMP-2 were not influenced by treatment with neutralizing Transforming growth factor (TGFβ1) antibodies. Only the transcript levels of MMP-3 showed a minor reduction upon treatment with neutralizing TGFβ1 antibodies. Thus, MMP-2, MMP-3 and MMP-9 appear to be of importance for the removal of extracellular matrix during regeneration from cerulein pancreatitis in rats. At least in this model TGFβ does not seem to be of major importance for the regulation of extracellular (ECM) removal by MMPs.

2.7 Conclusion

The pathophysiology of acute pancreatitis is still not fully understood. It includes the activation and release of pancreatic enzymes in the interstitium, the autodigestion of the pancreas, and multiple organ dysfunction following their release in the systemic circulation. The initial phase of the disease originates from the activation of trypsinogen to trypsin within the acinar cells, which in turn activates various enzymes such as elastase and phospholipase and the complement and kinin systems. Proteases and protease inhibitors undoubtedly play a crucial role in acute pancreatitis.

3. CHRONIC PANCREATITIS

3.1 Introduction

Chronic pancreatitis is a progressive inflammatory disorder ultimately leading to irreversible structural changes resulting in functional impairment of exocrine and/or endocrine physiology. It is relatively frequent and the prevalence has been estimated at 50–75 cases per 100 000 inhabitants. The mortality rate approaches 50% within 20 years after diagnosis (Etemad and Whitcomb 2001). It is an important problem as most patients with chronic pancreatitis require frequent and intensive medical care because of relapsing attacks of incapacitating abdominal pain. In the Western world, alcohol abuse is generally considered as a substantial aetiological factor for the development of chronic pancreatitis. In addition, other aetiological factors such as heredity, cigarette smoking, anatomical variations, and various metabolic disorders have been identified. In up to 30% of patients, association with any of the aforementioned risk factors is lacking and the disease is classified as idiopathic (Strate *et al* 2003).

In the past several decades, four major theories have emerged to explain the pathogenesis of chronic pancreatitis: toxic-metabolic, oxidative stress, stone and duct obstruction, and necrosis-fibrosis. Each of these models provides a mechanism to explain the pathogenic sequence. Moreover, a great deal of new knowledge has accumulated in recent years regarding the cellular, genetic, and molecular mechanisms of pancreatic fibrosis, and new pathogenic models are being generated.

Whitcomb and colleagues have proposed an interesting hypothesis for chronic pancreatitis pathogenesis (the sentinel acute pancreatitis event hypothesis) that incorporates these recent advances while unifying many of the previous theories (Whitcomb 1999, 2000, 2001, 2003). In at-risk individuals the pancreatic acinar cells are under stimulation by alcohol, oxidative stress, and other insults. Fibrosis does not yet occur because a pro-fibrotic cellular infiltrate is not yet present. Through unregulated trypsin activation, the first episode of acute pancreatitis occurs (sentinel event). The sentinel event produces a massive inflammatory response, of both early and late phases. The early phase consists of pro-inflammatory cells (neutrophils, lymphocytes, *etc.*). Cytokines (TGF-beta, TNF-alpha, IL-6, others) released during the early inflammatory phase attract a distinct, later, anti-inflammatory cellular infiltrate. Pro-fibrotic cells, including stellate cells constitute the late phase of acute pancreatitis. The attraction and activation of stellate cells sets the stage for the development of pancreatic fibrosis. If inciting factors (alcohol and oxidative stress) are removed, the pancreas heals to its baseline, normal state. However if the acinar cells continue to secrete cytokines in response to oxidative stress, recalcitrant alcohol use, or recurrent bouts of acute pancreatitis, activated stellate cells are now present to respond to those cellular signals. The stellate cells are directly stimulated by cytokines, alcohol, and oxidative stress to deposit collagen, leading to periacinar fibrosis and eventual chronic pancreatitis.

The sentinel acute pancreatitis event (SAPE) hypothesis is fascinating because it incorporates much of the recent knowledge about the molecular and cellular mechanisms of pathogenesis, while unifying previous theories (necrosis-fibrosis, toxic-metabolic, oxidative stress). Moreover, it provides a "final common pathway" for the many aetiologies of pancreatitis. More studies are needed to confirm various aspects of this hypothesis as well as the role of proteases in chronic pancreatitis.

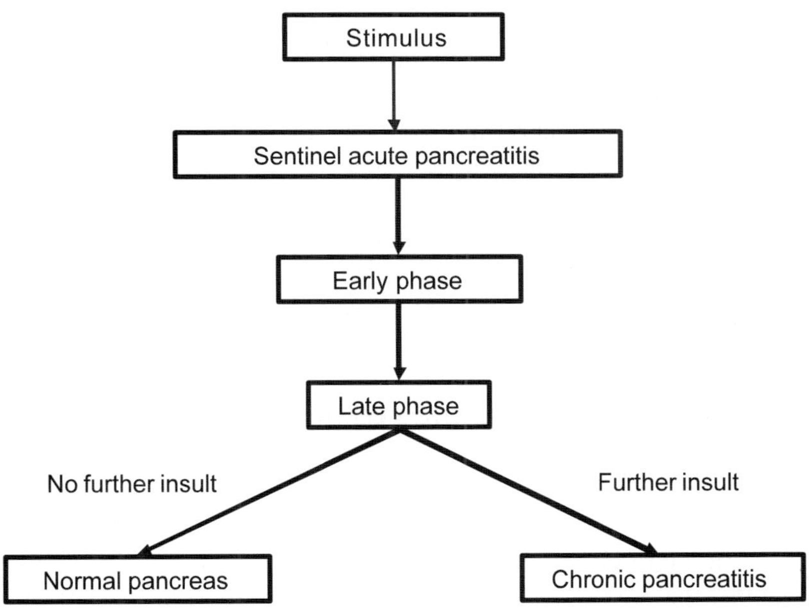

Figure 3: SAPE hypothesis.

3.2 Trypsin and chronic pancreatitis

Inappropriate activation of trypsinogen within the pancreas leads to the development of pancreatitis. Once trypsin is activated, it is capable of activating many other digestive pro-enzymes. These activated pancreatic enzymes further enhance autodigestion of the pancreas. Trypsin also activates cells via the trypsin receptor PAR-2. Both acinar cells and duct cells express abundant PAR-2 (Ikeda *et al* 2003).

Trypsin activity in the pancreas is mainly controlled by serine protease inhibitor Kazal type 1 (SPINK1). SPINK1 is synthesized in the acinar cells of the pancreas and acts as a potent natural inhibitor of trypsin in order to prevent the occurrence of pancreatitis. When trypsinogen is activated into trypsin in the pancreas, SPINK1 immediately binds to trypsin to prevent further activation of pancreatic enzymes. The protease also blocks the further activation of pancreatic cells via the trypsin receptor, PAR-2. Several gene mutations in trypsinogen have been identified and are presumed to be pathogenic in patients with hereditary pancreatitis through the enhancement of intrapancreatic trypsin activity (Applebaum-Shapiro *et al* 2001; Charnley 2003; Trunninger *et al* 2001; Pfutzer and Whitcomb 2001; Howes *et al* 2005). To clarify the relationship between the expression of PAR-2 and fibrosis, the immunohistochemical expression of PAR-2 in chronic pancreatitis tissue was also examined by Ikeda *et al.* (Ikeda *et al* 2003). Strong expression of PAR-2 was also observed in acinar cells of the pancreatitis tissue with severe fibrosis. These tendencies of PAR-2 expression in pancreatic cancers and chronic pancreatitis strongly suggest that the activation of PAR-2 is related to induction of fibrosis.

3.3 Proteases, fibrosis and cell death in chronic pancreatitis

In chronic pancreatitis fibrosis is the most impressive morphological finding. The current model of molecular pathogenesis of fibrosis demonstrates the central role of activated pancreatic stellate cells. Chronic pancreatitis is characterized by destruction of acinar cells and islet cells, activation of pancreatic stellate cells and replacement by connective tissue. This connective tissue results from an increased deposition and disorganization of extracellular matrix proteins including fibronectin, laminin, and collagens type I, III and IV (Kennedy *et al* 1987). It has been shown that these alterations of ECM-proteins are accompanied by an increase in the transcription levels of genes coding for collagens I , III and IV, fibronectin and laminin in human chronic pancreatitis (Gress *et al* 1994).

The biological cause of fibrosis is the accumulation of excessive amounts of extracellular matrix (ECM) which leads to tissue dysfunction and organ failure. A strong correlation can be found between pancreatic diseases and fibrotic processes, in particular chronic pancreatitis and pancreatic cancer. There is growing evidence that pancreatic fibrosis represents a dysregulation of the normal repair processes after injury. This concept is based on the findings that fibrosis and tissue repair involve similar biological reactions regulated by the same group of molecules. The best characterised examples for these regulatory molecules are the members of the transforming growth factor beta family (TGFbeta). TGFbeta1 represents the prototype of this family of highly similar growth factors, with the unique ability to stimulate the expression and deposition of extracellular matrix and to inhibit its degradation. Growth factor-induced fibrotic events are targeted by a myofibroblast-like cell called pancreatic stellate cell (PSC). These cells show enhanced expression of all-important ECM proteins after TGFβ stimulation including collagen, fibronectin and proteoglycans. At the same time TGFβ inhibits the degradation of ECM by blocking the secretion of proteases and stimulating the production of naturally occurring protease inhibitors.

Matrix metalloproteinases (MMPs) are the proteases involved in the degradation of the extracellular matrix. MMP-1 is thought to be one of the key enzymes in fibrolysis, a process closely related to tissue remodelling. MMP-1 secretion from human pancreatic periacinar myofibroblasts in response to pro-inflammatory cytokines IL-1β and TNF-alpha has been investigated. Tasaki *et al.* (Tasaki *et al* 2003) attempted to clarify the intracellular signalling pathways mediating the cytokine-induced MMP-1 secretion. MMP-1 secretion was measured by an enzyme-linked immunosorbent assay. MMP-1 molecules were analyzed by western blotting. MMP-1 mRNA expression was evaluated by northern blotting. IL-1β and TNF-alpha stimulated the MMP-1 secretion in a dose- and time-dependent manner. Ninety percent of MMP-1 was secreted as inactive form (pro-MMP-1). They concluded that, in human pancreatic periacinar myofibroblasts, MMP-1 secretion was regulated by the pro-inflammatory cytokines via the MEK/ERK cascade. Thus, human pancreatic periacinar myofibroblasts may play an important role in the remodelling of damaged pancreatic tissue in chronic pancreatitis via MMP-1 secretion.

It is suggested that caspases play an important role in apoptosis, but recent observations could show that caspase-1 might also be involved in cellular proliferation. Ramadani and colleagues (Ramadani *et al* 2001) investigated the expression of caspase-1 in 38 chronic pancreatitis tissues, six pancreatitis tissues from patients with pancreatic carcinoma and nine normal pancreatic tissues by immunohistochemistry. Western blot analysis was used to confirm the immunohistochemical findings. They found a clear expression of caspase-1 in chronic pancreatitis, but not in normal pancreatic tissues.

Interestingly, they found expression of caspase-1 in three distinct morphologic compartments: (i) in atrophic acinar cells (31 of 35; 89%), (ii) proliferating cells of ductal origin (33 of 38; 87%), and (iii) in acinar cells redifferentiating to form tubular structures (26 of 31; 83%). These immunohistochemical findings were confirmed by western blot analysis, which showed an expression of caspase-1 in 85% of the tissues. No correlation was found between any of the examined clinicopathologic features and the caspase-1 expression in chronic pancreatitis. The investigators claim that the expression of caspase-1 is a frequent event in chronic pancreatitis and its distribution pattern may reflect two functions of this protease: on one hand its participation in the apoptotic pathway in atrophic acinar cells and, on the other hand, its role in proliferation and differentiation in proliferating duct cells.

3.4 Conclusion

A comprehensive literature review highlighted how little is known about the role of proteasaes in chronic pancreatitis. We can only hypothesise as to the paucity of work done in this particular field. Perhaps the lack of an adequate animal model or even the close overlap at a molecular level between the initial events in both acute pancreatitis and chronic pancreatitis could well be responsible.

4. PROTEASES AND PANCREATIC CANCER

4.1 Introduction

The incidence of pancreatic cancer varies among populations, being the fourth or fifth cause of cancer death in the west. Moreover pancreatic cancer is generally regarded to respond poorly to current oncologic chemotherapy, radiotherapy and immunotherapy (Imamura *et al* 2004; Wilkowski *et al* 2004; Sasson *et al* 2003; Ghaneh *et al* 2004; Xiong *et al* 2004). Outcome therefore in the main remains bleak and opinions divided over the optimal management of the condition. At present the only curative treatment of pancreatic cancer is surgical removal of the tumour. Considerable progress has been made over the last two decades in the field of surgical resection for cancer of the pancreas. Operative mortality has fallen to as low as 1.4-5% in large centres and 5-year survival rates risen to as high as 25% in patients with negative resection margins and negative lymph nodes (Yeo *et al* 1997; Nagakawa *et al* 2004). However most newly diagnosed patients have unresectable tumour at the time of diagnosis. The reason for the poor prognosis associated with pancreatic cancer is thought to be due to the propensity of pancreatic cancer to invade into adjacent blood vessels and metastasis very early in the disease process. Cancer invasion and metastasis results from several complex processes including:

1. detachment of cancer cells from their original location;
2. cancer cell migration;
3. invasion of cancer cells into the surrounding tissue, requiring adhesion to and degradation of extracellular matrix components;
4. access of cancer cells to blood and lymphatic vessels;
5. adhesion to and invasion through the endothelium, allowing colonization at distant sites.

Tumour cell invasion is a key step of this process that is believed to involve a controlled, protease-driven degradation of the tumour cell-associated adhesion molecules, extracellular matrix (ECM) and basement membrane. Proteolytic enzymes, which degrade the extracellular matrix and basement membrane, have been reported as essential for this process (Vassalli and Pepper 1994, Mignatti and Rifkin 1993). Most proteolytic enzymes with such characteristics have been divided into two families. The first family includes the serine proteases, and in particular, the plasminogen/ plasmin system. The other family consists of the matrix metalloproteases (MMPs).

4.2 Trypsin and pancreatic cancer

It is well known that pancreatic acinar cells are the major source of trypsinogen, zymogen of trypsin. Trypsinogen has been reported to be produced in many cancers (Oyama *et al* 2000; Hedstrom *et al* 2001; Uchima *et al* 2003; Miyata *et al* 1998; Williams *et al* 2001). Several studies have suggested that tumour derived trypsin contributes to growth and invasion of cancer cells (Miyata *et al* 1998; Yamamoto *et al* 2001), and is involved in cancer aggressiveness through the potent proteolytic activity which can degrade ECM and activate latent forms of various matrix metalloproteases and serine proteases (Paju *et al* 2001; Imai *et al* 1995) . Recently it has been reported that the action of trypsin can be mediated not only by its classical ability to catalyze the hydrolysis of various proteins, but also through specific cleavage and activation of a cell surface receptor proteinase-activated receptor-2 (PAR-2) (Ikeda *et al* 2003; Kaufmann *et al* 1998; Ohta *et al* 2003; Shimamoto *et al* 2004, Yada *et al* 2005). These past reports and findings about PAR-2 expression in pancreatic cancer cell lines lead us to believe that PAR-2 is cleaved and activated by trypsin produced by cancer itself and/or surrounding acinar cell, and activating PAR-2 is involved in some function of cancer cells.

Ikeda *et al.* (Ikeda *et al* 2003) also observed PAR-2 expression in all 21 paraffin embedded specimens from pancreatic cancer that they examined. PAR-2 expression was found to be higher in the cases of infiltrative growth pattern than others of expansive growth pattern. Moreover, significantly higher expression of PAR-2 was observed in the tissues which were accompanied with severe fibrosis. Even in the same specimen, the expression of PAR-2 was higher in the part with severe fibrosis than that with mild fibrosis. These tendencies of PAR-2 expression in pancreatic cancers and chronic pancreatitis strongly suggest that the activation of PAR-2 is related to induction of fibrosis.

Fibrosis is one of the morphological hallmarks of several human tumours. Intratumoral fibrosis has been reported to be closely correlated with cancer progression and poor prognosis (Hasebe *et al* 2000, 2001). The higher expression PAR-2 in pancreatic cancer showing infiltrative growth and higher degree of fibrosis observed in this study may indicate that the activation of PAR-2 is involved in cancer invasion and the induction of fibrosis in human pancreatic cancer.

Extra-pancreatic production of trypsin i.e tumour-associated trypsinogen (TAT), has been reported to be produced by several cancer cell lines, including acinar cells (Uchima *et al* 2003). Over-expression of exogenous trypsinogen cDNA in human gastric cancer cells has been reported to increase their tumourigenicity in nude mice. Uchima *et al.* (Uchima *et al* 2003), showed that not only TAT but also pancreatic acinar trypsinogen (PAT) played an important role in pancreatic cancer invasion and metastasis. Trypsinogen activity stimulating factor (TASF), secreted by pancreatic cancer cells, was associated with u-PA. Both PAT and TAT are activated by urokinase plasminogen activator (u-PA) as the first step in invasion by cancer cells. Once activated, TAT and PAT can degrade extracellular matrix components and they both can also directly further activate TAT, PAT, pro-u-PA, and pro-MMPs (except for pro-MMP-2), even at a neutral pH.

4.3 The effect of proteases on cell adhesion molecules

Several classes of proteins are participating when cells exhibit an invasive or metastatic phenotype. This includes cell-cell adhesion molecules (CAMs) like members of the immunoglobulin and calcium-dependent cadherin families and integrins. Alterations of cell adhesion molecule expression in the immunoglobulin superfamily also appear to play critical role in invasion and metastasis (Skubitz 2003). Clearly neural cell adhesion molecule (N-CAM) undergoes a switch in expression from a highly adhesive isoform to poorly adhesive forms and its down regulation leads to invasive pancreatic cancer (Fogar *et al* 1997). Furthermore, differential expression of the cell adhesion molecules intercellular adhesion molecule-1 (ICAM-1), vascular cell adhesion molecule-1 (VCAM-1), and endothelial leukocyte adhesion molecule-1 (ELAM-1) in human pancreatic cancer has recently been studied (Tempia-Caliera *et al* 2002). Northern blot analysis revealed a 5.4-fold increase of ICAM-1 and a 3.7-fold increase in VCAM-1 mRNA expression in cancer samples in comparison with normal controls. In contrast, ELAM-1 mRNA levels did not show significant differences between cancer and normal tissues. Therefore, it is likely that enhanced ICAM-1 and VCAM-1 expression plays a role in human pancreatic cancer pathogenesis, where they likely contribute to cancer cell migration and the spread of cancer cells to distant organs, or both (Tempia-Caliera *et al* 2002).

Notably, all of these "adherence" interactions convey regulatory signals to the cell (Aplin *et al* 1998). One widely observed alteration in cell-to-environment interaction in pancreatic cancer involves E-cadherin, which couples adjacent cells by E-cadherin bridges. As a result the transmission of antigrowth signals is mediated via cytoplasmic contacts with catenin to intracellular signalling circuits (Christofori and Semb 1999). E-cadherin function is lost in a majority of pancreatic tumours (Karayiannakis *et al* 2001; Menke *et al* 2001; Li and Ji 2003).

E-cadherin is a 120-kDa transmembrane glycoprotein involved in the calcium dependent adhesion of epithelial cells. Soluble E-cadherin was first reported by Damsky and colleagues studying MCF-7 human carcinoma cells (Damski *et al* 1983). This 80 kDa peptide is thought to be a degradation product of the 120 kDa E-cadherin molecule generated by a calcium ion dependent proteolytic process (Wheelock *et al* 1987; Takeichi 1988). Healthy individuals produce E-cadherin continuously and low levels of soluble E-cadherin, independent of age and sex, are found in serum (Katayama *et al* 1994). Soluble E-cadherin levels are elevated in patients with certain malignancies (Chan *et al* 2001; Cioffi *et al* 1999; Durkan *et al* 1999; Gofuku *et al* 1999; Griffiths *et al* 1996; Sundfeldt 2001). Metalloproteinases have been shown to be capable of cleaving the extracellular portion of E-cadherin (Noe *et al* 2001). In a recent study (Steinhusen *et al* 2001) it was reported that during apoptosis fragments of E-cadherin with apparent molecular masses of 24, 29, and 84 kDa were generated by two distinct proteolytic activities. In addition to a caspase-3-mediated cleavage releasing the cytoplasmic domain of E-cadherin, a metalloproteinase shed the extracellular domain from the cell surface during apoptosis.

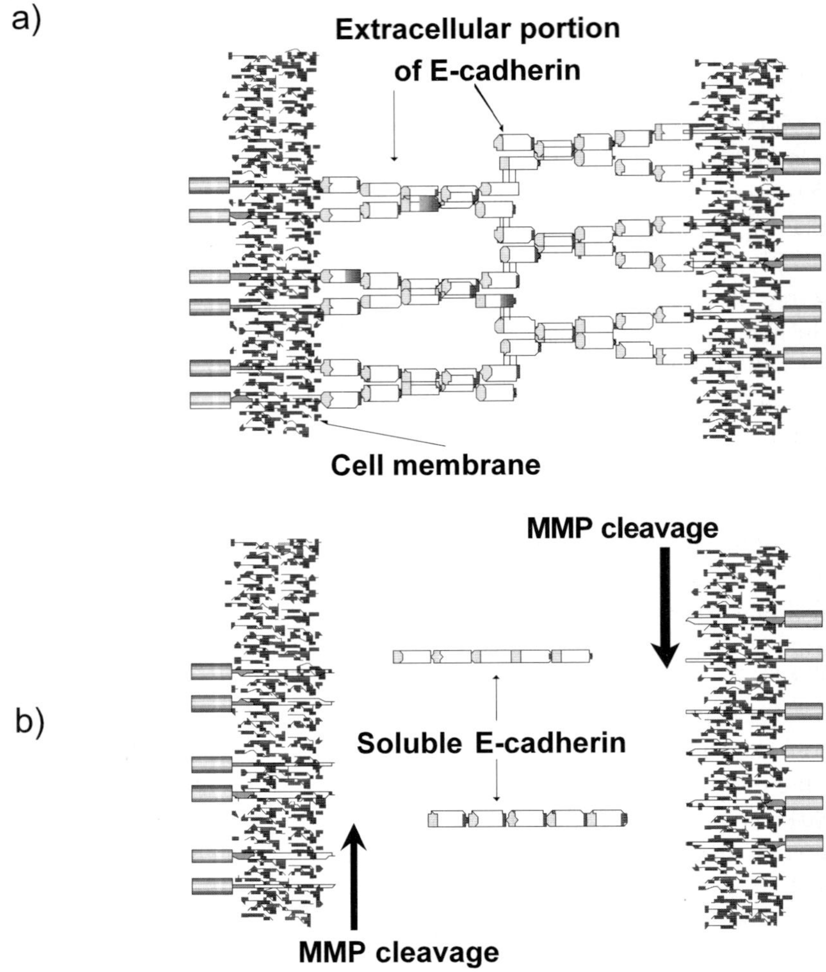

Figure 4: a) The zipper model for cadherin interaction showing homophilic interactions between E-cadherin molecules expressed on the cell membranes. b) MMPs cleave off the extracellular portion of the E-cadherin fragment generating soluble E-cadherin and cells lose E-cadherin function.

4.4 The role of MMPs and their inhibitors in pancreatic cancer

Recent studies of the activity of MMPs and their tissue inhibitors (TIMPS) in invasive neoplasms have indicated that these enzymes play an important role in the degradation of connective tissue which is associated with the development of tumor metastases (Kleiner and Stetler-Stevenson 1999).

The matrix metalloproteases comprise a family of secreted or transmembrane proteins. Currently at least 15 structurally related members with a broad spectrum of proteolytic activities against components of the extracellular matrix have been identified. Based on their substrate specificities, MMPs have been categorized into five groups: collagenases, gelatinases, stromelysins, metalloelastases and the newly identified membrane-type MMP. In particular, MMP-2 and MMP-9 (gelatinase A and gelatinase B) are involved in the systemic dissemination of tumours. The importance of MMPs during tumour metastasis may be related to their proteolytic activity against type IV collagen, which is a major component of epithelial basement membranes (Kleiner and Stetler-Stevenson 1999).

The proteolytic acitivity of MMPs is regulated at different levels, including regulation of mRNA transcription by biologically active agents such as growth factors, hormones and oncogenes, as well as regulation at the level of mRNA stability and translation. Most of the MMPs are produced in the form of biologically inactive pro-enzymes and need to become activated. For example, activation of MMP-2 involves the action of a membrane-type 1 matrix metalloproteinase (MT-1-MMP) which cleaves a portion of the carboxy terminus of pro-MMP-2 (Cornelius *et al* 1998). Once MMP-2 is active, it is susceptible for inhibition by a family of so called specific tissue inhibitors of metalloproteinases (TIMPS). There is strong experimental evidence that MMPs play a major role in local and systemic growth of pancreatic cancer (Matsuyama *et al* 2002). Furthermore, high expression of MT1-MMP and MT2-MMP, MMP-2, and MMP-9, as well as TIMP-1 and TIMP-2 was found in pancreatic cancer (Gress *et al* 1995).

Recent studies suggested that members of the MMPs also enhance tumour angiogenesis by triggering the angiogenic switch (Bergers *et al* 2000). Jones *et al.* (Jones *et al* 2004) found that MMP-15 was expressed at significantly lower levels in the tumour by real-time polymerase chain reaction (RT-PCR), but were unable to confirm this by immunohistochemistry. They also found that MMPs 7, 8, 9, 11 and TIMPs 1 and 3 were expressed at significantly higher levels in the tumour as shown by immunohistochemistry and RT-PCR. Of most significance, both MMPs 7 and 11 predicted survival. In the case of MMP-7, this was of independent prognostic significance. Studies of MMP-7 in pancreatic cancer have shown that it is present at higher levels in cancers than in the normal pancreas (Yamamoto *et al* 2001; Crawford *et al* 2002). Yamamoto *et al.* (Yamamoto *et al* 2001) found that MMP-7 expression in pancreatic adenocarcinoma correlated with a poor prognosis and was a significant independent prognostic factor for overall survival.

In another study, it was reported that 6 of 21 (29%) cases of pancreatic cancer expressed MMP-11 in the epithelial tumour cells with 17 of 21 (81%) cases displaying expression in the adjacent stromal cells (von Marschall *et al* 1998). Data from Jones *et al.* suggest that the majority of MMP-11 expression is derived from the tumour epithelial cells themselves, with 52 of 75 (69%) cases staining these cells. They also observed adjacent staining of malignant stromal cells in 22 of 75 (29%) of cases (Jones *et al* 2004).

Membrane-bound MMP-14 has previously been found expressed exclusively localised in the tumour epithelial cells (Bramhall *et al* 1997). In contrast to Jones *et al.* (Jones *et al* 2004), using *in situ* hybridization, investigators found that MMP-14 mRNA was not localized to the tumour epithelial cells, but was present in cellular elements within the tumour stroma (Imamura *et al* 1998; Ellenrieder *et al* 2000). It has been suggested that MMP-14 may activate pro-MMP-2 (Hernandez-Barrantes *et al* 2000). Although it is clear that the activation and inhibition of MMPs and TIMPs is a complex issue, it has been suggested previously that there is a link between MMP-14 and pro-MMP-2 activation (Bramhall *et al* 1997). There are currently only five studies in which expression of MMP-15 in cancer has been described (Jones *et al* 2004; Kim *et al* 2001; Ohira *et al* 2002; Cho *et al* 2004; Sheu *et al* 2003). In recent studies, MMP-15 mRNA was found at higher levels in hepatocellular carcinoma cell lines (Kim *et al* 2001) and by micro-array analysis in lung cancer tissues from patients who had received chemotherapy (Ohira *et al* 2002). By contrast, Jones *et al.* (Jones *et al* 2004) found that MMP-15 mRNA levels were significantly lower ($P = 0.0026$) in tumour tissue compared with normal tissue.

In breast carcinoma TIMP mRNA expression was found to be higher in the carcinoma than the surrounding normal breast tissue (Bramhall *et al* 1997). Bramhall *et al* (Bramhall *et al* 1997) showed by northern blot analysis that seven (7 of 7) pancreatic cancer cell lines and all (17 of 17) of the pancreatic tumour samples expressed detectable TIMP-1 mRNA. TIMP-3 in pancreatic cancer has been less well studied.

4.5 The plasminogen activator/plasmin system

In addition to the MMP family, the plasminogen activator/plasmin system has been implicated in tumour invasion and metastasis. Plasmin participates in tissue degradation and is activated from the inactive precursor plasminogen by two types of plasminogen activators – uPA (urokinase plasminogen activator) and tPA (tissue plasminogen activator) (Wang 2001). The proteolytic activity of uPA plays a dominant role in cell migration, angiogenesis, and tumour metastases and is tightly regulated by proteolytic cleavage. It is released from various cell types as an inactive proenzyme (pro-uPA) which upon cleavage by proteinases becomes enzymatically active (Wang 2001). uPA binds to a specific cell surface receptor the urokinase plasminogen activator receptor (uPAR). Upon binding, uPA converts the zymogen plasminogen to plasmin, an enzyme which degrades fibrin and numerous other components of the extracellular matrix, such as type IV collagen, fibronectin and laminin enabling tumour cells to migrate through tissue barriers (Wang 2001). Evidence that the expression of active uPA by malignant cells correlates with their invasive potential was provided by Bramhall *et al.* (Bramhall *et al* 1997). Elevated levels of uPA/uPAR have been reported in numerous tumours, including pancreatic cancer (Cantero *et al* 1997). In patients with pancreatic cancer concomitant over-expression of uPA and uPAR was found to be associated with a shorter post-operative survival compared with those patients in whom only uPA or its receptor were overexpressed (Cantero *et al* 1997). In a recent study, the u-PA/u-PA receptor proteolytic system has been reported to be involved in the hepatocyte growth factor (HGF)-stimulated motility of pancreas cancer cells (Paciucci *et al* 1998). HGF-induced cell motility is significantly reduced by inhibitors of u-PA proteolytic activity, such as antibodies neutralizing u-PA activity, plasminogen activator inhibitor 1 and amiloride (Paciucci *et al* 1998). Additionally, anti-uPA antibodies injected into mice together with tumour cells caused a significant inhibition of metastasis formation, providing strong evidence for the involvement of this enzymatic system in tumour invasion and metastases.

4.6 Proteases and angiogenesis in pancreatic cancer

Oxygen and nutrients supplied by the vasculature are crucial for cell function and survival. Thus, the formation of new blood vessels (angiogenesis) is required for local and systemic expansion of the tumour mass and can be induced by multiple molecules that are released by both cancer cells and stromal cells (Bergers *et al* 1999). Angiogenesis itself encompasses a cascade of sequential processes emanating from micro-vascular endothelial cells, which are stimulated to proliferate and degrade the endothelial basement membrane of parental vessels, migrate, and penetrate into host stroma and initiate a capillary sprout.

Pancreatic tumours are avascular tumours, suggesting that they may produce angiogenesis inhibitors that suppress the growth of the vasculature to the tumour and metastases. Brammer *et al.* (Brammer *et al* 2005) sought evidence for the angiogenesis inhibitor, endostatin, in normal and cancerous pancreatic tissue. Using western blotting, they found mature 20 kDa endostatin in cancer tissue but not in normal tissue. Extracts from normal tissue were able to degrade exogenous endostatin, whereas extracts from cancer were without effect. The trypsin/chymotrypsin inhibitor, glycine max, did not prevent the degradation of endostatin by normal pancreatic extracts but elastatinal, a specific inhibitor of elastase, reduced the rate of degradation. Extracts of pancreatic tumours did not express any detectable elastase activity, but an elastase was expressed by extracts of normal pancreas. They concluded that endostatin was present and stable in pancreatic cancer tissues, which may explain their avascular nature, but that normal pancreatic tissue expresses enzymes, including elastase, which rapidly degrade endostatin.

Integrin signalling also contributes to tumour neo-angiogenesis. Quiescent vessels express one class of integrins, whereas sprouting capillaries express another. Interference with signalling from the latter class of integrins can inhibit angiogenesis underscoring the important contribution of cell adhesion to the angiogenic program which has also been shown for pancreatic cancer (Varner and Cheresh 1996). Furthermore, extracellular proteases are physically and functionally connected with pro-angiogenic integrins, and both help to dictate the invasive capability of angiogenic endothelial cells (Joyce *et al* 2004; Niedergethmann *et al* 2000). Joyce *et al* (Joyce *et al* 2004) used a broad-spectrum cysteine cathepsin inhibitor was used to pharmacologically knock out cathepsin function at different stages of tumourigenesis, impairing angiogenic switching in progenitor lesions, as well as tumour growth, vascularity, and invasiveness (Joyce *et al* 2004).

4.7 Conclusion

The involvement of proteases in various malignancies, including pancreatic cancer is still being unravelled. They are attractive potential pharmacological or genetic targets for anti-tumoural therapies. It remains to be determined whether some targeted agents are more likely to be effective when used in earlier stages of rapidly progressing diseases such as pancreatic cancer. Despite the negative studies of MMPIs and FTIs in advanced disease, phase II studies of EGFR- and VEGF based approaches, COX-2 inhibitors, and different immunotherapeutic strategies have been encouraging. Results of the ongoing and completed phase III trials of cetuximab and erlotinib (monoclonal antibody immunotherapies targeting epidermal growth factor receptor) are expected within the next few years. In addition, the oncology community is likely to witness the discovery and development of many other targeted agents that will eventually be used alone or in combination with currently available treatment modalities, and this may ultimately improve the prognosis of patients with pancreatic cancer.

REFERENCES

Adams JM, 2003, Ways of dying: multiple pathways to apoptosis. *Genes Dev.* **17:** 2481-2495.

Altznauer F, Conus S, Cavalli A, Folkers G, Simon HU, 2004, Calpain-1 regulates Bax and subsequent Smac-dependent caspase-3 activation in neutrophil apoptosis. *J Biol Chem.* **279:** 595947-57.

Aplin AE, Howe A, Alahari SK, Juliano RL, 1998, Signal transduction and signal modulation by cell adhesion receptors: the role of integrins, cadherins, immunoglobulin-cell adhesion molecules, and selectins. *Pharmacol Rev.* **50:** 197-263.

Applebaum-Shapiro SE, Finch R, Pfutzer RH, Hepp LA, Gates L, Amann S, Martin S, Ulrich CD 2nd, Whitcomb DC, 2001, Hereditary pancreatitis in North America: the Pittsburgh-Midwest Multi-Center Pancreatic Study Group Study. *Pancreatology.* **1**: 439-443.

Banerjee AK, 1995, An audit of fatal acute pancreatitis. *Postgraduate Med J.* **71:** 472-475.

Bergers G, Brekken R, McMahon G, Vu TH, Itoh T, Tamaki K, Tanzawa K, Thorpe P, Itohara S, Werb Z, Hanahan D, 2000, Matrix metalloproteinase-9 triggers the angiogenic switch during carcinogenesis. *Nature Cell Biol.* **2:** 737-744.

Bergers G, Javaherian K, Lo KM, Folkman J, Hanahan D, 1999, Effects of angiogenesis inhibitors on multistage carcinogenesis in mice. *Science.* **284:** 808-812.

Bramhall SR, Neoptolemos JP, Stamp GW, Lemoine NR,, 1997, Imbalance of expression of matrix metalloproteinases (MMPs) and tissue inhibitors of the matrix metalloproteinases (TIMPs) in human pancreatic carcinoma. *J Pathol.* **182:** 347-355.

Brammer RD, Bramhall SR, and Eggo MC, 2005, Endostatin expression in pancreatic tissue is modulated by elastase.[see comment]. *Br J Cancer.* **92:** 89-93.

Campo E, Merino MJ, Liotta L, Neumann R, Stetler-Stevenson W, 1992, Distribution of the 72-kd type IV collagenase in nonneoplastic and neoplastic thyroid tissue. *Human Pathol.* **23:** 1395-1401.

Cantero D, Friess H, Deflorin J, Zimmermann A, Brundler MA, Riesle E, Korc M, Buchler MW, 1997, Enhanced expression of urokinase plasminogen activator and its receptor in pancreatic carcinoma. *Br J Cancer.* **75:** 388-395.

Chan AO, Lam SK, Chu KM, Lam CM, Kwok E, Leung SY, Yuen ST, Law SY, Hui WM, Lai KC, Wong CY, Hu HC, Lai CL, Wong J, 2001, Soluble E-cadherin is a valid prognostic marker in gastric carcinoma. *Gut.* **48**: 808-811.

Chappell MC, Diz DI, and Jacobsen DW, 1992, Pharmacological characterization of angiotensin II binding sites in the canine pancreas. *Peptides.* **13:** 313-318.

Chappell MC, Millsted A, Diz DI, Brosnihan KB, Ferrario CM, 1991, Evidence for an intrinsic angiotensin system in the canine pancreas. *J Hypertension.* **9:** 751-759.

Charnley RM, 2003, Hereditary pancreatitis. *World J Gastroenterol.* **9:** 1-4.

Cho NH, Hong KP, Hong SH, Kang S, Chung KY, Cho SH, 2004, MMP expression profiling in recurred stage IB lung cancer. *Oncogene.* **23:** 845-851.

Cioffi M, Gazzerro P, Di Finizio B, Vietri MT, Di Macchia C, Puca GA, Molinari AM, 1999, Serum-soluble E-cadherin fragments in lung cancer. *Tumori.* **85:** 32-34.

Corfield AP, Cooper MJ, and Williamson RCN, 1985, Acute pancreatitis: a lethal disease of increasing incidence. *Gut.* **26:** 724-729.

Cornelius LA, Nehring LC, Harding E, Bolanowski M, Welgus HG, Kobayashi DK, Pierce RA, Shapiro SD, 1998, Matrix metalloproteinases generate angiostatin: effects on neovascularization. *J Immunol.* **161:** 6845-6852.

Crawford HC, Scoggins CR, Washington MK, Matrisian LM, Leach SD, 2002, Matrix metalloproteinase-7 is expressed by pancreatic cancer precursors and regulates acinar-to-ductal metaplasia in exocrine pancreas.[see comment]. *J Clin Invest.* **109:** 1437-1444.

Creighton J, Lyall R, Wilson DI, Curtis A, Charnley R, 1999, Mutations of the cationic trypsinogen gene in patients with chronic pancreatitis.[see comment]. *Lancet.* **354:** 42-43.

Christofori G and Semb H, 1999, The role of the cell-adhesion molecule E-cadherin as a tumour-suppressor gene. *Trends Biochem Sci.* **24**: 73-76.

Damsky CH, Richa J, Solter D, Knudsen K, Buck CA, 1983, Identification and purification of a cell surface glycoprotein mediating intercellular adhesion in embryonic and adult tissue. *Cell.* **34:** 455-466.

de Beaux AC, Palmer KR, Carter DC, 1995, Factors influencing morbidity and mortality in acute pancreatitis; an analysis of 279 cases. *Gut.* **37:** 121-126.

Durkan GC, Brotherick I, and Mellon JK, 1999, The impact of transurethral resection of bladder tumour on serum levels of soluble E-cadherin. *Bju International.* **83:** 424-428.

Ellenrieder V, Alber B, Lacher U, Hendler SF, Menke A, Boeck W, Wagner M, Wilda M, Friess H, Buchler M, Adler G, Gress TM, 2000, Role of MT-MMPs and MMP-2 in pancreatic cancer progression. *Int J Cancer.* **85:** 14-20.

Etemad B and Whitcomb DC, 2001, Chronic pancreatitis: diagnosis, classification, and new genetic developments. *Gastroenterology.* **120:** 682-707.

Fitz R, 1989, Acute pancreatitis: a consideration of pancreatic haemorrhage, haemorrhagic, supporative and gangrenous pancreatitis, and of disseminated fat necrosis. *Boston Med J.* **120:** 181-187, 205-207, 229-235.

Fogar P, Basso D, Pasquali C, De Paoli M, Sperti C, Roveroni G, Pedrazzoli S, Plebani M, 1997, Neural cell adhesion molecule (N-CAM) in gastrointestinal neoplasias. *Anticancer Res.* **17:** 1227-1230.

Frossard JL, Saluja A, Bhagat L, Lee HS, Bhatia M, Hofbauer B, Steer ML, 1999, The role of intercellular adhesion molecule 1 and neutrophils in acute pancreatitis and pancreatitis-associated lung injury. *Gastroenterol.* **116:** 694-701.

Gallagher SF, Yang J, Baksh K, Haines K, Carpenter H, Epling-Burnette PK, Peng Y, Norman J, Murr MM, 2004, Acute pancreatitis induces FasL gene expression and apoptosis in the liver. *J Surg Res.* **122:** 201-209.

Ghaneh P and Neoptolemos JP, 2004, Conclusions from the European Study Group for Pancreatic Cancer adjuvant trial of chemoradiotherapy and chemotherapy for pancreatic cancer. *Surg Oncol Clin North Am.* **13:** 567-87.

Gofuku J, Shiozaki H, Doki Y, Inoue M, Hirao M, Fukuchi N, Monden M, 1998, Characterization of soluble E-cadherin as a disease marker in gastric cancer patients. *Br J Cancer.* **78:** 1095-1101.

Gress TM, Muller-Pillasch F, Lerch MM, Friess H, Buchler M, Adler G, 1995, Expression and in-situ localization of genes coding for extracellular matrix proteins and extracellular matrix degrading proteases in pancreatic cancer. *Int J Cancer.* **62:** 407-413.

Gress TM, Muller-Pillasch F, Lerch MM, Friess H, Buchler M, Beger HG, Adler G, 1994, Balance of expression of genes coding for extracellular matrix proteins and extracellular matrix degrading proteases in chronic pancreatitis. *Z Gastroenterol.* **32:** 221-225.

Griendling KK, Minieri CA, Ollerenshaw JD, Alexander RW, 1994, Angiotensin II stimulates NADH and NADPH oxidase activity in cultured vascular smooth muscle cells. *Circ Res.* **74:** 1141-1148.

Griffiths TR, Brotherick I, Bishop RI, White MD, McKenna DM, Horne CH, Shenton BK, Neal DE, Mellon JK, 1996, Cell adhesion molecules in bladder cancer: soluble serum E-cadherin correlates with predictors of recurrence. *Br J Cancer.* **74:** 579-584.

Guice KS, Oldham KT, Caty MG, Johnson KJ, Ward PA, 1989, Neutrophil-dependent, oxygen-radical mediated lung injury associated with acute pancreatitis. *Ann Surg.* **210:** 740-747.

Gukovskaya AS, Gukovsky I, Jung Y, Mouria M, Pandol SJ, 2002, Cholecystokinin induces caspase activation and mitochondrial dysfunction in pancreatic acinar cells. Roles in cell injury processes of pancreatitis. *J Biol Chem.* **277:** 22595-22604.

Gukovskaya AS, Perkins P, Zaninovic V, Sandoval D, Rutherford R, Fitzsimmons T, Pandol SJ, Poucell-Hatton S, 1996, Mechanisms of cell death after pancreatic duct obstruction in the opossum and the rat.[see comment]. *Gastroenterol.* **110:** 875-884.

Halangk W, Lerch MM, Brandt-Nedelev B, Roth W, Ruthenbuerger M, Reinheckel T, Domschke W, Lippert H, Peters C, Deussing J, 2000, Role of cathepsin B in intracellular trypsinogen activation and the onset of acute pancreatitis. *J Clin Invest.* **106:** 773-781.

Hartwig W, Werner J, Warshaw AL, Antoniu B, Castillo CF, Gebhard MM, Uhl W, Buchler MW, 2004, Membrane-bound ICAM-1 is upregulated by trypsin and contributes to leukocyte migration in acute pancreatitis. *Am J Physiol Gastrointest Liver Physiol.* **287:** G1194-G1199.

Hasebe T, Sasaki S, Imoto S, Ochiai A, 2000, Proliferative activity of intratumoral fibroblasts is closely correlated with lymph node and distant organ metastases of invasive ductal carcinoma of the breast. *Am J Pathol.* **156:** 1701-1710.

Hasebe T, Sasaki S, Sugitoh M, Ono M, Saitoh N, Ochiai A, 2001, Highly proliferative intratumoral fibroblasts and a high proliferative microvessel index are significant predictors of tumor metastasis in T3 ulcerative-type colorectal cancer. *Human Pathol.* **32:** 401-409.

Hernandez-Barrantes S, Toth M, Bernardo MM, Yurkova M, Gervasi DC, Raz Y, Sang QA, Fridman R, 2000, Binding of active (57 kDa) membrane type 1-matrix metalloproteinase (MT1-MMP) to tissue inhibitor of metalloproteinase (TIMP)-2 regulates MT1-MMP processing and pro-MMP-2 activation. *J Biol Chem.* **275:** 12080-12089.

Hedstrom J, Haglund C, Leinonen J, Nordling S, Stenman UH, 2001, Trypsinogen-1, -2 and tumour-associated trypsin-inhibitor in bile and biliary tract tissues from patients with biliary tract diseases and pancreatic carcinomas. *Scand J Clin Laboratory Invest.* **61:** 111-118.

Hofbauer B, Saluja AK, Lerch MM, Bhagat L, Bhatia M, Lee HS, Frossard JL, Adler G, Steer ML, 1998, Intra-acinar cell activation of trypsinogen during caerulein-induced pancreatitis in rats. *Am J Physiol.* **275:** G352-G362.

Hori Y, Takeyama Y, Ueda T, Shinkai M, Takase K, Kuroda Y, 2000, Macrophage-derived transforming growth factor-beta1 induces hepatocellular injury via apoptosis in rat severe acute pancreatitis. *Surgery.* **127:** 641-649.

Howes N, Greenhalf W, Stocken DD, Neoptolemos JP, 2005, Cationic trypsinogen mutations and pancreatitis. *Clin Laboratory Med.* **25:** 39-59.

Ikeda O, Egami H, Ishiko T, Ishikawa S, Kamohara H, Hidaka H, Mita S, Ogawa M, 2003, Expression of proteinase-activated receptor-2 in human pancreatic cancer: a possible relation to cancer invasion and induction of fibrosis. *Int J Oncol.* **22:** 295-300.

Imai K, Yokohama Y, Nakanishi I, Ohuchi E, Fujii Y, Nakai N, Okada Y, 1995, Matrix metalloproteinase 7 (matrilysin) from human rectal carcinoma cells. Activation of the precursor, interaction with other matrix metalloproteinases and enzymic properties. *J Biol Chem.* **270:** 6691-6697.

Imamura T, Ohshio G, Mise M, Harada T, Suwa H, Okada N, Wang Z, Yoshitomi S, Tanaka T, Sato H, Arii S, Seiki M, Imamura M, 1998, Expression of membrane-type matrix metalloproteinase-1 in human pancreatic adenocarcinomas. *J Cancer Res Clin Oncol.* **124:** 65-72.

Imamura M, Doi R, Imaizumi T, Funakoshi A, Wakasugi H, Sunamura M, Ogata Y, Hishinuma S, Asano T, Aikou T, Hosotani R, Maetani S, 2004, A randomized multicenter trial comparing resection and radiochemotherapy for resectable locally invasive pancreatic cancer. *Surgery.* **136:** 1003-1011.

Jaffray C, Yang J, Carter G, Mendez C, Norman J, 2000, Pancreatic elastase activates pulmonary nuclear factor kappa B and inhibitory kappa B, mimicking pancreatitis-associated adult respiratory distress syndrome. *Surgery.* **128:** 225-231.

Johnson CD and Abu-Hilal M, 2004, Persistent organ failure during the first week as a marker of fatal outcome in acute pancreatitis. *Gut.* **53:** 1340-1344.

Johnson GB, Brunn GJ, and Platt JL, 2004, Cutting edge: an endogenous pathway to systemic inflammatory response syndrome (SIRS)-like reactions through Toll-like receptor 4. *J Immunol.* **172:** 20-24.

Jones LE, Humphreys MJ, Campbell F, Neoptolemos JP, Boyd MT, 2004, Comprehensive analysis of matrix metalloproteinase and tissue inhibitor expression in pancreatic cancer: increased expression of matrix metalloproteinase-7 predicts poor survival. *Clin Cancer Res.* **10:** 2832-2845.

Joyce JA, Baruch A, Chehade K, Meyer-Morse N, Giraudo E, Tsai FY, Greenbaum DC, Hager JH, Bogyo M, Hanahan D, 2004, Cathepsin cysteine proteases are effectors of invasive growth and angiogenesis during multistage tumorigenesis.[see comment]. *Cancer Cell.* 5: 443-453.

Kaiser AM, Saluja AK, and Steer ML, 1999, Repetitive short-term obstructions of the common bile-pancreatic duct induce severe acute pancreatitis in the opossum. *Digest Dis Sci.* **44:** 1653-1661.

Karayiannakis AJ, Syrigos KN, Polychronidis A, Simopoulos C, 2001, Expression patterns of alpha-, beta- and gamma-catenin in pancreatic cancer: correlation with E-cadherin expression, pathological features and prognosis. *Anticancer Res.* **21:** 4127-4134.

Katayama M, Hirai S, Kamihagi K, Nakagawa K, Yasumoto M, Kato I, 1994, Soluble E-cadherin fragments increased in circulation of cancer patients. *Br J Cancer.* **69:** 580-585.

Kaufmann P, Smolle KH, Brunner GA, Demel U, Tilz GP, Krejs GJ, 1999, Relation of serial measurements of plasma-soluble intercellular adhesion molecule-1 to severity of acute pancreatitis. *Am J Gastroenterol.* **94:** 2412-2416.

Kaufmann P, Demel U, Tilz GP, Krejs GJ, 1999, Time course of plasma soluble intercellular adhesion molecule-1 (sICAM-1) is related to severity of acute pancreatitis. *Hepato-Gastroenterol.* **46:** 2565-2571.

Kaufmann R, Schafberg H, and Nowak G, 1998, Proteinase-activated receptor-2-mediated signaling and inhibition of DNA synthesis in human pancreatic cancer cells. *Int J Pancreatol.* **24:** 97-102.

Kennedy RH, Bockman DE, Uscanga L, Choux R, Grimaud JA, Sarles H, 1987, Pancreatic extracellular matrix alterations in chronic pancreatitis. *Pancreas.* **2:** 61-72.

Kim JH, Kim TH, Jang JW, Jang YJ, Lee KH, Lee ST, 2001, Analysis of matrix metalloproteinase mRNAs expressed in hepatocellular carcinoma cell lines. *Molecules Cells.* **12:** 32-40.

Kleiner DE and Stetler-Stevenson WG, 1999, Matrix metalloproteinases and metastasis. *Cancer Chemother Pharmacol* **43(Suppl.):** S42-S51.

Klonowski-Stumpe H, Luthen R, Han B, Sata N, Haussinger D, Niederau C, 1998, Inhibition of cathepsin B does not affect the intracellular activation of trypsinogen by cerulein hyperstimulation in isolated rat pancreatic acinar cells. *Pancreas.* **16:** 96-101.

Kohli V, Madden JF, Bentley RC, Clavien PA, 1999, Calpain mediates ischemic injury of the liver through modulation of apoptosis and necrosis. *Gastroenterology.* **116:** 168-78.

Lerch MM, Halangk W, and Kruger B, 2000, The role of cysteine proteases in intracellular pancreatic serine protease activation. *Adv Exp Med Biol.* **477:** 403-411.

Leung PS, Chan WP, and Nobiling R, 2000, Regulated expression of pancreatic renin-angiotensin system in experimental pancreatitis. *Mol Cell Endocrinol.* **166:** 121-128.

Leung PS, Chan WP, Wong TP, Sernia C, 1999, Expression and localization of the renin-angiotensin system in the rat pancreas. *J Endocrinol.* **160:** 13-19.

Leung PS, Chan HC, and Wong PY, 1998, Immunohistochemical localization of angiotensin II in the mouse pancreas. *Histochem J.* **30:** 21-25.

Leung PS, Chan HC, Fu LX, Wong PY, 1997, Localization of angiotensin II receptor subtypes AT1 and AT2 in the pancreas of rodents. *J Endocrinol.* **153:** 269-274.

Luthen R, Owen RL, Sarbia M, Grendell JH, Niederau C, 1998, Premature trypsinogen activation during cerulein pancreatitis in rats occurs inside pancreatic acinar cells. *Pancreas.* **17:** 38-43.

Luthen RE, Niederau C, and Grendell JH, 1993, Effects of bile and pancreatic digestive enzymes on permeability of the pancreatic duct system in rabbits. *Pancreas.* **8:** 671-681.

Li YJ and Ji XR, 2003, Relationship between expression of E-cadherin-catenin complex and clinicopathologic characteristics of pancreatic cancer. *World J Gastroenterol.* **9:** 368-372.

Mandi Y, Farkas G, Takacs T, Boda K, Lonovics J, 2000, Diagnostic relevance of procalcitonin, IL-6, and sICAM-1 in the prediction of infected necrosis in acute pancreatitis. *Int J Pancreatol.* **28:** 41-49.

Matsuyama Y, Takao S, and Aikou T, 2002, Comparison of matrix metalloproteinase expression between primary tumors with or without liver metastasis in pancreatic and colorectal carcinomas. *J Surg Oncol.* **80:** 105-110.

McCachren SS, 1991, Expression of metalloproteinases and metalloproteinase inhibitor in human arthritic synovium. *Arthritis Rheumat.* **34:** 1085-1093.

Menke A, Philippi C, Vogelmann R, Seidel B, Lutz MP, Adler G, Wedlich D, 2001, Down-regulation of E-cadherin gene expression by collagen type I and type III in pancreatic cancer cell lines. *Cancer Res.* **61:** 3508-3517.

Mignatti P and Rifkin DB, 1993, Biology and biochemistry of proteinases in tumor invasion. *Physiol Rev.* **73:** 161-195.

Mirkovic D, 2000, The role of phospholipase A2 in the pathogenesis of respiratory damage in hemorrhagic necrotizing pancreatitis--assessment of a new experimental model. *Vojnosanitetski Pregled.* **57:** 625-633.

Miyata S, Miyagi Y, Koshikawa N, Nagashima Y, Kato Y, Yasumitsu H, Hirahara F, Misugi K, Miyazaki K, 1998, Stimulation of cellular growth and adhesion to fibronectin and vitronectin in culture and tumorigenicity in nude mice by overexpression of trypsinogen in human gastric cancer cells. *Clin Exp Metast.* **16:** 613-622.

Muhs BE, Patel S, Yee H, Marcus S, Shamamian P, 2001, Increased matrix metalloproteinase expression and activation following experimental acute pancreatitis. *J Surg Res.* **101:** 21-28.

Muller-Pillasch F, Gress TM, Yamaguchi H, Geng M, Adler G, Menke A, 1997, The influence of transforming growth factor beta 1 on the expression of genes coding for matrix metalloproteinases and tissue inhibitors of metalloproteinases during regeneration from cerulein-induced pancreatitis. *Pancreas.* **15:** 168-175.

Nagakawa T, Sanada H, Inagaki M, Sugama J, Ueno K, Konishi I, Ohta T, Kayahara M, Kitagawa H, 2004, Long-term survivors after resection of carcinoma of the head of the pancreas: significance of histologically curative resection. *J Hepatobiliary Pancreat Surg.* **11:** 402-408.

Neoptolemos JP, Raraty M, Finch M, Sutton R, 1998, Acute pancreatitis: The substantial human and financial costs. *Gut.* **42:** 886-891.

Niederau C, Fronhoffs K, Klonowski H, Schulz HU, 1995, Active pancreatic digestive enzymes show striking differences in their potential to damage isolated rat pancreatic acinar cells. *J Lab Clin Med.* **125:** 265-275.

Niederau C and Grendell JH, 1988, Intracellular vacuoles in experimental acute pancreatitis in rats and mice are an acidified compartment. *J Clin Invest.* **81:** 229-236.

Niederau C and Luthen R, 1999, Events inside the pancreatic acinar cell in acute pancreatitis: role of secretory blockade, calcium release, and dehydration in the initiation of trypsinogen activation and autodigestion. Pancreatic disease: state of the art and future aspects of research., ed. Lankisch PG and Di Magno EP. Springer: Berlin. 14-23.

Niedergethmann M, Hildenbrand R, Wolf G, Verbeke CS, Richter A, Post S, 2000, Angiogenesis and cathepsin expression are prognostic factors in pancreatic adenocarcinoma after curative resection. *Int J Pancreatol.* **28:** 31-39.

Noe V, Fingleton B, Jacobs K, Crawford HC, Vermeulen S, Steelant W, Bruyneel E, Matrisian LM, Mareel M, 2001, Release of an invasion promoter E-cadherin fragment by matrilysin and stromelysin-1. *J Cell Sci.* **114:** 111-118.

Norman J, 1998, The role of cytokines in the pathogenesis of acute pancreatitis. *Am J Surg.* **175:** 76-83.

Ogawa M, 1998, Acute pancreatitis and cytokines: "second attack" by septic complication leads to organ failure. *Pancreas.* **16:** 312-315.

Ohira T, Akutagawa S, Usuda J, Nakamura T, Hirano T, Tsuboi M, Nishio K, Taguchi F, Ikeda N, Nakamura H, Konaka C, Saijo N, Kato H, 2002, Up-regulated gene expression of angiogenesis factors in post-chemotherapeutic lung cancer tissues determined by cDNA macroarray. *Oncol Reports.* **9:** 723-728.

Ohta T, Shimizu K, Yi S, Takamura H, Amaya K, Kitagawa H, Kayahara M, Ninomiya I, Fushida S, Fujimura T, Nishimura G, Miwa K, 2003, Protease-activated receptor-2 expression and the role of trypsin in cell proliferation in human pancreatic cancers. *Int J Oncol.* **23:** 61-66.

O'Neill S, O'Neill AJ, Conroy E, Brady HR, Fitzpatrick JM, Watson RW, 2000, Altered caspase expression results in delayed neutrophil apoptosis in acute pancreatitis. *J Leukocyte Biol.* **68:** 15-20.

Oyama K, Ohta T, Nishimura GI, Elnemr A, Yasui T, Fujimura T, Fushida S, Kitagawa H, Kayahara M, Terada T, Miwa K, 2000, Trypsinogen expression in colorectal cancers. *Int J Mol Med.* **6:** 543-548.

Paciucci R, Vila MR, Adell T, Diaz VM, Tora M, Nakamura T, Real FX, 1998, Activation of the urokinase plasminogen activator/urokinase plasminogen activator receptor system and redistribution of E-cadherin are associated with hepatocyte growth factor-induced motility of pancreas tumor cells overexpressing Met. *Am J Pathol.* **153:** 201-212.

Paju A, Sorsa T, Tervahartiala T, Koivunen E, Haglund C, Leminen A, Wahlstrom T, Salo T, Stenman UH, 2001, The levels of trypsinogen isoenzymes in ovarian tumour cyst fluids are associated with promatrix metalloproteinase-9 but not promatrix metalloproteinase-2 activation. *Br J Cancer.* **84:** 1363-1371.

Peppin GJ and Weiss SJ, 1986, Activation of the endogenous metalloproteinase, gelatinase, by triggered human neutrophils. *Proc Natl Acad Sci U S A.* **83:** 4322-4326.

Pfutzer RH and Whitcomb DC, 2001, SPINK1 mutations are associated with multiple phenotypes. *Pancreatology.* **1:** 457-460.

Poch B, Gansauge F, Rau B, Wittel U, Gansauge S, Nussler AK, Schoenberg M, Beger HG, 1999, The role of polymorphonuclear leukocytes and oxygen-derived free radicals in experimental acute pancreatitis: mediators of local destruction and activators of inflammation. *FEBS Letters.* **461:** 268-272.

Ramadani M, Yang Y, Gansauge F, Gansauge S, Beger HG, 2001, Overexpression of caspase-1 (interleukin-1beta converting enzyme) in chronic pancreatitis and its participation in apoptosis and proliferation. *Pancreas.* **22:** 383-387.

Reber HA, 1991, Acute pancreatitis: another piece of the puzzle? *N Engl J Med.* **325:** 423-424.

Salomone T, Tosi P, Raiti C, Guariento A, Tomassetti P, Migliori M, Saieva C, Romboli M, Gullo L, 2002, Apoptosis in the peripheral blood mononuclear cells as a self-limitation process in human acute pancreatitis. *Pancreatology.* **2:** 204-210.

Saluja A, Saluja M, Villa A, Leli U, Rutledge P, Meldolesi J, Steer M, 1989, Pancreatic duct obstruction in rabbits causes digestive zymogen and lysosomal enzyme colocalization. *J Clin Invest.* **84:** 1260-1266.

Saluja AK, Donovan EA, Yamanaka K, Yamaguchi Y, Hofbauer B, Steer ML, 1997, Cerulein-induced in vitro activation of trypsinogen in rat pancreatic acini is mediated by cathepsin B. *Gastroenterol.* **113:** 304-310.

Sasson AR, Wetherington RW, Hoffman JP, Ross EA, Cooper H, Meropol NJ, Freedman G, Pingpank JF, Eisenberg BL, 2003, Neoadjuvant chemoradiotherapy for adenocarcinoma of the pancreas: analysis of histopathology and outcome. *Int J Gastrointest Cancer.* **34:** 121-128.

Satoh A, Masamune A, Kimura K, Kaneko K, Sakai Y, Yamagiwa T, Satoh M, Kikuta K, Asakura T, Shimosegawa T, 2003, Nuclear factor kappa B expression in peripheral blood mononuclear cells of patients with acute pancreatitis. *Pancreas.* **26:** 350-356.

Sheu BC, Lien HC, Ho HN, Lin HH, Chow SN, Huang SC, Hsu SM, 2003, Increased expression and activation of gelatinolytic matrix metalloproteinases is associated with the progression and recurrence of human cervical cancer. *Cancer Res.* **63:** 6537-6542.

Shimamoto R, Sawada T, Uchima Y, Inoue M, Kimura K, Yamashita Y, Yamada N, Nishihara T, Ohira M, Hirakawa K, 2004, A role for protease-activated receptor-2 in pancreatic cancer cell proliferation. *Int J Oncol.* **24:** 1401-1406.

Skubitz AP, 2002, Adhesion molecules. *Cancer Treatment Res.* **107:** 305-329.

Steer ML, 1999, Early events in acute pancreatitis. *Bailliere's Best Pract Clin Gastroenterol.* **13:** 213-225.

Steinhusen U, Weiske J, Badock V, Tauber R, Bommert K, Huber O, 2001, Cleavage and shedding of E-cadherin after induction of apoptosis. *J Biol Chem.* **276:** 4972-4980.

Strate T, Knoefel WT, Yekebas E, Izbicki JR, 2003, Chronic pancreatitis: etiology, pathogenesis, diagnosis, and treatment. *Int J Colorect Dis.* **18:** 97-106.

Sundfeldt K, Ivarsson K, Rask K, Haeger M, Hedin L, Brannstrom M, 2001, Higher levels of soluble E-cadherin in cyst fluid from malignant ovarian tumours than in benign cysts. *Anticancer Res.* **21:** 65-70.

Sunamura M, Yamauchi J, Shibuya K, Chen HM, Ding L, Takeda K, Kobari M, Matsuno S, 1998, Pancreatic microcirculation in acute pancreatitis. *J Hepatobiliary-Pancreat Surg.* **5:**62-68.

Tahmasebi M, Puddefoot JR, Inwang ER, Vinson GP, 1999, The tissue renin-angiotensin system in human pancreas. *J Endocrinol.* **161:** 317-322.

Takeichi M, 1988, The cadherins: cell-cell adhesion molecules controlling animal morphogenesis. *Development.* **102:** 639-655.

Tasaki K, Shintani Y, Saotome T, Andoh A, Fujiyama Y, Hozawa S, Bamba T, 2003, Pro-inflammatory cytokine-induced matrix metalloproteinase-1 (MMP-1) secretion in human pancreatic periacinar myofibroblasts. *Pancreatology.* **3:** 414-421.

Tempia-Caliera AA, Horvath LZ, Zimmermann A, Tihanyi TT, Korc M, Friess H, Buchler MW, 2002, Adhesion molecules in human pancreatic cancer. *J Surg Oncol.* **79:** 93-100.

Truninger K, Kock J, Wirth HP, Muellhaupt B, Arnold C, von Weizsacker F, Seifert B, Ammann RW, Blum HE, 2001, Trypsinogen gene mutations in patients with chronic or recurrent acute pancreatitis. *Pancreas.* **22:** 18-23.

Uchima Y, Sawada T, Nishihara T, Umekawa T, Ohira M, Ishikawa T, Nishino H, Hirakawa K, 2003, Identification of a trypsinogen activity stimulating factor produced by pancreatic cancer cells: its role in tumor invasion and metastasis. *Int J Mol Med.* **12:** 871-878.

Uehara S, Honjyo K, Furukawa S, Hirayama A, Sakamoto W, 1989, Role of the kallikrein-kinin system in human pancreatitis. *Adv Exp Med Biol.* **247B:** 643-648.

Van Acker GJ, Saluja AK, Bhagat L, Singh VP, Song AM, Steer ML, 2002, Cathepsin B inhibition prevents trypsinogen activation and reduces pancreatitis severity. *Am J Physiol Gastrointest Liver Physiol.* **283:** G794-G800.

Varner JA and Cheresh DA, 1996, Integrins and cancer. *Curr Opinion Cell Biol.* **8:** 724-730.

Vassalli JD and Pepper MS, 1994, Tumour biology. Membrane proteases in focus.[comment]. *Nature.* **370:** 14-15.

von Marschall Z, Riecken EO, and Rosewicz S, 1998, Stromelysin 3 is overexpressed in human pancreatic carcinoma and regulated by retinoic acid in pancreatic carcinoma cell lines. *Gut.* **43:** 692-698.

Wang Y, 2001, The role and regulation of urokinase-type plasminogen activator receptor gene expression in cancer invasion and metastasis. *Med Res Rev.* **21:** 146-170.

Wang XP, Zhang R, and Wu K, 2004, Angiotensin II Mediates Acinar Cell Apoptosis During the Development of Rat Pancreatic Fibrosis by AT1R. *Pancreas.* **29:** 264-270.

Wang KK, 2000, Calpain and caspase: can you tell the difference?[erratum appears in Trends Neurosci 2000 Feb;23(2):59]. *Trends Neurosci.* **23:** 20-26.

Wheelock M, Buck C, and Bechtol K, 1987, Soluble 80-kd fragment of cell-CAM 120/80 disrupts cell-cell adhesion. *Cell Biochem.* **34:** 187-202.

Whitcomb DC, 1999, Hereditary pancreatitis: new insights into acute and chronic pancreatitis. *Gut.* **45:** 317-322.

Whitcomb DC, 2000a, New insights into hereditary pancreatitis.[see comment]. *Curr Gastroenterol Reports.* **1:** 154-160.

Whitcomb DC, 2000b, Genetic predispositions to acute and chronic pancreatitis. *Med Clin North Am.* **84:** 531-547.

Whitcomb DC, 2001, Hereditary pancreatitis: a model for understanding the genetic basis of acute and chronic pancreatitis. *Pancreatology.* **1:** 565-570.

Whitcomb DC, 2003, Genetic predisposition to alcoholic chronic pancreatitis. *Pancreas.* **27:** 321-326.

Whitcomb DC, Gorry MC, Preston RA, Furey W, Sossenheimer MJ, Ulrich CD, Martin SP, Gates LK Jr, Amann ST, Toskes PP, Liddle R, McGrath K, Uomo G, Post JC, Ehrlich GD, 1996, Hereditary pancreatitis is caused by a mutation in the cationic trypsinogen gene.[see comment]. *Nature Genet.* **14:** 141-145.

Wilkowski R, Thoma M, Schauer R, Wagner A, Heinemann V, 2004, Effect of chemoradiotherapy with gemcitabine and cisplatin on locoregional control in patients with primary inoperable pancreatic cancer. *World J Surg.* **28:** 1011-1018.

Williams SJ, Gotley DC, and Antalis TM, 2001, Human trypsinogen in colorectal cancer. *Int J Cancer.* **93:** 67-73.

Witt H, Luck W, Becker M, Bohmig M, Kage A, Truninger K, Ammann RW, O'Reilly D, Kingsnorth A, Schulz HU, Halangk W, Kielstein V, Knoefel WT, Teich N, Keim V, 2001, Mutation in the SPINK1 trypsin inhibitor gene, alcohol use, and chronic pancreatitis. *JAMA.* **285:** 2716-2717.

Yada K, Shibata K, Matsumoto T, Ohta M, Yokoyama S, Kitano S, 2005, Protease-activated receptor-2 regulates cell proliferation and enhances cyclooxygenase-2 mRNA expression in human pancreatic cancer cells. *J Surg Oncol.* **89:** 79-85.

Yamada T, Horiuchi M, and Dzau VJ, 1996, Angiotensin II type 2 receptor mediates programmed cell death. *Proc Natl Acad Sci U S A.* **93:** 156-160.

Yamaguchi Y, Matsuno K, Goto M, Ogawa M, 1993, In situ kinetics of acinar, duct, and inflammatory cells in duct ligation-induced pancreatitis in rats. *Gastroenterol.* **104:** 1498-1506.

Yamamoto H, Iku S, Itoh F, Tang X, Hosokawa M, Imai K. 2001, Association of trypsin expression with recurrence and poor prognosis in human esophageal squamous cell carcinoma. *Cancer.* **91:** 1324-1331.

Yamamoto H, Itoh F, Iku S, Adachi Y, Fukushima H, Sasaki S, Mukaiya M, Hirata K, Imai K, 2001a, Expression of matrix metalloproteinases and tissue inhibitors of metalloproteinases in human pancreatic adenocarcinomas: clinicopathologic and prognostic significance of matrilysin expression. *J Clin Oncol.* **19:** 1118-1127.

Yang J, Gallagher SF, Haines K, Epling-Burnette PK, Bai F, Gower WR Jr, Mastorides S, Norman JG, Murr MM, 2004, Kupffer cell-derived Fas ligand plays a role in liver injury and hepatocyte death. *J Gastrointest Surg.* **8:** 166-174.

Yeo CJ, Cameron JL, Sohn TA, Lillemoe KD, Pitt HA, Talamini MA, Hruban RH, Ord SE, Sauter PK, Coleman J, Zahurak ML, Grochow LB, Abrams RA, 1997, Six hundred fifty consecutive pancreaticoduodenectomies in the 1990s: pathology, complications, and outcomes. *Ann Surg.* **226:** 248-257.

Xie MJ, Motoo Y, Su SB, Sawabu N, 2001, Expression of tumor necrosis factor-alpha, interleukin-6, and interferon-gamma in spontaneous chronic pancreatitis in the WBN/Kob rat. *Pancreas.* **22:** 400-408.

Xiong HQ, Rosenberg A, LoBuglio A, Schmidt W, Wolff RA, Deutsch J, Needle M, Abbruzzese JL, 2004, Cetuximab, a monoclonal antibody targeting the epidermal growth factor receptor, in combination with gemcitabine for advanced pancreatic cancer: a multicenter phase II Trial. *J Clin Oncol.* **22:** 2610-2616.

Chapter 5

PAR in the Pathogenesis of Pain in Pancreatic Disease

Pankaj J. Pasricha
Enteric Neuromuscular Disorders and Pain Group, Division of Gastroenterology and Hepatology, Department of Internal Medicine, University of Texas Medical Branch, Galveston, TX

1. INTRODUCTION

Pancreatitis, is a significant contributor to the "burden of gastrointestinal disease" in this country, according to a recent survey conducted by the American Gastroenterological Association (2001). In 1998 there were about 1.2 million prevalent cases, with 327,000 inpatient and 530,000 physician office visits. The estimated total direct cost for this group of diseases was $2.1 billion in 1998.

The cardinal manifestations of chronic pancreatitis are glandular (endocrine as well as exocrine insufficiency) and pain. Modern medicine has brought the former under reasonable control by replacement therapy (insulin, enzymes) but the latter continues to provide a major clinical challenge- "painful chronic pancreatitis is poorly understood and its management is controversial" (DiMagno 1999). Our lack of knowledge about what causes pain in pancreatitis has been a serious obstacle to improvement of the care of these patients, leading to various empirical approaches that are often based on purely anatomical grounds, are generally highly invasive and at best of marginal value (1998). Despite a wide variety of approaches covering innocuous (enzyme therapy), minimally invasive (endoscopic decompression, nerve blocks) and highly aggressive (surgical decompression, pancreatectomy), no consensus has emerged and no form of treatment can be considered satisfactory at the present time.

U. Lendeckel and Nigel M. Hooper (eds.), Proteases in Gastrointestinal Tissue, 123-130.

2. CURRENT THEORIES ON THE PATHOGENESIS OF PAIN IN PANCREATITIS

As with other organs, pain signaling from the pancreas involves at least three levels of neurons: the first is the primary nociceptor with its peripheral nerve endings located within the gland and its cell body located in the dorsal root ganglia. The central ends of these nociceptors terminate in the dorsal horn of the spinal cord where they make contact with neurons in the gray matter. Postsynaptic (i.e., second-order) neurons then travel cephalad within ascending pathways to synapse in several thalamic and reticular nuclei on their way to the sensory cortex. Signal transduction presents a unique challenge for nociceptors because unlike other sensory stimuli (such as light), noxious stimuli can take one of a variety of diverse forms including heat, pressure and chemical injury. In general, nociceptors convert noxious stimuli to an electrical response via specialized receptors such as the vanilloid receptor, TRPV1 and a variety of others.

A minority of patients with chronic pancreatitis and pain have readily identifiable lesions such as pseudocysts that are relatively easy to treat surgically or endoscopically. In the others, pain has traditionally been thought to result from a variety of causes including elevated intrapancreatic pressures, ischemia and fibrosis. However, it is likely that these phenomena, while clearly associated with the disease, are not the root cause of the pain. Instead, they probably are inciting factors on a background of neuronal sensitization induced by damage to the perineurium and subsequent exposure of the nerves to mediators and products of inflammation. The evidence for neuroimmune interactions in the pathogenesis of pain in humans with chronic pancreatitis has recently been reviewed (Di Sebastiano *et al* 2003). In general, the data is in keeping with evidence from the somatic literature that the persistent pain associated with peripheral tissue injury or inflammation results from long-term changes in nociceptive processing that can involve both primary sensory neurons (peripheral sensitization), as well as neurons in the spinal cord and higher structures (central sensitization). The gain of the entire system is therefore reset upwards, with the result that noxious stimuli now elicit a pain response that is much greater when compared with the normal state (hyperalgesia). A further characteristic of the sensitized state is called allodynia, a term that refers to the phenomenon in which innocuous or physiological stimuli are perceived as painful. Conceptually, one can therefore postulate that patients with pancreatic neuronal sensitization may experience mechanical allodynia: pain in response to physiological changes in intraductal pressure (which would otherwise have not been perceived). Similarly, subsequent minor flare-ups of inflammation in such patients could also cause the associated pain to be felt as severe, rather than mild (hyperalgesia).

3. A POTENTIAL ROLE FOR TRYPSIN IN PANCREATIC PAIN

Nociceptive sensitization results from both early posttranslational changes as well as later transcription-dependent changes in effector genes, with both processes occurring in the peripheral terminals of the nociceptor and in dorsal horn neurons (Woolf and Costigan 1999). In turn these processes alter the sensitivity of the system with augmentation of the response to peripheral stimuli. Many of the elements of the "inflammatory soup" described in somatic pain models (including ions (K+, H+), amines (5-HT, histamine), kinins (bradykinin), prostanoids (PGE_2), purines (ATP), cytokines (TNF, IL-1, IL-6), nitric oxide and caloric activity (heat)) are likely to result in early sensitization of pancreatic nociceptors in patients with pancreatitis as well. However, in addition to these ubiquitous elements, pancreatitis is also uniquely associated with a significant release and activation of endogenous proteases such as trypsin. Activated forms of these enzymes are detected in the pancreatic parenchyma and pancreatic juice of patients with pancreatitis (Steer 1993). Although activated enzymes are usually implicated in the pathogenesis of acute pancreatitis, they are probably also important in chronic pancreatitis, especially in the early stages. Perhaps the most conclusive evidence for the importance of the role of trypsin has come from the study of hereditary pancreatitis, which is a rare condition that leads to serial attacks of acute pancreatitis eventually followed by the development of chronic pancreatitis. Patients with hereditary pancreatitis have a mutation in the trypsinogen gene, which results in failure of cleavage and persistent tryptic activity, causing a pancreatitis that is very similar in its clinical picture to nonhereditary forms of chronic pancreatitis (Whitcomb *et al* 1996; Whitcomb 1999).

Given the importance of trypsin and other proteases in the pathogenesis of pancreatitis, we hypothesized that they may also be key players in early forms of neuronal sensitization in this condition an effect mediated by specific receptors such as the protease activated receptors (PARs), a unique family of G-protein coupled receptors (Dery and Bunnett 1999).

4. PROTEASE-ACTIVATED RECEPTORS

Proteases abound in the body in both humoral (thrombin, factor Xa) and cellular compartments (trypsin, tryptase and other tryptic enzymes from mast cells), and are capable of a wide variety of biological functions, that extend beyond simple protein degradation. They can also act as biological signals, interacting with specific receptors in the form of either traditional receptor-ligand coupling (such as those involving the coagulation factor Xa and urokinase) or through a recently described, novel method of receptor activation, requiring proteolytic cleavage. The latter is exemplified by the interactions of thrombin, trypsin, tryptase and perhaps other serine proteases, with what are called protease (or proteinase) -activated receptors (PARs). This is a growing family of G-protein-coupled-receptors (Dery and Bunnett 1999) that are biologically unique in that they are tethered to their own ligands under resting conditions. Upon exposure to certain serine proteases (e.g. thrombin for PAR1, PAR3 and PAR4 or trypsin for PAR1, PAR-2, PAR4), this ligand is "released" by proteolytic cleavage, subsequently binding and activating the receptor, which triggers a rise in intracellular calcium via phospholipase C activation and possibly, other mechanisms. Synthetic peptides (SLIGRL in the case of rat PAR-2) corresponding to the tethered ligand can also activate the receptor without the need for proteolysis.

The original, and best studied protease activated receptor is the thrombin-sensitive PAR-1 which is thought to play a role in inflammation and cell growth(Vergnolle *et al* 1999). Much less is known about PAR-2 and its role in health and disease. However, it is expressed in a variety of gastrointestinal organs and tissues including enterocytes, pancreatic ductal epithelium, colonic and vascular smooth muscle and the enteric nervous system where it is speculated that it may be important in mediating the cytoprotective, vascular, secretory and motility responses to inflammation (Coelho *et al* 2003; Cottrell *et al* 2003; Amadesi and Bunnett 2004).

5. THE PROTEASE ACTIVATED RECEPTOR-2 AND NOCICEPTION

Recently, others and we have begun exploring a role for protease-PAR-2 signaling in primary afferent nociceptors. We first demonstrated the presence of PAR-2 mRNA and protein expression in adult rat thoracic DRG, as well as an increase in intracellular calcium in response to treatment of cultured DRG neurons with either trypsin or the PAR-2 agonist activating peptide (AcPeP) (Hoogerwerf *et al* 2001). Others have also shown that PAR-2 is expressed by a subset of peripheral nociceptive (peptidergic) neurons in the rat (Steinhoff *et al* 2000). Its activation results in the release of substance P and CGRP and the development of edema, suggesting a role for PAR-2 in the neurogenic component of inflammation. Further, PAR-2 activation can mediate both thermal and mechanical hyperalgesia (Vergnolle *et al* 2001; Kawabata *et al* 2001).

6. PAR-2 AND PANCREATIC NOCICEPTION

Studies with the specific activating peptide, as described above, convincingly demonstrate that activation of PAR-2 may play a role in nociception. Sources of proteases capable of activating PAR-2 during inflammation include leukocytes and in particular, mast cells (rich in tryptase). However, in the context of pancreatitis, trypsin is an obvious endogenous candidate ligand for PAR-2 (see discussion above) and we have begun exploring the role of this system in pancreatic pain.

The gene c-fos and its protein product fos are expressed in the spinal cord after various types of noxious stimuli, leading to its widely accepted use as a surrogate marker for nociceptive activation in response to peripheral stimulation (Harris 1998). We therefore determined whether the PAR-2 agonist, AcPep (SLIGRL-NH_2) could activate pancreatic nociceptors by studying the effect of intraductal pancreatic AcPep injections on Fos expression (Hoogerwerf *et al* 2001). AcPeP was able to directly activate pancreas-specific afferent neurons in vivo. As previously discussed noxious stimuli can either activate nociceptors or sensitize them, or both. The mechanisms and pathways involved may be separate. Sensitization is assessed by observing the effects of the proposed agent on the pain response to other forms of stimulation (chemical, mechanical or thermal in nature).

We therefore tested the sensitizing effects, if any, of PAR-2 activation on the pancreatic nociceptive response to capsaicin, a potent and noxious agonist of the TRPV1 receptor. The TRPV1 (vanilloid) receptor is a key integrator of noxious thermal and chemical stimuli expressed by nociceptive neurons (Caterina and Julius 2001). We examined PAR-2 and TRPV1 expression in dorsal root ganglia receiving innervation from the pancreas (thoracic segments, T8-T13). Ninety eight percent (259/263) of all TRPV1-IR neurons demonstrate PAR-2 IR. Conversely, 60% (259/434) of PAR-2 IR neurons also show TRPV1-IR (Hoogerwerf *et al* 2004). After intraductal injection of AcPeo and enhanced spinal Fos response to capsaicin was observed, suggesting that PAR-2 activation may sensitize the nociceptors to stimulation by capsaicin. Examination of pancreatic histology did not reveal any evidence of pancreatitis, ruling out the possibility that the Fos response was secondary to induction of inflammation in response to intraductal infusion of AcPep.

The natural agonist for PAR-2 includes trypsin and tryptase, with the former the obvious candidate in the setting of pancreatitis. We therefore tested the the effect of different doses of intraductal pancreatic trypsin injections on FOS expression was studied *in vivo* and showed that it significantly increased FOS expression over boiled trypsin in a dose-dependent manner in spinal segments receiving signals from the pancreas (Hoogerwerf *et al* 2004). We also examined whether infusion of trypsin into the pancreatic duct could provoke a behavioral pain response in awake rats. To test this we used a surrogate assay for visceral pain, the visceromotor reflex (VMR). Acute visceral pain can cause reflex contractions of somatotopically-innervated skeletal muscle, which can be measured by electromyography (EMG). Infusion of trypsin as well as AcPep into the pancreatic duct significantly increased EMG activity of the acromiotrapezius muscle suggesting that trypsin can induce a behavioral nocisponsive effect in conscious rats. To determine whether direct activation of PAR-2 produces a similar nocisponsive effect as trypsin, the PAR-2 agonist, AcPep (1 mM), was injected into the pancreas. We examined cross de-sensitization of the nocisponsive effect to provide evidence that trypsin and PAR-2 AcPep activate the same receptor. Infusion of the pancreatic duct with AcPep significantly decreased subsequent responses to trypsin.

7. CONCLUSIONS

The studies described above have led the development of a plausible model in which PAR-2 contributes to nociceptive signaling and sensitization and may provide a novel link between inflammation and pain in pancreatitis (Figure 1). Activated trypsin in the inflamed pancreas may stimulate PAR-2 on peripheral sensory neurons, resulting in their excitation and central release of neurotransmitters such as substance P (SP) and CGRP in the spinal cord. This, in turn, can cause excitation of second-order neurons in the dorsal horn to activate ascending pathways that can relay nociceptive information to the brain. Thus, suppression of trypsin activity appears to be a legitimate target for the relief of pain in pancreatitis, independent of its effects on inflammation. If validated, these findings have major implications for the pathogenesis of pain in chronic pancreatitis and will provide novel targets for analgesic therapy.

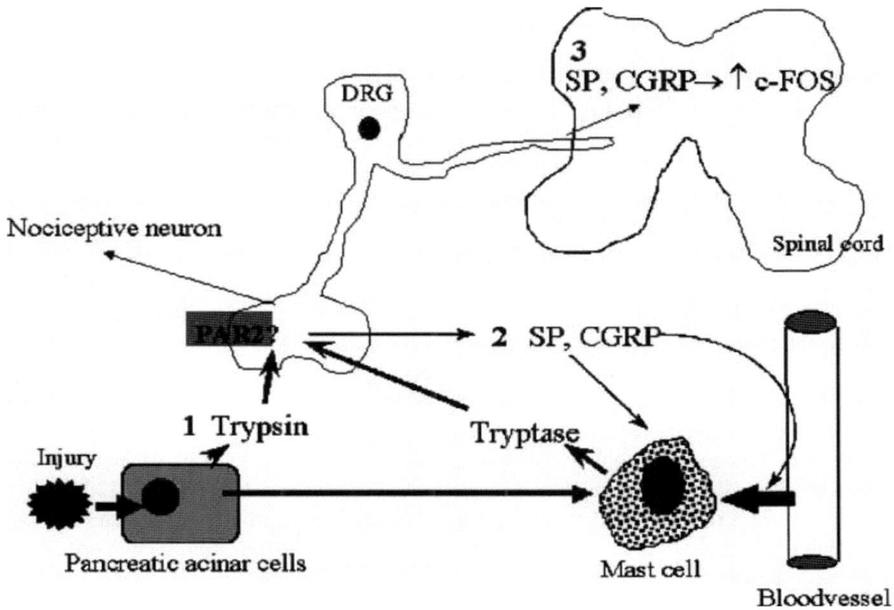

Figure 1: Proposed involvement of PAR-2 in nociceptive signaling in pancreatitis. 1. In pancreatitis, PAR-2 receptors on sensory neurons are activated by proteases such as trypsin released from injured pancreatic epithelial cells. Degranulation of mast cells releases tryptase that also acts on PAR-2 receptors. 2. PAR-2 stimulated release of CGRP and SP occurs peripherally, which further amplifies inflammation and mast cell degranulation. 3. Central release of these neurotransmitters leads to activation of nociceptivepathways and an increase in Fos expression. DRG = dorsal root ganglion. From Hoogerwerf *et al* 2001 with permission.

REFERENCES

American Gastroenterological Association Medical Position Statement, 1998, Treatment of pain in chronic pancreatitis. *Gastroenterology*. **115:** 763-4.

The Burden of Gastrointestinal Diseases, 2001, Bethesda, AGA Publications.

Amadesi S, Bunnett N, 2004, Protease-activated receptors: protease signaling in the gastrointestinal tract. *Curr Opin Pharmacol*. **4:** 551-6.

Caterina MJ, Julius D, 2001, The vanilloid receptor: a molecular gateway to the pain pathway. *Annu Rev Neurosci*. **24:** 487-517.

Coelho AM, Ossovskaya V, Bunnett NW, 2003, Proteinase-activated receptor-2: physiological and pathophysiological roles. *Curr Med Chem Cardiovasc Hematol Agents*. **1:** 61-72.

Cottrell GS, Amadesi S, Amadesi S, Schmidlin F, Bunnett N, 2003, Protease-activated receptor 2: activation, signalling and function. *Biochem Soc Trans.* **31:** 1191-1197.

Dery O, Bunnett NW, 1999, Proteinase-activated receptors: a growing family of heptahelical receptors for thrombin, trypsin and tryptase. *Biochem Soc Trans.* **27:** 246-254.

Di Sebastiano P, di Mola FF, Bockman DE, Friess H, Buchler MW, 2003, Chronic pancreatitis: the perspective of pain generation by neuroimmune interaction. *Gut.* **52:** 907-911.

DiMagno EP, 1999, Toward understanding (and management) of painful chronic pancreatitis. *Gastroenterol.* **116:** 1252-1257.

Harris JA, 1998, Using c-fos as a neural marker of pain. *Brain Res Bullet.* **45:** 1-8.

Hoogerwerf WA, Shenoy M, Winston JH, Xiao SY, He Z, Pasricha PJ, 2004, Trypsin mediates nociception via the proteinase-activated receptor 2: a potentially novel role in pancreatic pain. *Gastroenterol.* **127:** 883-891.

Hoogerwerf WA, Zou L, Shenoy M, Sun D, Micci MA, Lee-Hellmich H, Xiao SY, Winston JH, Pasricha PJ, 2001, The proteinase-activated receptor 2 is involved in nociception. *J Neurosci*. **21:** 9036-9042.

Kawabata A, Kawao N, Kuroda R, Tanaka A, Itoh H, Nishikawa H, 2001, Peripheral PAR-2 triggers thermal hyperalgesia and nociceptive responses in rats. *Neuroreport.* **12:** 715-719.

Steer ML, 1993, Etiology and Pathophysiology of Acute Pancreatitis. The Pancreas: Biology, Pathobiology and Disease. VLW Go, EP DiMagno, JD Gardner et al. New York, Raven Press: 581-92.

Steinhoff M, Vergnolle N, Young SH, Tognetto M, Amadesi S, Ennes HS, Trevisani M, Hollenberg MD, Wallace JL, Caughey GH, Mitchell SE, Williams LM, Geppetti P, Mayer EA, Bunnett NW, 2000, Agonists of proteinase-activated receptor 2 induce inflammation by a neurogenic mechanism. *Nat Med.* **6:** 151-158.

Vergnolle N, Bunnett NW, Sharkey KA, Brussee V, Compton SJ, Grady EF, Cirino G, Gerard N, Basbaum AI, Andrade-Gordon P, Hollenberg MD, Wallace JL, 2001, Proteinase-activated receptor-2 and hyperalgesia: A novel pain pathway. *Nat Med.* **7:** 821-826.

Vergnolle N, Hollenberg MD, Wallace JL, 1999, Pro- and anti-inflammatory actions of thrombin: a distinct role for proteinase-activated receptor-1 (PAR1). *Br J Pharmacol.* **126:** 1262-1268.

Whitcomb DC, 1999, Hereditary pancreatitis: new insights into acute and chronic pancreatitis. *Gut.* **45:** 317-322.

Whitcomb DC, Gorry MC, Preston RA, Furey W, Sossenheimer MJ, Ulrich CD, Martin SP, Gates LK Jr, Amann ST, Toskes PP, Liddle R, McGrath K, Uomo G, Post JC, Ehrlich GD, 1996, Hereditary pancreatitis is caused by a mutation in the cationic trypsinogen gene [see comments]. *Nat Genet.* **14:** 141-145.

Woolf CJ and Costigan M, 1999, Transcriptional and posttranslational plasticity and the generation of inflammatory pain. *Proc Natl Acad Sci U S A.* **96:** 7723-7730.

Chapter 6

Importance of the Local Renin-Angiotensin System in Pancreatic Disease

Po Sing Leung
Department of Physiology, Faculty of Medicine, The Chinese University of Hong Kong, Shatin, New Territories, Hong Kong

1. INTRODUCTION

The pancreas is structurally made up of two organs in one: the exocrine gland, consisting of acinar cells and duct cells that produce digestive enzymes and sodium bicarbonate, respectively; the endocrine gland, consisting of four islet cells, namely α-, β-, δ- and PP- cells that produce glucagon, insulin, somatostatin and pancreatic polypeptide, respectively. The exocrine pancreas' major function is to secrete digestive enzymes, including amylase, lipase and proteases that are responsible for the normal digestion of our daily foodstuff; while sodium bicarbonate is critical for the neutralization of gastric chyme entering the duodenum. The endocrine pancreas' major function is to secrete the four islet hormones that maintain glucose homeostasis in our body. The exocrine and endocrine functions are finely regulated by neurocrine, endocrine, paracrine and/or intracrine mechanisms (Solomon 1994; Cluck *et al* 2005; Toskes 1998). Dysregulation of these pathways thus leads to such pancreatic diseases as pancreatitis, cystic fibrosis, pancreatic cancer and diabetes mellitus.

The local mechanisms that regulate pancreatic exocrine and endocrine physiology and pathophysiology remain poorly understood. However, a recently-identified local pancreatic renin-angiotensin system (RAS) is of considerable interest due to its involvement in major pancreatic functions. Components of this pancreatic RAS are subject to upregulation by various

U. Lendeckel and Nigel M. Hooper (eds.), Proteases in Gastrointestinal Tissue, 131-152.

physiological and pathological conditions such as hypoxia, pancreatitis, type 2 diabetes mellitus (T2DM), and islet transplantation (Leung and Carlsson 2001; Leung and Chappell 2003). Emerging data from our laboratory and others indicate that activation of the pancreatic RAS could influence cell inflammatory responses, driving apoptosis, fibrosis, and generation of reactive oxygen species observed in pancreatitis, islet transplantation and T2DM (Leung 2005; Leung and Carlsson 2005). The elucidation of the regulatory pathways of pancreatic RAS activation and the consequent oxidative stress-induced pancreatic cell dysfunction has the potential to significantly improve our understanding of pancreatic physiology and pathophysiology. Ultimately, understanding the local pancreatic RAS should lead to new insights into the development of novel therapeutic strategies in the prevention and treatment of patients with pancreatitis, pancreatic cancer, islet transplantation and T2DM.

2. THE RENIN-ANGIOTENSIN SYSTEM

2.1 Circulating RAS

The circulating RAS is an endocrine system best known for its regulation of blood pressure and fluid homeostasis (Peach 1977; Reid *et al* 1978). These regulatory functions are mediated largely by potent actions on the vascular smooth muscle and on renal reabsorption of electrolyte and water via direct tubule actions and via the stimulation of aldosterone and vasopressin (Lumber 1999; Matsusaka and Ichikawa 1997). This classic RAS consists of several components: the liver-derived precursor angiotensinogen, two critical enzymes for the system, namely kidney renin and membrane-bound pulmonary angiotensin-converting enzyme (ACE). The sequential actions of these two enzyme generate plasma angiotensin I (1-10) and angiotensin II (1-8), respectively, the latter being the physiologically active element of the RAS. In addition, alternate enzymes to renin and ACE produce a number of bioactive peptides including angiotensin III (2-8), angiotensin IV (3-8) and angiotensin (1-7). Angiotensin II and these bioactive peptides mediate their specific functions via respective cellular transmembrane receptors of target tissues and organs (Leung 2004). Figure 1 summarizes the biosynthetic cascade for the RAS using renin and ACE and other alternate enzymes, which are linked by the bioactive peptide products along with their respective receptors.

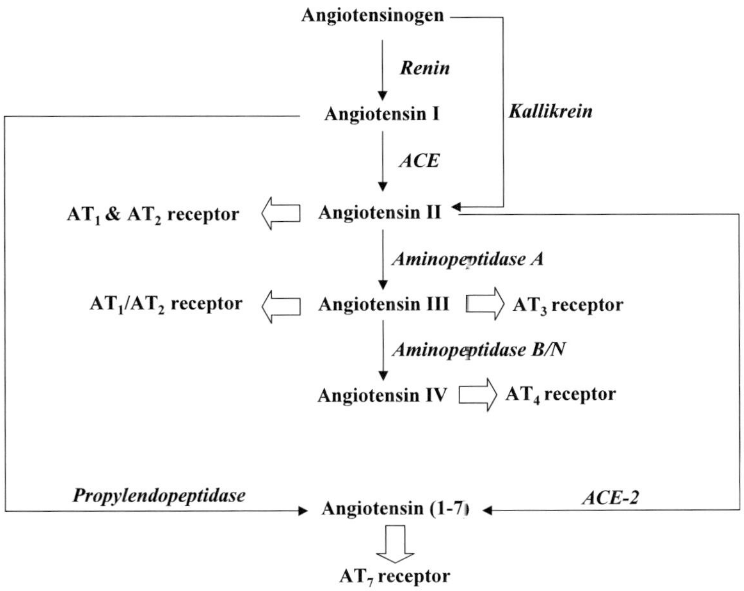

Figure 1: An outline of the RAS depicting its biologically active peptides generated by various angiotensin-processing peptidases, along with their respective receptors.

2.2 Renin and angiotensin-converting enzyme

Renin (EC 3.4.23.15) is an aspartyl protease, one of the key enzymes of the RAS. It is synthesized as a zymogen prorenin and subsequently activated by proteolytic cleavage. The gene coding for renal renin has 10 exons in human and 9 in rodents. A high degree of sequence homology is found among these renin isoforms (Hardman *et al* 1984; Hobart *et al* 1984). Active renin cleaves its substrate angiotensinogen to angiotensin I; however, the inactive renin, i.e. preprorenin and prorenin are the precursors of active renin and they are found in circulating blood plasma, amniotic fluid and kidney (Lumbers 1971; Day and Luetscher 1975; Nielsen and Poulsen 1988). The afferent arteriolar juxtaglomerular cells of kidney act as the site of renin production for the RAS (Hackenthal 1990). The preprorenin synthesized is rapidly hydrolyzed by signal protease to give prorenin. The prorenin is then converted to active renin and is secreted via a regulated pathway (Pratt *et al* 1983). The renin gene is expressed in many tissues besides the kidneys, including the vascular endothelium and islet beta cells of the pancreas (Leung *et al* 1999; Tahmasebi *et al* 1999) and may show species selectivity, as evidenced by its expression in the submandibular glands of the mouse but not the rat (Morris *et al* 1980).

ACE (EC 3.4.15.1) is a membrane-bound zinc ectoenzyme that functions as dipeptidyl carboxypeptidase (also called peptidyl-dipeptidase A, kininase II, peptidase P, and carboxycathepsin). Its major function is to process angiotensin I to angiotensin II and degrade bradykinin by removal of a dipeptide from the C-terminus. Other bioactive peptides such as metenkephalin, substance P, tachykinins, and prohormone convertase are also substrates for ACE (Coates 2003). Two isoforms of ACE are expressed in mammals: a germinal isoform (gACE) required for male fertility, and a somatic isoform (sACE) which plays a critical for the RAS (Corvol *et al* 1995). Until now, the clinical application of ACE inhibitors (e.g. captopril and ramipril) has been for the treatment of hypertension, diabetic nephropathy and heart failure (Dell'Italia *et at* 2002). In the pancreas, ACE has been identified in islet cells and in the vascular endothelium of pancreatic islets (Reddy *et al* 1995; Carlsson *et al* 1998). ACE activity and ACE mRNA have also been detected in the rat pancreas (Ip *et al* 2003a).

2.3 Other angiotensin-processing peptidases

Apart from renin and ACE, a raft of angiotensin-processing peptidases is involved in the generation and metabolism of active angiotensin peptides. These enzymes include, to name but a few, the chymase, cathepsin G, chymotrypsin, trypsin, tonin, kallikrein, ACE-2 and other exopeptidases as well as endopeptidases. The existence of these enzymes has expanded the classic view of RAS to a more contemporary model of "angiotensin-generating systems" that recognizes the contribution of alternate pathways (Sernia 2001). These peptidases act directly on angiotensin I and/or angiotensin II as well as the precursor angiotensinogen to generate a number of bioactive peptides with varying physiological activities, such as angiotensin (1-7), angiotensin III and angiotensin IV (Campbell 2003). Of particular interest in this context is the discovery of a novel peptidase termed ACE-2, which is the first human homologue of ACE. Like ACE, ACE-2 acts as a carboxypeptidase; however, ACE-2 hydrolyzes a single residue either from angiotensin II (Pro^7-Phe^8) or angiotensin I (His^9-Leu^{10}) to generate angiotensin (1-7) and angiotensin (1-9), respectively (Rice *et al* 2004). ACE-2 also cleaves other peptides, such as dynorphin, apelin and bradykinin. A physiological role for ACE-2 has been implicated in hypertension, heart function and diabetes and, perhaps more importantly, as a receptor of the severe acute respiratory syndrome coronarvirus (Warner *et al* 2004). Figure 2 depicts the peptide linkages that are cleaved by the angiotensin-processing peptidases. In the pancreas, kallikrein has been isolated in the dog and rat (Hojima *et al* 1977). It is a peptidase capable of generating angiotensin II directly from its precursor angiotensinogen (Arakawa and Maruta 1980;

Arakawa 1996). In addition, a number of serine proteases capable of forming angiotensin II from angiotensin I and/or angiotensinogen have been identified in the pancreas (Sasaguri *et al* 1999).

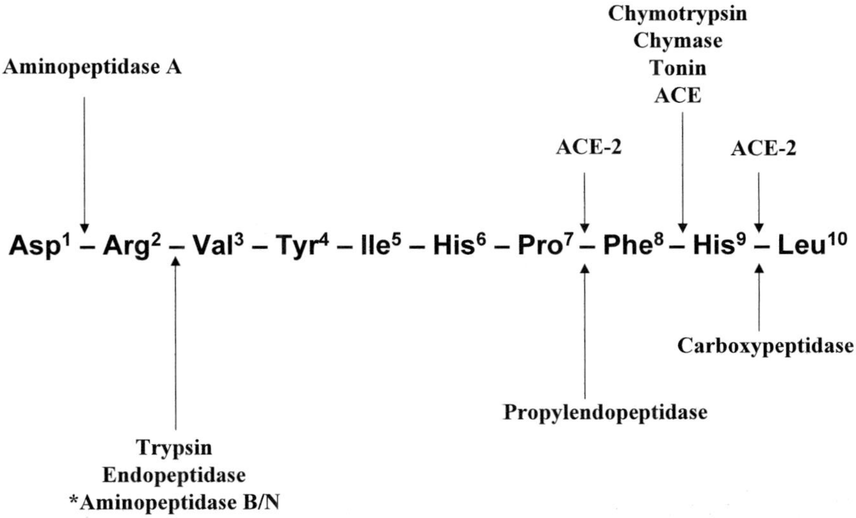

Figure 2: Different angiotensin-processing peptidases including endopeptidase, aminopeptidase and carboxypeptidase that cleave peptide linkages from the interior, aminoterminal and carboxy-terminus of angiotensin I and angiotensin II. * denotes that upon removal of Asp by aminopeptidase A, the resultant peptide can be metabolized by aminopeptidase B and N.

2.4 Angiotensin receptors

Most of the major functions, if not all, of the RAS are mediated by the physiologically active peptide angiotensin II. The actions are mediated by its two angiotensin II receptor subtypes, AT_1 receptor and AT_2 receptor (De Gasparo *et al* 2000). Both receptor subtypes belong to the seven transmembrane-spanning G-protein-coupled receptors. AT_1 receptor comprises 359 amino acids while AT_2 receptor is 363 amino acids, and they share about 30 % sequence similarity (Speth *et al* 1995). Apart from its well-established regulation of blood pressure and fluid homeostasis, AT_1 and AT_2 receptors have been recently proposed to participate in novel and cell-specific functions in tissue organs such as the pancreas and liver (Leung 2004). These functions include stimulation and inhibition of cell proliferation; induction of apoptosis; generation of reactive oxygen species; regulation of hormone secretion; and proinflammatory and profibrogenic actions (Leung and Chappell 2003).

On the other hand, proteolytic fragments of angiotensin II also have biological activity via these and other receptors (Thomas and Mendelsohn 2003). In this regard, angiotensin II can be metabolized into angiotensin III which acts either on the AT_1 and AT_2 receptors or on a specific receptor for angiotensin III, i.e. AT_3 receptor (Chaki and Inagami 1992). Angiotensin III has been proposed to be involved in chemokine production and cell growth regulation (Ruiz-Ortega *et al* 2000); it also plays a role in the control of blood pressure, thus serving as a putative target for the treatment of hypertension (Reaux-Le Goazigo *et al* 2005). However, the role for angiotensin III is still largely undefined. Angiotensin III can be further metabolized into a hexapeptide called angiotensin IV, a bioactive ligand of the AT_4 receptor. The AT_4 receptor has a wide distribution in a range of tissues, particularly located in the brain (Chai *et al* 2000). Interestingly, the AT_4 receptor has been recently identified as the transmembrane enzyme, insulin-regulated membrane aminopeptidase (IRAP), which is predominantly found in GLUT4 vesicles in insulin-responsive cells. Although the role of AT_4 receptor/IRAP has yet to be determined, it has been suggested to mediate memory and glucose uptake; the former might be attributed to the action of IRAP that prolongs the action of endogenous neuropeptides whereas the latter could be due to the action of glucose uptake by modulating trafficking of GLUT4 (Chai *et al* 2004). Finally, a high affinity binding site for angiotensin (1-7) has been reported (Tallant *et al* 1997). By using a specific analogue for angiotensin (1-7), it has been possible to selectively block the binding site for angiotensin (1-7) but not ACE. Several studies support the concept that angiotensin (1-7) induces vasodilation via activation of AT_7 receptor (Tom *et al* 2003). However, solid evidence for the existence of AT_7 receptor in human remains unavailable. In this context, it is quite intriguing that a "cross-talk" among AT_2 receptor, bradykinin type 2 receptor (BK_2 receptor) and AT_7 receptor may exist in the RAS (Leung and Chappell 2003). Figure 3 illustrates some of the proposed functions of angiotensin receptors (AT_1, AT_2, AT_3, AT_4 and AT_7 receptors) and their site of potential cross-talk in the RAS.

3. THE PANCREATIC RENIN-ANGIOTENSIN SYSTEM

3.1 Local renin-angiotensin systems

Apart from the well-known circulating RAS in our body, we have recently started to recognize the existence of local angiotensin-generating systems which seem to be of considerable importance in clinical applications (Montgomery *et al* 2003). These functional local RAS have been found in such diverse tissues and organs as from the brain to placenta (McKinley *et al* 2003; Leung *et al* 2001), from heart to bone marrow (Dostal 2000; Haznedaroglu and Ozturk 2003), from adipose tissue to carotid body (Crandall *et al* 1994; Lam *et al* 2004), from adrenal gland to liver (Vinson *et al* 1998; Leung *et al* 2003) and, last but not least, from kidney to pancreas (Nobiling 2001; Leung and Carlsson 2001). The roles of the local RAS are varied and tissue and organic specific (Figure 3).

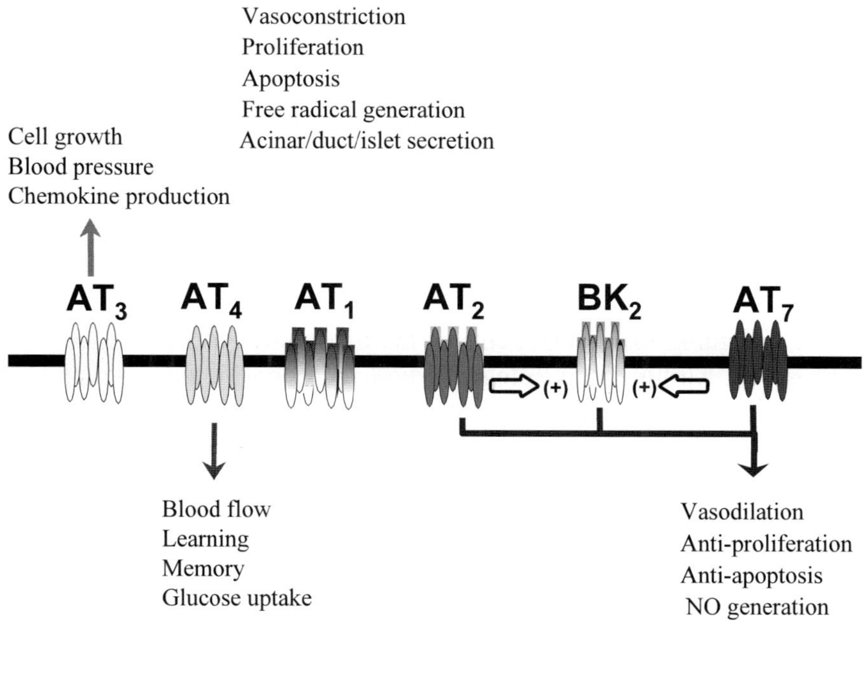

Figure 3: A schematic representation showing several proposed functions of different angiotensin receptors.

3.2 Expression and localization of pancreatic RAS

Several RAS components at the protein and gene levels have been found to express in the dog pancreas (Chappell *et al* 1991). The fundamental premise for the existence of a local RAS is based on the expression and localization of angiotensinogen, the mandatory component for an intrinsic angiotensin-generating system in the rat pancreas (Leung *et al* 1999). Besides angiotensinogen, renin mRNA is also expressed in the rat pancreas, indicating that a renin-dependent RAS may be operating, at least in this species (Leung *et al* 1999). However, neither angiotensin I nor renin activity has been identified in the dog pancreas (Chappell *et al* 1991). In view of this, the biosynthetic pathway of the pancreatic RAS needs further investigations. On the other hand, binding sites for angiotensin II receptors have also been localized and characterized in the endocrine and exocrine portions of pancreas (Chappell *et al* 1992 & 1995; Ghiani and Masini 1995). By detailed immunohistochemistry, AT_1 and AT_2 receptors and angiotensin II have been specifically localized to different cell types of the pancreas (Leung *et al* 1997; Leung *et al* 1998). Consistently, mRNA for AT_1 receptor subtypes (AT_{1a} and AT_{1b}) and AT_2 receptor has also been found in the rat pancreas (Leung *et al* 1999). In the human pancreas, AT_1 receptors and (pro)renin have been localized by immunohistochemistry and *in situ* hybridization, not only to the exocrine cells but also to the beta cells of the endocrine pancreas (Tahmasebi *et al* 1999). All these studies support the existence of a local RAS in the pancreas, implicating its involvement in the regulation of pancreatic exocrine and endocrine functions.

3.3 Regulation of pancreatic RAS

It is intriguing that components of the pancreatic RAS are responsive to changes by various physiological and pathophysiological conditions, including hypoxia, pancreatitis, islet transplantation, T2DM and pancreatic cancer (Leung 2004). In chronic hypoxia, several major components of the pancreatic RAS are significantly activated (Chan *et al* 2000), closely associated with a parallel upregulation of its counterpart circulating RAS. These changes may be responsible for the physiological and pathophysiological aspects of a biological system under chronic hypoxia stress (Ip *et al* 2002). Of great interest in this context is the reversibility and adaptability of RAS activation by chronic hypoxia, a further indication of its physiological relevance to the pancreas (Ip *et al* 2003b).

Hypoxia causes a decrease of blood flow or ischemia in several tissues, including the pancreas and leads to enhanced tissue inflammation and injury (Kuwahira *et al* 1993). The upregulation of RAS by hypoxia could be contributing to the ischemia via vasoconstriction of the pancreatic microcirculation (Carlsson *et al* 1998). In another situation of inflammation due to acute pancreatitis, the expression of several components of the pancreatic RAS is significantly activated (Leung *et al*. 2000). Pancreatic ACE activity is markedly increased by acute pancreatitis as well as chronic hypoxia; and the addition of captopril, a specific inhibitor for ACE, completely blocks the response (Ip *et al* 2003a). Little information exists on the expression of pancreatic RAS in pancreatic tumour although it has been previously implicated in pancreatic cancer cells (Reddy *et al* 1995). However, a recent study has clearly supported the existence of a local RAS in a pancreatic endocrine tumour (Lam and Leung 2002). Several RAS components are regulated by islet transplantation and diabetes; among them, there is a markedly increased expression of the AT_1 receptor in islets retrieved from 4-week-old islet transplants (Lau *et al* 2004) and in islets or pancreas from animal models of T2DM (Leung *et al* 2005; Tikellis *et al* 2004). The up-regulation of the pancreatic RAS by these conditions suggests that inhibitors of RAS may be useful in the treatment of pancreatic inflammation (*vide infra*).

3.4 Exocrine function

In the exocrine pancreas, recent studies have reported some novel roles of the pancreatic RAS in the regulation of pancreatic duct cell and acinar cell secretion. In the ductal epithelial cells, angiotensin II influences ductal anion secretion via the mediation of AT_1 receptors, an effect also seen in a cystic fibrosis pancreatic cell line (Chan *et al* 1997; Cheng *et al* 1999). By using isolated dog pancreatic epithelial cells together with cystic fibrosis pancreatic cell cultures, it has been shown that AT_1 receptor activation of calcium chloride channels is involved in bicarbonate secretion (Fink *et al* 2002).

In acinar cells, the rat pancreatic AR42J cells have been shown to express AT_1 receptors that mediate an angiotensin II dose-dependent secretion of amylase and production of inositol 1,3,4-triphosphate (Chappell *et al* 1995, Cheung *et al* 1999). The action of angiotensin II and angiotensin III is at least an order of magnitude more potent than angiotensin I on the release of amylase and could be blocked by losartan, a selective AT_1 receptor antagonist but not by CGP42112, a selective AT_2 receptor antagonist. Recently, several key RAS components (AT_1 and AT_2 receptors and angiotensinogen) have been found to be expressed in isolated pancreatic acinar cells (Tsang *et al* 2004a). Addition of angiotensin II to these cells stimulates a dose-dependent release of digestive enzyme secretion (α amylase and lipase) that could be inhibited by losartan but not PD123319 (Tsang *et al* 2004a).

All these data indicate that the pancreatic RAS plays a physiological role in ductal bicarbonate secretion and acinar digestive enzyme secretion.

3.5 Endocrine function

In endocrine pancreas, an islet RAS exists with a novel role on glucose homeostasis. In this context, pancreatic islet blood flow is suppressed by locally formed angiotensin II in perfused rat pancreas with a consequent suppression of the first phase of insulin release in response to glucose. This inhibitory effect was prevented by RAS blockers (Carlsson *et al* 1998). In another study, intravenous infusion of angiotensin II in a pressor dose (5.0 ng x kg^{-1} x min^{-1}) suppressed both basal and pulsatile insulin secretion. At a sub-pressor dose (1.0 ng x kg^{-1} x min^{-1}), this insulinemic response to an oral glucose load was significantly lower while the plasma glucose concentration was higher compared to the placebo group (Fliser *et al* 1997). In contrast, angiotensin II does not affect insulin release in response to a low glucose challenge (5.6 mM) in isolated rat islets (Dunning *et al* 1984) while it does affect release in isolated mouse islet at a high glucose concentration (16.7 mM) (Lau *et al* 2004). However at the highest concentration of 100 nM used, the glucose-stimulated insulin secretion was completely abolished (Figure 4A). This inhibitory action, partly due to a decreased (pro)insulin biosynthesis is fully reversible by pretreatment of the islets with losartan (Figure 4B). These data from isolated islets rule out the possibility that the inhibitory effect of angiotensin II on insulin release is exclusively due to its vasoconstrictor action on pancreatic islet blood flow, as demonstrated by previous perfusion study (Carlsson *et al* 1998).

AT_2 receptors have been found in isolated mouse islets; however, the specific antagonist PD123319 does not affect glucose-stimulated insulin secretion after application of angiotensin II (Lau *et al* 2004). AT_2 receptor has also been found at the outer region of islets and colocalized with somatostatin-producing cells in the endocrine pancreas and in immortalized rat pancreatic cell lines RIN-m and RIN-14B (Wong *et al* 2004). In RIN-14B cells angiotensin II stimulates somatostatin secretion in a dose-dependent manner. This action seems to be mediated by AT_2 receptors since the addition of CGP42112, a selective antagonist, abolished the response to angiotensin II, (Wong *et al* 2004). In summary, the data show that the pancreatic islet RAS has a functional role in regulating pancreatic islet insulin and somatostatin secretion, and thus implicating a physiological function in glucose homeostasis.

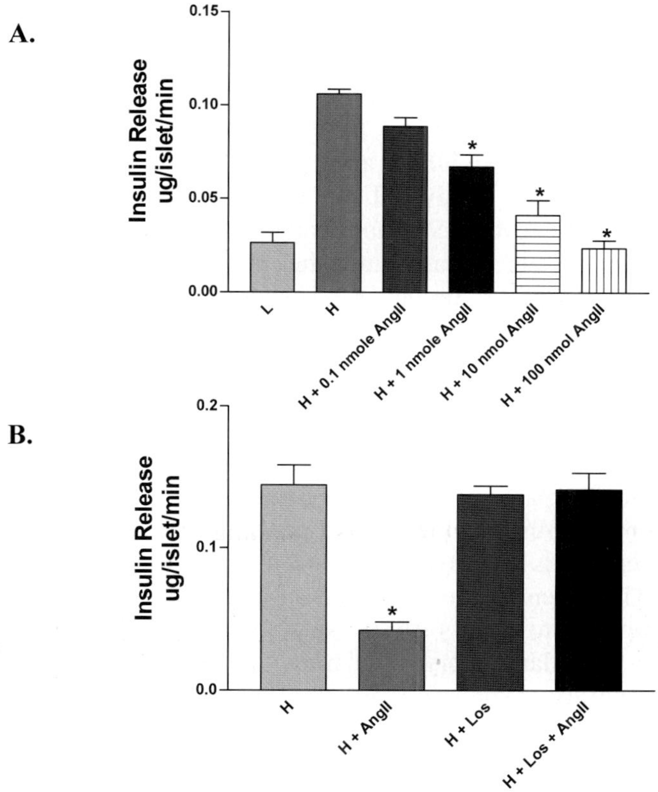

Figure 4 : (A) Insulin release from isolated mouse islets in the presence of 1.7 (low; L) or 16.7 mmol/l (high; H) glucose. Ang II was applied at concentrations of 0.1, 1, 10 and 100 nmol/l at the higher glucose concentration. (B) Effects of losartan (Los, 1μmol/l) and Ang II (100 nmol/l) on the glucose (16.7 mmol/l)-stimulated insulin release from isolated islets. All data are expressed as means ± SEM for four experiments in each group. * denotes $P < 0.05$ when compared to islets exposed to 16.7 mmol/l glucose only. Reproduced from Lau *et al.* (2004) with permission from *Diabetologia*.

4. PANCREATIC DISEASE AND THE RAS

4.1 Pancreatitis and RAS blockade

Pancreatitis refers to an inflammation of the pancreas that may be acute or chronic and may vary in duration and severity. Acute pancreatitis is characterized by edema, acinar cell necrosis, hemorrhage, and severe inflammation of the pancreas. Clinically, there is an elevation of pancreatic enzymes, such as amylase and lipase, in blood and urine. The release of pancreatic lipase causes fat necrosis in the pancreas. In severe conditions, it may lead to systemic inflammatory response syndrome and multi-organ dysfunction syndrome. The pancreatitis-induced systemic injury is the major culprit accounting for the high mortality rate. The most common causes of acute pancreatitis include gallstones (45 %), alcoholism (35 %), idiopathic cases (10 %), and others (Steinberg and Scott 1994). Although the etiology of acute pancreatitis is equivocal, it is thought to be multifactorial (Whitcomb 1999). However a common feature is the premature activation of trypsinogen prior to its release into the duodenum, thus precipitating autodigestion of pancreatic tissue (Wedgewood and Reber 1986). Some vasoactive peptides such as angiotensin II have been proposed as potential candidates for the development of pancreatitis via changes in pancreatic microcirculation that involve sequential vasoconstriction, capillary stasis, decreased oxygen tension and progressive ischemia (Knoefel *et al* 1994). Since angiotensin II plays a key mediator of tissue inflammatory reactions and injury (De Gasparo *et al* 2002; Suzuki *et al* 2003), a selective upregulation of the RAS by hypoxia and pancreatitis may also be clinically relevant to pancreatitis and hypoxia-induced tissue injury in the pancreas (*vide supra*). The potential mechanism(s) of angiotensin II in inflammation have been proposed to be (1) Direct activation of immune cells and (2) Production of proinflammatory mediators that alter hemodynamics and vascular permeability, expression of adhesion molecules, chemotaxis for leukocytes, activation of vascular pericytes, and repair via cellular growth and matrix synthesis (Suzuki *et al* 2003).

There is evidence for the involvement of reactive oxygen species (ROS) in the pathogenesis of acute pancreatitis (Czako *et al* 2000; Rau *et al* 2001; Telek *et al* 2001). The source of ROS in acute pancreatitis is not well characterized but it is believed that polymorphonuclear neutrophils, macrophages, and endothelial cells produce ROS through activation of the xanthine-xanthine oxidase system (Schulz *et al* 1999; Granell *et al* 2003). In this regard, activation of a pancreatic RAS may be an alternative source of ROS in acute pancreatitis due to the stimulation by angiotensin II of superoxide and hydrogen peroxide via activation of the NADPH oxidase system (Jaimes *et al* 1998; Dijkhorst-Oei *et al* 1999). The location of NADPH oxidase that may be targeted by angiotensin II and cytokines is neutrophils and vascular endothelial cells. (Griendling *et al* 2000). When stimulated, the enzyme subunits are activated and result in the generation of superoxide (Bendall *et al* 2002; Dang *et al* 2003; Li and Shah 2003). The association between RAS activation and NADPH oxidase-dependent generation of ROS suggests that RAS blockade might be effective in reducing pancreatic inflammation and injury.

To address this issue, we have recently studied the differential effects of RAS inhibitors and their potential use in the treatment of pancreatitis.

Intriguingly, prophylactic administration of saralasin, a nonspecific antagonist for AT_1/AT_2 receptor, has been found to be effective in improving pancreatitis-induced injury in the pancreas. However, ramiprilat, an ACE inhibitor, does not exhibit such a beneficial effect (Tsang *et al* 2003). The effect of saralasin can be explained by proposing an inhibition of RAS activation of ROS in acute pancreatitis (Ip *et al* 2003c). Prophylactic and therapeutic administration of AT_1 receptor blocker (losartan) and AT_2 receptor blocker (PD123319) also inhibit the pancreatitis-induced oxidative stress; presumably by preventing impaired microcirculation and from the inhibition of the AT_1 receptor-mediated NADPH oxidase-dependent production of ROS (Tsang *et al* 2004b). Histological examination of the pancreas shows that losartan alone is effective against pancreatitis-induced pancreatic injury (Figure 5). A recent study from another laboratory has shown that ACE inhibition attenuates chronic pancreatitis-induced injury and pancreatic fibrosis, possibly via the prevention of pancreatic stellate cell activation (Kuno *et al* 2003). In summary, available data support the potential clinical value of RAS blockade in treating pancreatic inflammation. However, a few reports indicate that ACE blockers induce acute pancreatitis in some patients. This may be attributed to the fact that such blockers prevent the breakdown of bradykinins, which in turn cause vasodilation and enhanced vascular permeability. It is therefore more likely that selective use of AT_1/AT_2 receptor blockers alone or in combination with ACE inhibitors will provide a more effective clinical strategy than ACE inhibitors alone.

4.2 Diabetes mellitus and RAS blockade

Diabetes mellitus (DM) is a disease of epidemic prevalence that is characterized by insufficient insulin secretion to promote glucose metabolism. This disorder is attributed, in most cases, to loss and/or dysfunction of pancreatic beta cells, the only cells in the human body that produce insulin. DM is divided into two categories: type 1 (T1DM) and type 2 (T2DM). T1DM (formerly called insulin-dependent diabetes mellitus) is due to absolute insulin deficiency, i.e. insulin is completely or almost completely absent from the pancreatic islets and the plasma. The pathogenesis of T1DM, which affects approximately 10% of diabetic patients, is primarily of autoimmune cause thus resulting in destruction of the pancreatic beta cells by the body's own white blood cells. In view of this clinical manifestation, patients with T1DM are treated with insulin injection (Nolte 1992). T2DM is due to relative insulin deficiency and accounts clinically for 90% cases of diabetes patients. The cause of T2DM constitutes a relatively complex spectrum of conditions with varying degree of pancreatic beta cell dysfunction and peripheral insulin resistance (Ferrannini *et al* 2003). Therefore, treatments of patients with T2DM lie in diet and exercise, if deemed, followed with antidiabetic drugs. In some severe forms, patients do require insulin administration (Bloomgarden 1995).

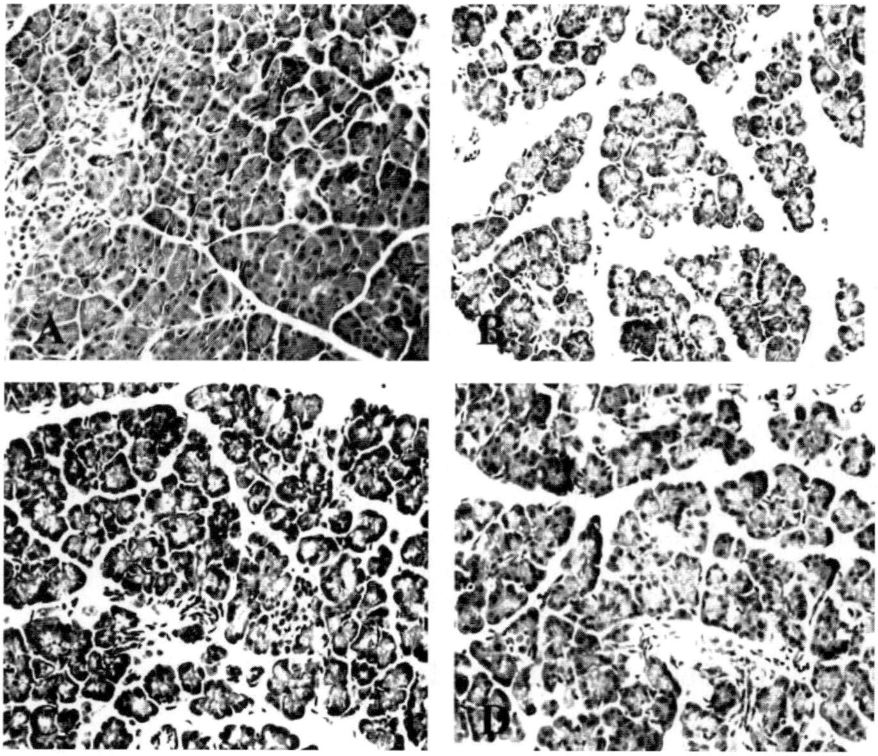

Figure 5: Histological examination of pancreatitis-induced cell injury with the treatment of losartan in the pancreas. (A) Normal pancreas. Intact histology of the pancreas is observed in this control pancreas; (B) Pancreatitis-induced pancreas. Substantial pancreatic cell injury characterized with interstitial edema and acinar cell necrosis are noted in this cerulean-induced pancreatitis pancreas; (C) Prophylactic treatment; (D) Therapeutic treatment. Both treatments with losartan ameliorate the morphological changes of cell injury when compared with pancreatitis-induced pancreas.

In several recent clinical trials, the Heart Outcomes Prevention Evaluation (HOPE, Yusuf *et al* 2000); the Losartan for Interventions for Endpoints in Hypertension (LIFE, Dahlof *et al* 2002); the Study of Cognition and Prognosis in the Elderly (SCOPE, Lithell *et al* 2003); the Nateglimide And Valsartan in Impaired Glucose Tolerance Outcomes Research (NAVIGATOR, Califf 2003); and the Captopril Prevention Project (CAPP, Hansson *et al* 1999), blockade of the RAS has been shown to reduce the incidence of diabetes in “at risk” patients with hypertension. In these studies, beneficial effects are largely attributed to improvements in peripheral insulin sensitivity. T2DM is, however, not likely to develop in patients as long as the pancreatic beta cells can secrete sufficient quantities of insulin (Hellerstrom 1984; Hjelmesaeth and Carlsson 2002. It remains a controversy on whether the impaired insulin secretion in T2DM is due to reduced beta cell mass or to an intrinsic defect in the secretory machinery of beta cells, and/or a combination of both conditions (Donath and Halban 2004). However, reduced glucose sensitivity in beta cells seems, initially at least, to predominate over insulin resistance in the generation of impaired glucose tolerance (Ferrannini *et al* 2003). Thus, therapies aimed at increasing insulin sensitivity offer only partial solutions for, once established, a progressive destruction of islet cells that contributes to disease progression. The benefits of RAS blockade in T2DM and its association with a reduced risk of developing diabetes have, until now, been hard to explain. Nevertheless, the recently-identified islet RAS appears to be implicated in the pathogenesis of the progressive islet destruction noted in T2DM (Leung and Carlsson 2005).

In this context, our preliminary results have shown that AT_1 receptor is significantly upregulated in db/db mice, a commonly used model of obesity-induced T2DM. Blockade of its activation in isolated islets by losartan led to improved insulin release, probably via an alteration of (pro)insulin biosynthesis (Lau 2004). Two recent studies, using similar animal models of T2DM, have demonstrated functional improvements in the first phase of glucose-stimulated insulin secretion, when the animals were treated with ACE and AT_1 receptor blockers (Tikellis *et al* 2004; Ko *et al* 2004). In one of these studies, the pancreatic RAS was shown to be upregulated in the Zucker diabetic fatty rats; its blockade significantly attenuated islet damage and augmented beta cell mass, probably via a reduction in oxidative stress, apoptosis, and decrease in islet fibrosis (Tikellis *et al* 2004). Notwithstanding the involvement of the RAS in islet function, causal relationship between RAS-induced oxidative stress and progression of T2DM remains equivocal.

Recently, pancreatic islet transplantation has been promoted as a promising approach for the restoration of physiological secretion of insulin in patients with T1DM and some patients with severe forms of T2DM (Hirshberg *et al* 2003). Beta cell replacement therapy is, however, significantly hampered by a limited source of human islets from cadaveric donors and toxic immunosuppression. As far as the number of islets available is concerned, more than 9,000 islet equivalents/kg of body weight are required for achieving insulin independence (Shapiro *et al* 2000). For proper islet transplantation, it is therefore not only necessary to optimize islet isolation protocol but also to ensure maximal preservation in function of the islet graft. Transplanted islets are subjected to acute inflammatory reactions immediately after transplantation (Davalli *et al* 1996) and it possible that RAS is activated as part of the inflammatory cascade (Suzuki *et al* 2003), as it is in the development of acute pancreatitis (Leung 2005). Interestingly, several major RAS components, notably the AT_1 receptor, are upregulated during islet transplantation (Lau *et al* 2004). In a recent report, AT_1 receptor blockade has been shown to significantly improve the blood perfusion, oxygen tension and first phase of glucose-stimulated insulin secretion in islet grafts (Kampf *et al* 2005). Thus inhibition of the RAS may provide an alternative strategy for enhancing the graft survival and function in islet transplantation.

5. CONCLUSIONS

The underlying mechanisms that regulate pancreatic physiology and pathophysiology are still poorly understood. However, a recently-identified local RAS appears to offer some important insights. The local pancreatic RAS is upregulated by hypoxia, pancreatitis, islet transplantation and T2DM. Activation of this local RAS may drive cell inflammatory response, apoptosis, islet fibrosis, and may additionally reduce pancreatic blood flow, oxygen tension and hormonal secretions. RAS activation may mediate oxidative stress-induced pancreatic beta cell dysfunction and apoptosis via the stimulation of ROS, and thereby contribute to beta cell dysfunction in T2DM. Further investigation of pancreatic RAS activation by pancreatitis and T2DM should elucidate the underlying mechanisms and contribute to the development of novel therapeutic strategies, based on RAS inhibition, for the prevention and treatment of pancreatitis and diabetes mellitus.

ACKNOWLEDGEMENTS

This work was supported by the Competitive Earmarked Research Grant from the Research Grants Council of Hong Kong (Project No. CUHK 4364/04M, CUHK 4116/01M, CUHK 4075/00M), and by the Chinese University of Hong Kong.

REFERENCES

Arakawa K, Maruta H, 1980, Ability of kallikrein to generate angiotensin II-like pressor substance and a proposed kinin-tensin enzyme system. *Nature* **288:** 705-706.

Arakawa K, 1996, Serine protease angiotensin II systems. *J Hyperten.* **14:** S3-S7.

Bendall JK, Cave AC, Heymes C, Gall N, Shah AM, 2002, Pivotal role of a gp91(phox)-containing NADPH oxidase in angiotensin II-induced cardiac hypertrophy in mice. *Circulation.* **105:** 293-296.

Bloomgarden ZT, 1995, NIDDM treatment. *Diabetes Care.* **18:** 425-428.

Califf RM, 2003, Insulin resistance: a global epidemic in need of effective therapies. *Eur Heart J.* **5**(Supplement C): 13-18.

Campbell DJ, 2003, The renin-angiotensin and the kallikrein-kinin systems. *Int J Biochem Cell Biol.* **35:** 784-791.

Carlsson PO, Berne C, Jansson L, 1998, Angitoensin II and the endocrine pancreas: effects on islet blood flow and insulin secretion in rats. *Diabetologia.* **41:** 127-133.

Chai SY, Fernando R, Peck G, Ye SY, Mendelsohn FA, Jenkins TA, Albiston AL, 2004, The angiotensin IV/AT4 receptor. *Cell Mol Life Sci.* **61:** 2728-2737.

Chai SY, Bastias MA, Clune EF, Matsacos DJ, Mustafa T, Lee JH, McDowall SG, Paxinos G, Mendelsohn FA, Albiston AL, 2000, Distribution of angiotensin IV binding sites (AT4 receptor) in the human forebrain, midbrain and ponsasvisualised by in vitro receptor autoradiography. *Chem Neuroanat.* **20:** 339-348.

Chaki S, Inagami T, 1992, A newly found angiotensin II receptor subtype mediates cyclic GMP formation in differentiated Neuro-2A cells. *Eur J Pharmacol.* **225:** 355-356.

Chan HC, Law SH, Leung PS, Wong PYD, 1997, Angiotensin II receptor type I-regulated anion secretion in cystic fibrosis pancreatic duct cells. *J Memb Biol.* **156:** 241-250.

Chan WP, Fung ML, Nobiling R, Leung PS, 2000, Activation of local renin-angiotensin system by chronic hypoxia in rat pancreas. *Mol Cell Endocrinol.* **160:** 107-114.

Chappell MC, Milsted A, Diz DI, Brosnihan KB, Ferrario CM, 1991, Evidence for an intrinsic angiotensin system in the canine pancreas. *J Hypertens.* **9:** 751-759.

Chappell MC, Diz DI, Jacobsen DW, 1992, Pharmacological characterization of angiotensin II binding sites in the canine pancreas. *Peptides.* **13:** 311-318.

Chappell MC, Jacobsen DW, Tallant EA, 1995, Characterization of angiotensin II receptor subtypes in pancreatic acinar AR42J cells. *Peptides.* **16:** 741-747.

Cheng HS, So SC, Law SH, Chan HC, 1999, Angiotensin II-mediated signal transduction in cystic fibrosis pancreatic cells. *Biochem et Biophys Acta.* **1449:** 254-260.

Cheung WT, Yeung SY, Yiu AKL, Ip TM, Wan DCC, Luk SKS, Ho WKK, 1999, Characterization of a functional AT_{1A} angiotensin receptor in pancreatoma AR4-2J cells. *Peptides.* **20:** 829-836.

Cluck MW, Chan CY, Adrian TE, 2005, The regulation of amylin and insulin gene expression and secretion. *Pancreas.* **30:** 1-14.

Coates D, 2003, The angiotensin converting enzyme (ACE). *Int J Biochem Cell Biol.* **35:** 769-773.

Corvol P, Williams TA, Soubrier F, 1995, Peptidyl dipeptidase an angiotensin-I converting enzyme. In Proteolytic Enzymes: Aspartic and Metallo Peptidases, pp. 283-305, Edited by AJ Barrett, Academic Press, San Diego.

Crandall DL, Herzlinger HE, Saunders BD, Kral JG, 1994, Developmental aspects of the adipose-tissue renin-angiotensin system: therapeutic implications. *Drug Dev Res.* **32:** 117-125.

Czako L, Takacs T, Varga IS, Tiszlavicz L, Hai DQ, Hegyi P, Matkovics B, Lonovics J, 2000, Oxidative stress in distant organs and the effects of allopurinol during experimental acute pancreatitis. *Int J Pancreatol.* **27:** 209-16.

Dahlof B, Devereux RB, Kjeldsen SE, Julius S, Beevers G, de Faire U, Fyhrquist F, Ibsen H, Kristiansson K, Lederballe-Pedersen O, Lindholm LH, Nieminen MS, Omvik P, Oparil S, Wedel H, 2002, Cardiovascular morbidity and mortality in the Losartan Intervention For Endpoints reduction in hypertension study (LIFE): a randomised trial against atenolol. *Lancet.* **359:** 995-1003.

Dang PM, Morel F, Gougerot-Pocidalo MA, Benna JE, 2003, Phosphorylation of the NADPH oxidase component p67(PHOX) by ERK2 and P38MAPK: selectivity of phosphorylated sites and existence of an intramolecular regulatory domain in the tetratricopeptide-rich region. *Biochemistry.* **42:** 4520-4526.

Davalli AM, Scaglia L, Zangen DH, Hollister J, Bonner-Weir S, Weir GC, 1996, Vulnerability of islets in the immediate posttransplantation period. Dynamic changes in structure and function. *Diabetes.* **45:** 1161-1167.

Day RP, Luetscher JA, 1975, Occurrence of big renin in human plasma, amniotic fluid and kidney extracts. *J Clin Endo Metab.* **40:** 1078-1084.

De Gasparo M, Catt KJ, Inagami T, Wright JW, Unger TH, 2000, The angiotensin II receptors. *Pharmacol Rev.* **52:** 415-472.

De Gasparo M, 2002, Angiotensin II and nitric oxide interaction. *Heart Fail Rev.* **7:** 347-358.

Dell'Italia LJ, Rocic P, Lucchesi PA, 2002, Use of angiotensin-converting enzyme inhibitors in patients with diabetes and coronary artery disease. *Curr Prob Cardiol.* **27:** 6-36.

Dijkhorst-Oei LT, Stroes ES, Koomans HA, Rabelink TJ, 1999, Acute simultaneous stimulation of nitric oxide and oxygen radicals by angiotensin II in humans in vivo. *J Cardiovasc Pharmacol.* **33:** 420-424.

Donath MY, Halban PA, 2004, Decreased beta-cell mass in diabetes: significance, mechanisms and therapeutic implications. *Diabetologia.* **47:** 581-589.

Dostal DE, 2000, The cardiac renin-angiotensin system: novel signalling mechanisms related to cardiac growth and function. *Regul Pept.* **91:** 1-11.

Dunning BE, Moltz JH, Fawcett CP, 1984, Actions of neurohypophysial peptides on pancreatic hormone release. *Am J Physiol.* **246:** E108-E114.

Ferrannini E, Gastaldelli A, Miyazaki Y, Matsuda M, Pettiti M, Natali A, Mari A, DeFronzo RA, 2003, Predominant role of reduced beta-cell sensitivity to glucose over insulin resistance in impaired glucose tolerance. *Diabetologia.* **46:** 1211-1219.

Fink AS, Wang Y, Mendez T, Worrell RT, Eaton D, Nguyen TD, Lee SP, 2002, Angiotensin II evokes calcium-mediated signaling events in isolated dog pancreatic epithelial cells. *Pancreas* **25:** 290-295.

Fliser D, Schaefer F, Schmid D, Veldhuis JD, Ritz E, 1997, Angiotensin II affects basal, pulsatile and glucose-stimulated insulin secretion in humans. *Hypertension.* **30:** 1156-1161.

Ghiani BU, Masini MA, 1995, Angiotensin II binding sites in the rat pancreas and their modulation after sodium loading and depletion. *Comp Biochem Physiol.* **111A:** 439-444.

Granell S, Gironella M, Bulbena O, Panes J, Mauri M, Sabater L, Aparisi L, Gelpi E, Closa D, 2003, Heparin mobilizes xanthine oxidase and induces lung inflammation in acute pancreatitis. *Crit Care Med.* **31:** 525-530.

Griendling KK, Sorescu D, Ushio-Fukai, 2000, NADPH oxidase: role in cardiovascular biology and disease. *Circ Res.* **86:** 494-501.

Hackenthal E, Paul M, Ganten D, Taugner R, 1990, Morphology, physiology, and molecular biology of renin secretion. *Physiol Rev.* **70:** 1067-1116.

Hansson L, Lindholm DH, Niskanen L, Lanke J, Hedner T, Niklason A, 1999, Effects of angiotensin-converting-enzyme inhibition compared with conventional therapy oncardiovascular morbidity and mortality in hypertension: the Captopril Prevention Project (CAPP) randomised trial. *Lancet.* **353:** 611-616.

Hardman JA, Hort Y, Cartanzaro DF, 1984, Primary structure of human renin gene. *DNA* **3:** 457-468.

Haznedaroglu IC, Ozturk MA, 2003, Towards the understanding of local hematopoitic bone marrow renin-angiotensin system. *Int J Biochem Cell Biol.* **35:** 867-880.

Hellerström C, 1984, The life story of the pancreatic B cell. *Diabetologia.* **26:** 393-400.

Hirshberg B, Rother KI, Digon III BJ, Venstrom J, Harlan DM, 2003, State of the art: islet transplantation for the cure of type 1 diabetes mellitus. *Rev Endocr Metab Disord.* **4:** 381-389.

Hjelmesaeth J, Carlsson PO, 2002, Losartan for cardiovascular disease in patients with and without diabetes in the LIFE study. *Lancet.* **359:** 2201-2202.

Hobart PM, Fogliano M, O'connor BA, Schaefer IM, Chirgwin JM, 1984, Human renin gene: structure and sequence analysis. *Proc Natl Acad Sci U S A.* **81:** 5026-5030

Hojima Y, Yamashita N, Ochi N, Moriwaki C, Moriya H, 1977, Isolation and properties of dog and rat pancreatic kallikreins. *J Biochem.* **81:** 599-610.

Ip SP, Kwan PC, Williams CH, Pang S, Hooper NM, Leung PS, 2003a, Changes of angiotensin-converting enzyme activity in the pancreas of chronic hypoxia and acute pancreatitis. *Int J Biochem Cell Biol.* **35:** 944-954.

Ip SP, Wong TP, Tsai SJ, Leung PS, 2003b, The recovery of some components of the renin-angiotensin system in the rat pancreas after chronic exposure to hypoxic condition. *J Mol Endocrinol.* **31:** 563-571.

Ip SP, Tsang SW, Wong TP, Che CT, Leung PS, 2003c, Saralasin, a non-specific angiotensin II receptor antagonist, attenuates oxidative stress and tissue injury in cerulien-induced acute pancreatitis. *Pancreas.* **26:** 224-229.

Ip SP, Chan YW, Leung PS, 2002, Effects of chronic hypoxia on the circulating and pancreatic renin-angiotensin system. *Pancreas.* **25:** 296-300.

Jaimes EA, Galceran JM, Raij L,1998, Angiotensin II induces superoxide anion production by mesangial cells. *Kidney Int.* **54:** 775-84.

Kampf C, Lau T, Olsson R, Leung PS, Carlsson PO, 2005, Angiotensin II type 1 receptor inhibition markedly improves the blood perfusion, oxygen tension and first phase of glucose-stimulated insulin secretion in revascularized syngeneic mouse islet grafts. *Diabetologia.* **48:** 1159-1167.

Knoefel WT, Kollias N, Warshaw AL, Waldner H, Nishioka NS, Rattner DW, 1994, Pancreatic microcirculatory changes in experimental pancreatitis of graded severity in rat. *Surgery.* **116:** 904-913.

Ko SH, Kwon HS, Kim SR, Moon SD, Ahn YB, Song KH, Son HS, Cha BY, Lee KW, Son HY, Kang SK, Park CG, Lee IK, Yoon KH, 2004, Ramipril treatment suppresses islet fibrosis in Otsuka Long-Evans Tokushima fatty rats. *Biochem Biophys Res Commum.* **316:** 114-122.

Kuno A, Yamada T, Kasuda K, Ogawa K, Sogawa M, Nakamura S, Ohara H, NomuraT, Joh T, Shirai T, Itoh M, 2003, Angiotensin-converting enzyme inhibitor attenuates pancreatic inflammation and fibrosis in male Wistar Bonn/Kobori rats. *Gastroenterology.* **124:** 1010-1019.

Kuwahira I, Gonzalez NC, Heisler N, Piipet, 1993, Changes in regional blood flow distribution and oxygen supply during hypoxia in conscious rats. *J Appl Physiol.* **74:** 211-214.

Lam SY, Fung ML, Leung PS, 2004, Regulation of the angiotensin-converting enzyme activity by a time-course hypoxia in the carotid body. *J Appl Physiol.* **96:** 809-813.

Lam KY, Leung PS, 2002, Regulation and expression of renin-angiotensin system in human pancreas and pancreatic endocrine tumours. *Eur J Endocrinol.* **146:** 567-572.

Lau T, 2004, Pancreatic islet renin-angiotensin system: its role in insulin secretion and in islet transplantation. Thesis, The Chinese University of Hong Kong.

Lau T, Carlsson PO, Leung PS, 2004, Evidence for a local angiotensin-generating system and dose-dependent inhibition of glucose-stimulated insulin release by angiotensin II in isolated pancreatic islets. *Diabetologia.* **47:** 240-248.

Leung PS, 2005, Roles of the renin-angiotensin system and its blockade in pancreatic inflammation. *Int J Biochem Cell Biol.* **37:** 237-238.

Leung PS, Carlsson PO, 2005, Pancreatic islet angiotensin system: its novel roles in islet function and in diabetes mellitus. *Pancreas.* **30:** 293-298.

Leung PS, Chu KY, Suen PM, 2005, Angiotensin II type 1 receptor inhibition improves beta-cell function and glucose tolerance in type 2 diabetic mice. In Abstract Book, 65th Scientific Sessions, June 10-14, 2005, San Diego, California, USA.

Leung PS, 2004, The peptide hormone angiotensin II: its new functions in tissues and organs. *Curr Protein Pept Sci.* **5:** 267-273.

Leung PS, Chappell MC, 2003, A local pancreatic renin-angiotensin system: endocrine and exocrine roles. *Int J Biochem Cell Biol.* **35:** 838-846.

Leung PS, Suen PM, Ip SP, Yip CK, Chen G, Lai PBS, 2003, Expression and localization of AT_1 receptors in hepatic Kupffer cells: its potential role in regulating a fibrogenic response. *Regul Pept.* **116:** 61-69.

Leung PS, Carlsson PO, 2001, Tissue renin-angiotensin system: its expression, localization, regulation and potential role in the pancreas. *J Mol Endocrinol.* **26:** 155-164.

Leung PS, Tsai SJ, Wallukat G, Leung TN, Lau TK, 2001, The upregulation of angiotensin II receptor AT_1 in human preeclamptic placenta. *Mol Cell Endocrinol.* **184:** 95-102.

Leung PS, Chan WP, Nobiling R, 2000, Regulated expression of pancreatic renin-angiotensin system in experimental pancreatitis. *Mol Cell Endocrinol.* **166:** 121-128.

Leung PS, Chan WP, Wong TP, Sernia C, 1999, Expression and localization of the renin-angiotensin system in the rat pancreas. *J Endocrinol.* **160:** 13-19.

Leung PS, Chan HC, Wong PYD, 1998, Immunohistochemical localization of angiotensin II in the mouse pancreas. *Histochemical J.* **30:** 21-25.

Leung PS, Chan HC, Fu LX M, Wong PYD, 1997, Localization of angiotensin II receptor subtypes AT_1 and AT_2 in the pancreas of rodents. *J Endocrinol.* **153:** 269-274.

Li JM, Shah AM, 2003, Mechanism of endothelial cell NADPH oxidase activation by angiotensin II: role of the p47phox subunit. *J Biol Chem.* **278:** 12094-12100.

Lithell H, Hansson L, Skoog I, Elmfeldt D, Hofman A, Olofsson B, Trenkwalder P, Zanchetti A, 2003, The study on Cognition and Prognosis in the Elderly (SCOPE): principal results of a randomized double-blind intervention trial. *J Hypertens.* **21:** 875-886.

Lumbers ER, 1999, Angiotensin and aldosterone. *Regul Pept.* **80:** 91-100.

Lumbers ER, 1971, Activation of renin in human amniotic fluid by low pH. *Enzymologia* **40:** 329-336.

Matsusaka T, Ichikawa I, 1997, Biological functions of angiotensin and its receptors. *Annu Rev Physiol.* **59:** 395-412.

McKinley MJ, Albiston AL, Allen AM, Mathai ML, May CN, McAllen RM, Oldfield BJ, Mendelsohn FAO, Chai SY, 2003. The brain renin-angiotensin system: location and physiological roles. *Int J Biochem Cell Biol.* **35:** 901-919.

Montgomery H, Humphries SE, Leung PS, 2003, Renin-angiotensin system: the new frontier. *Int J Biochem Cell Biol.* **35:** 758.

Morris BJ, De Zwart RT, Young JA, 1980, Renin in mouse but not in rat submandibular glands. *Experientia.* **36:** 1333-1334.

Nielsen AH, Poulsen K, 1988, Is prorenin of physiological and clinical importance? *Hypertension.* **6:** 949-958.

Nobiling R, 2001, The renin-angiotensin system: from the renal basis to an organ-specific subsystem in the pancreas. *JOP.* **2:** 9-12.

Nolte MS, 1992, Insulin therapy in insulin-dependent (type I) diabetes mellitus. *Endocrinol Metab Clin North Am.* **21:** 281-312.

Peach M, 1977, Renin-angiotensin system: biochemistry and mechanism of action. *Physiol Rev.* **57:** 313-370.

Pratt RE, Ouellette AJ, Dzau VJ, 1983, Biosynthesis of the renin: multiplicity of active and intermediate forms. *Proc Natl Acad Sci U S A.* **80:** 6909-6813.

Rau B, Bauer A, Wang A, Gansauge F, Weidenbach H, Nevalainen T, Poch B, Beger HG, Nussler AK, 2001, Modulation of endogenous nitric oxide synthase in experimental acute pancreatitis: role of anti-ICAM-1 and oxygen free radical scavengers. *Ann Surg.* **233:** 195-203.

Reaux-Le Goazigo A, Iturrioz X, Fassot C, Claperon C, Roques BP, Llorens-Cortes C, 2005, Role of angiotensin III in hypertension. *Curr Hypertens Rep.* **7:** 128-134.

Reddy MK, Baskaran K, Moiteni A, 1995, Inhibitors of angiotensin-converting enzyme modulate mitosis and gene expression in pancreatic cancer cells. *Proc Soc Exp Biol Med.* **210:** 221-226.

Reid IA, Morris BJ, Ganong WF, 1978, The renin-angiotensin system. *Annu Rev Physiol.* **40:** 377-410.

Rice GI, Thomas DA, Grant PJ, Turner AJ, Hooper NM, 2004, Evaluation of angiotensin-converting enzyme (ACE), its homologue ACE2 and neprilysin in angiotensin peptide metabolism. *Biochem J.* **383:** 45-51.

Ruiz-Ortega M, Lorenzo O, Egido J, 2000, Angiotensin III increases MCP-1 and activates NF-kappa B and AP-1 in cultured mesangial and mononuclear cells. *Kid Int.* **57:** 2285-2298.

Sasaguri M, Noda K, Tsuji E, Koga M, Kinoshita A, Ideishi M, Ogata S, Arakawa K, 1999, Structure of a kallikrein-like enzyme and its tissue localization in the dog. *Immunopharmacology.* **44:** 15-19.

Sernia C, 2001, A critical appraisal of the intrinsic pancreatic angiotensin-generating system. *JOP* **2:** 50-55.

Schulz HU, Niederau C, Klonowski-Stumpe H, Halangk W, Luthen R, Lippert H, 1999, Oxidative stress in acute pancreatitis. *Hepato-gastroenterol.* **46:** 2736-2750.

Shapiro AM, Lakey JR, Ryan EA, Korbutt GS, Toth E, Warnock GL, Kneteman NM, Rajotte RV, 2000, Islet transplantation in seven patients with type 1 diabetes mellitus using a glucocorticoid-free immunosuppressive regimen. *N Engl J Med.* **343:** 230-238.

Solomon TE, 1994, Control of exocrine pancreatic secretion. In Physiology of the Gastrointestinal Tract, pp. 1499-1529, Edited by LR Johnson, Raven Press, New York. Speth RC, Thompson SM, Johns SJ, 1995, Angiotensin II receptors: structural and functional considerations. In Tissue Renin-Angiotensin Systems, pp. 169-192, Edited by AK Mukhopadhyay and MK Raizada, Plenum Press, New York.

Speth RC, Thompson SM, Hohns SJ, 1995, Angiotensin II receptors: structural and functional considerations. *Adv Exp Med Biol.* **377:** 169-192.

Steinberg W, Scott T, 1994, Medical progress: acute pancreatitis. *N Engl J Med.* **330:** 1198-1210.

Suzuki Y, Ruiz-Ortega M, Lorenzo O, Ruperez M, Esteban V, Egido J, 2003, Inflammation and angiotensin II. *Int J Biochem Cell Biol.* **35:** 881-900.

Tahmasebi M, Puddefoot JR, Inwang ER, Vinsion GP, 1999, The tissue renin-angiotensin system in human pancreas. *J Endocrinol.* **161:** 317-322.

Tallant EA, Lu X, Weiss RB, Chappell MC, Ferrario CM, 1997, Bovine aortic endothelial cells contain an angiotensin (1-7) receptor. *Hypertension.* **29:** 388-393.

Telek G, Regoly-Merei J, Kovacs GC, Simon L, Nagy Z, Hamar J, Jakab F, 2001, The first histological demonstration of pancreatic oxidative stress in human acute pancreatitis. *Hepatogastroenterol.* **48:** 1252-1258.

Thomas WG, Mendelsohn FAO, 2003, Angiotensin receptors: form and function and distribution. *Int J Biochem Cell Biol.* **35:** 774-779.

Tikellis C, Wookey, PJ, Candido, R, Andrikopoulos S, Thomas MC, Cooper ME, 2004, Improved islet morphology after blockade of the renin-angiotensin system in the ZDF rat. *Diabetes.* **53:** 989-997.

Tom B, Dendorfer A, Danser AHJ, 2003, Bradykinin, angiotensin-(1-7), and ACE inhibitors: how they interact. *Int J Biochem Cell Biol.* **35:** 792-801.

Toskes PP, 1998, Pancreas. Current Medicine, Philadelphia. Tsang SW, Cheng CHK, Leung PS, 2004a, The role of the pancreatic renin-angiotensin system in acinar digestive enzyme secretion and in acute pancreatitis. *Regul Pept.* **119:** 213-219.

Tsang SW, Ip SP, Leung PS 2004b, Prophylactic and therapeutic treatments with AT_1 and AT_2 receptor antagonists and their effects on changes in the severity of pancreatitis. *Int J Biochem Cell Biol.* **36:** 330-339.

Tsang SW, Ip SP, Wong TP, Che CT, Leung PS, 2003, Differential effects of saralasin and ramiprilat, the inhibitors of renin-angiotensin system, on cerulein-induced acute pancreatitis. *Regul Pept.* **111:** 47-53.

Vinson GP, Teja R, Ho MM, Hinson JP, Puddefoot JR, 1998, The role of the tissue renin-angiotensin system in the response of the rat adrenal to exogenous angiotensin II. *J Endocrinol.* **158:** 153-159.

Warner FJ, Smith AI, Hooper NM, Turner AJ, 2004, Angiotensin-converting enzyme-2: a molecular and cellular perspective. *Cell Mol Life Sci.* **61:** 2704-2713.

Wedgewood K, Reber HA, 1986, Acute pancreatitis: the concepts of pathogenesis. In Surgical Diseases of the Pancreas, pp. 12-25, Edited by J Howard, G Jordan and HA Reber, Lea and Febiger, Philadelphia.

Whitcomb DC, 1999, Acute pancreatitis: mechanisms of cell injury. In Pancreatic Disease, pp. 3-13, Edited by PG Lankisch and EP DiMagno, Springer Verlag, Berlin.

Wong PF, Lee SS, Cheung WT, 2004, Immunohistochemical colocalization of type II angiotensin receptors with somatostatin in rat pancreas. *Regul Pept.* **117:** 195-205.

Yusuf S, Sleight P, Pogue J, Bosch J, Davies R, Dagenais G, 2000, The Heart Outcomes Prevention Evaluation Study: effects of an angiotensin-converting enzyme inhibitor ramipril on cardiovascular events in high-risk patients. *N Engl J Med.* **342:** 145-153.

Chapter 7

Hepatitis C Viral Proteases And Inhibitors

Mingjun Huang, Avinash Phadke and Atul Agarwal
Achillion Pharmaceuticals, New Haven, Connecticut 06511, USA

1. INTRODUCTION

The hepatitis C virus (HCV) is the major cause of blood transfusion-related hepatitis. An estimated 170 million people worldwide have been infected by HCV, a number more than four times as many as HIV; 5 million in Europe and 4 million in USA (WHO 1997; Alter *et al* 1999; Cohen J 1999; Lauer and Walker 2001; CDC 2004). The acute phase of HCV infection is usually associated with mild symptoms. However, only 15%~20% of the infected people will clear HCV from the bloodstream, leaving 75~85% to develop into a long-term chronic infection status. Among this group of chronically infected people, 10~20% will progress to life-threatening conditions known as cirrhosis and another 1~5% will develop a liver cancer called hepatocellular carcinoma. Unfortunately, the entire infected population is at risk for these life-threatening conditions because no one can predict which individual will eventually progress to any of them.

Tremendous advances have been made in the past several years for HCV chemotherapy. It began with the interferon-alpha (IFN-α) monotherapy which was shown to be effective for treating hepatitis C patients (Hoofnagle *et al* 1986). Unfortunately, the sustained virological response (SVR) obtained with this regimen was very modest, 12 to 16%, especially in HCV genotype 1- infected patients. The combination of IFN and nucleoside analog D-ribavirin increases SVR almost three fold (McHutchison *et al* 1998; Poynard T *et al* 1998). Introduction of pegyleted IFN-α most recently into combination therapy yields a SVR of nearly 40% to 50% in genotype 1-infectected patients, and 80% to 90% in those infected with genotype 2 and 3 (Manns *et al* 2001; Fried *et al* 2002). Despite of these advances, the

U. Lendeckel and Nigel M. Hooper (eds.), Proteases in Gastrointestinal Tissue, 153-181.

current treatment regimen is ineffective in many patients, has significant side effects and is often poorly tolerated (Ahn and Flamm 2004).

Although treatment of viral infection with interferon and ribavirin for decades, the mechanisms underling their actions are still poorly understood but their nonspecific nature. Simply improvement in IFNs and ribavirin – like molecules may result in more effective and less toxic treatment options, but is unlikely to cure all HCV infection. Hence, there is a great demand for development of drugs specific against HCV.

Among specific anti-viral targets, viral proteases are often drawn most interest because they fit traditional criteria on development of antivirals: 1) They are usually essential for the viral replication; 2) They are viral specific proteins; 3) They are validated as antiviral targets in anti-HIV drug development history; and 4) In most case, they are well characterized biochemically and biophysically which makes rational drug design feasible.

In the chapter, we will discuss HCV viral proteases, focusing on the functions and structures of the proteases, and the development of inhibitors of the viral proteases.

2. HCV REPLICATION

HCV is an enveloped, positive-strand RNA virus belonging to hepacivirus genus of the flaviviridae family that contains the two other genera, pestivirus (such as bovine viral diarrhea virus, BVDV) and flavivirus (Lindenbach and Rice 2001).

The genome of HCV is about 9.6 kb containing a single open reading frame (ORF) of about 3000 amino acids (Figure 1). The ORF is flanked by 5' and 3' nontranslated region (NTR), which are essential for RNA replication. The 5' NTR also acts as an internal ribosomal entry site (IRES) for translation of the viral polyprotein which is organized in the order: NH_2-C-E1-E2-p7-NS2-NS3-NS4A-NS4B-NS5A-NS5B-COOH (Figure 1).

An additional protein, F (for frameshift protein) or ARFP (alternate reading frame protein), generated from an overlapping reading frame in the core (C) protein coding sequence, has been proposed (Xu *et al* 2001; Walewski *et al* 2001; Varaklioti *et al* 2002). The polyprotein undergoes a series of membrane associated co- and post-translational cleavages by viral and host cell proteases to yield the mature forms of the individual HCV proteins. The structural proteins, C (capsid protein), E1 (envelope protein 1) and E2 (envelope protein 2) are directed to the endoplasmic reticulum (ER)-Golgi complex and processed by cellular signal peptidases associated with the lumen of ER to generate the components for the assembly of progeny. The small hydrophobic p7 protein has been demonstrated to form ion channels in the host cell membrane, although the functional consequences of this observation are not clear (Griffin *et al* 2003). The region of polyprotein downstream of E2-p7 harbors nonstructural (NS) proteins and is processed by the two distinct viral protease activities. The integral membrane NS2 protein, together with the N-terminal region of the NS3 protein, constitutes the NS2/3 protease that catalyzes the cleavage between NS2 and NS3. The NS3 protein, in conjunction with the NS4A cofactor, serves as a serine protease for the cleavage of the remaining non-structural proteins. Once cleaved, the NS proteins assemble into the membrane associated HCV RNA replication complex (replicase). In fact, the RNA molecule (replicon) is able to replicate in cell cultures if it encodes the polyprotien of NS3-5B and contains the NTRs at its 5' and 3' (Blight *et al* 2000; Lohmann *et al* 2001). Hence, these nonstructural proteins (NS3, NS4A, NS4B, NS5A, and NS5B) have been defined as essential components of the replicase. In addition to NS3 aforementioned role in polyprotein processing, its C-terminal domain harbors an ATPase/helicase activity capable of unwinding double stranded nucleic acids, an activity likely utilized during replication. The small NS4A protein serves as a cofactor for both the protease and helicase activities of NS3. NS4B is an integral membrane protein that has a direct role in reorganization of cellular membranes to form the membranous web. Additionally, NS4B is a GTP-binding protein and the viability of the HCV replicon is abolished if the binding is blocked by introduction of mutations into the nucleotide-binding motif in NS4B (Einav *et al* 2004). NS5A is a phosphoprotein of unknown function although it is involved in regulation of viral replication and modulation of cellular processes ranging from innate immunity to dysregulated cell growth (Macdonald and Harris 2004). Recently, the structure of NS5A domain I at 2.5-A resolution was reported which will facilitate our understanding of its function (Tellinghuisen *et al* 2005). The NS5B protein is an RNA-dependent RNA polymerase that is responsible for viral RNA synthesis.

The lifecycle of HCV is outlined in Figure 2. Due to the lack of a robust cell culture for HCV propagation, the model is largely hypothetical. It is proposed based on the characterization of recombinant proteins, the analogies to other viruses of flaviviridae, and the successful establishment of HCV replicons (Lohmann *et al* 1999). Hepatocytes appear to be the major site of HCV replication but peripheral blood mononuclear cells (PBMC) are also natural host for HCV. The mechanism of cell entry (attachment and fusion) likely involves the interaction between E1 and E2 and host protein(s) acting as receptor(s). After uncoating of the nucleocapsid to liberate the genomic RNA, the viral polyprotein is translated from the genomic RNA under IRES direction on ER membrane. Following co-and post translational cleavage of polyprotein by cellular and viral proteases (NS2/3 and NS3/4A), the viral proteins assemble into a replicase which remains tightly associated with intracellular membrane and gives rise to a seemingly ER-derived membrane web. Within the complex, viral RNA synthesis occurs, first negative stand using the positive strand RNA genome as template and then positive strand using the negative strand RNA as template. The positive strand RNA genome interacts with multiple molecules of core proteins to form the nucleocapsid, which buds to ER to be enveloped. Finally the enveloped nucleocapsid (virion) is released from the cell via the cell secretory pathway.

Although any of the events (targets) in HCV life cycle as described above are in theory suitable for intervention, only a few are drawn most attention due to lack of proper *in vitro* systems to investigate the consequence resulting from intervention of the events and due to our limited understanding of the events. If the NS3/4A protease serves as an example for the further, the target drawn the most attention, the NS2/3 protease would be an opposite example though both of them in theory are suitable for intervention.

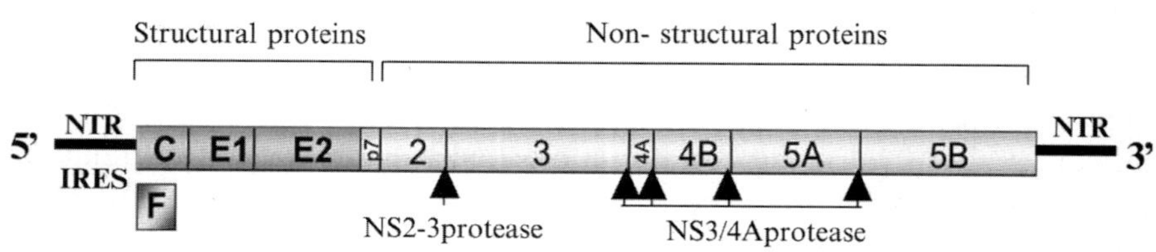

NTR	Non- translated region
IRES	Internal ribosomal entry site
C	nucleocapsid or core protein
F/ARFP	frameshift or alternative reading frame protein
El	envelope glycoprotein 1
E2	envelope glycoprotein 2
P7	ion channel protein
NS2	component of NS2-3 auto-protease
NS3	serine protease (aa1-180) and RNA helicase (aa 181-631)
NS4A	Co factor of NS3 serine protease
NS4B	GTP- binding integral membrane protein
NS5A	phosphoprotein related to interferon resistance
NS5B	RNA-dependent RNA polymerase

Figure 1: HCV genome organization. For details, see review Huang and Deshpande 2004.

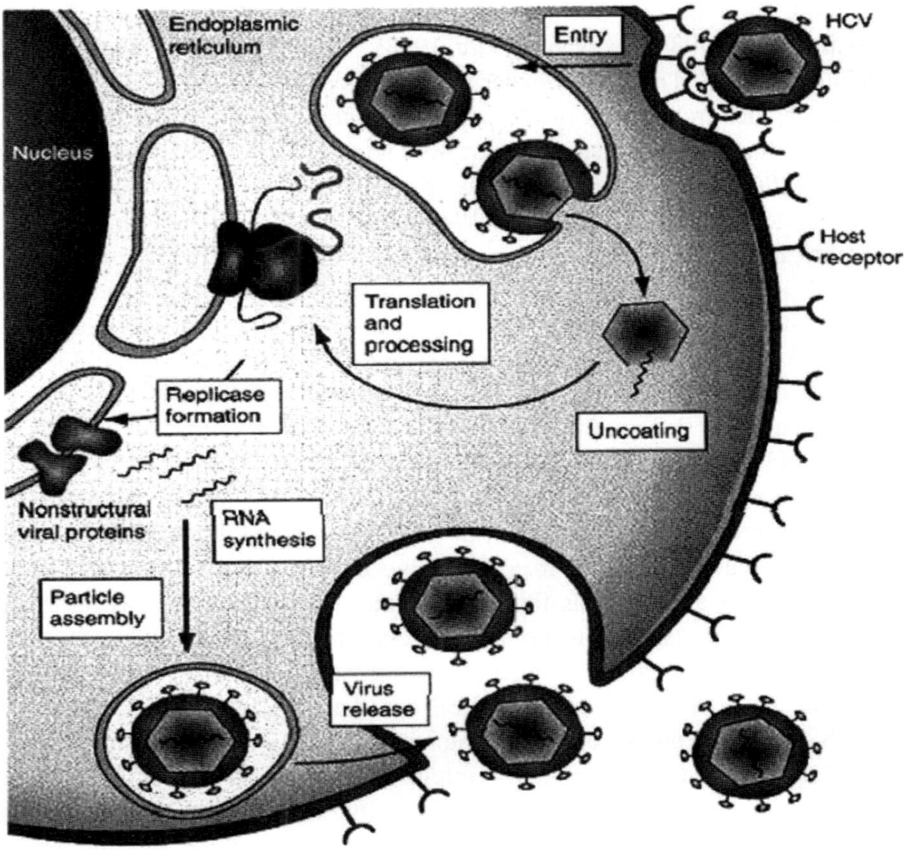

Figure 2: Hypothetical HCV life cycle. From Huang and Deshpande 2004.

3. NS2/3 PROTEASE

As described above, the matured N-terminus of NS3 is generated by intramolecular cleavage performed by the NS2/3 protease. In fact, NS2 in association with NS3 (NS2/NS3 protease) is the first activated viral protease within the HCV polypeptide responsible for the maturation of the remaining NS proteins. This NS2/NS3 autoprotease is essential for highly productive in vivo replication as a modified HCV genome (in which mutations ablating the activity of the NS2-3 protease were introduced into the NS2 sequence of HCV polypeptide) that abolished its infectivity in chimpanzees (Kolykhalov *et al* 2000).

The NS2 protein extends from amino acids 810 to 1026 and autocleavage of the NS2/3 junction is at amino acids 1026-1027 (Figure 3). The NS2/3 protease consists of the NS2 region and the minimal NS3 protease domain that flank the cleavage site (amino acids 810-1206) (Grakoui *et al* 1993; Hijikata *et al* 1993; Hirowatari *et al* 1993; Reed *et al* 1995; Pieroni *et al* 1997) (Figure 3). Truncation experiments indicated that the NS2/3 protease activity resides in a region of the polyprotein that spans from an N-terminal boundary located between residues 898 and 923 to a C-terminal end at residue 1206, even though constructs spanning only up to residue 1137 still show some residual activity (Grakoui *et al* 1993; Hijikata *et al* 1993; Santolini *et al* 1995). Furthermore, introduction of site-directed mutations into the catalytic residues of the NS3 protease domain had no effect on the activity of the NS2/3 protease (Grakoui *et al* 1993). Optimal processing at the NS2/3 junction thus appears to necessitate the presence of the NS3 serine protease domain (residues 1027 to 1206 of the HCV polyprotein) as a structural unit but does not require its serine protease activity.

The NS2 region shares no obvious sequence homology to known proteolytic enzymes. It is actually highly hydrophobic and associated with the cellular membrane (Santolini *et al* 1995). Studies with classical protease inhibitors have not resulted in a definitive classification, either. Since the NS2/3 protease activity was found to be stimulated by zinc and inhibited by chelating agents, it was tentatively classified as a metalloprotease, a hypothesis that has gained a wide acceptance (Hijikata at al 1993; Pieroni *et al* 1997). Biochemical and structural data have subsequently shown that the NS3 serine protease domain contains a tightly bound zinc ion that is absolutely required for its structural integrity (De Francesco *et al* 1996). The zinc dependence of the NS2/3 protease activity could therefore be related to the role of this metal ion in stabilizing the fold of NS3 and not to its participation in the catalytic mechanism. Nevertheless, a hydrolytic function of the zinc-binding site within NS3 cannot be ruled out. In fact, its possible spatial nearness to the NS2/3 junction in addition to the presence, in the zinc coordination sphere, of a well-defined water molecule has been discussed in terms of this metal binding site having a catalytic role in addition to its structural one (Wu *et al* 1998). On the other hand, site-directed mutagenesis experiments have shown that C993 and H952, contained within NS2, are absolutely required for NS2/3 processing, leading to the suggestion that these residues might constitute the catalytic dyad of a novel cysteine protease (Gorbalenya *et al* 1996; Wu *et al* 1998).

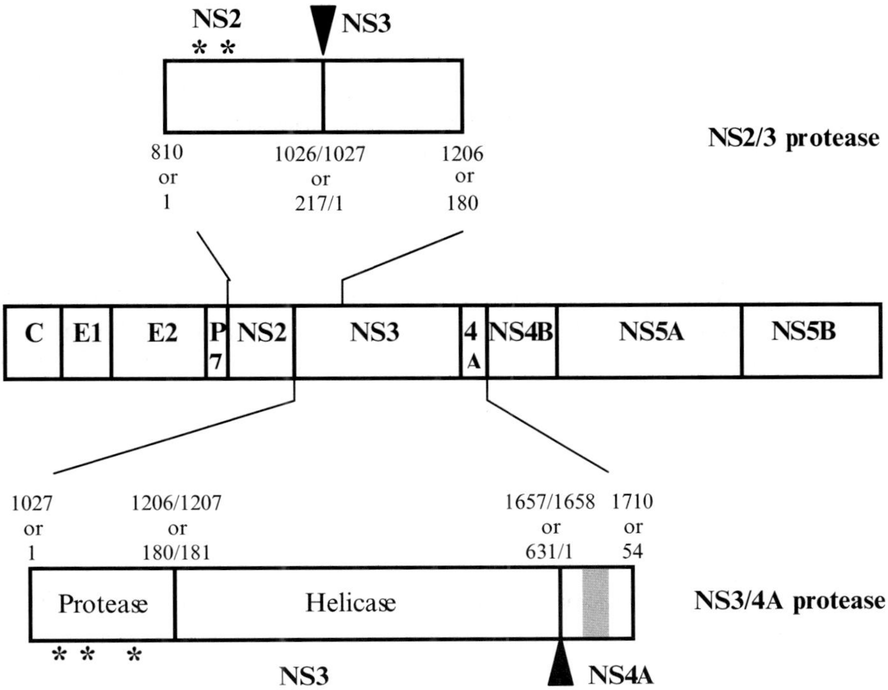

Figure 3: Schematic representation of the HCV NS2/3 and the NS3/4A protease. The NS2/3 and the NS3/4A protease are enlarged from the HCV polyprotein. The amino acid position for each domain and sub-domain is indicated as a number either starting from the 1st amino acid of the entire polyprotein (the number at the top) or starting from the 1st amino acid of the NS2, NS3 or NS4A (the number at the bottom). The black arrow indicates the autocleavage site. On the NS2/3protease, the residues His^{952} and $Cys^{993}$of the polyprotein (or His^{143} and Cys^{184} of the NS2), known to be essential for autocleavage between NS2 and NS3, are labeled as "*". On the NS3/4A protease, the catalytic triad, namely His-1083, Asp-1107 and Ser-1165 of the polyproteins (or His-57, Asp-81 and Ser-139 of the NS3), is also indicated as "*". The gray box in the NS4A indicates the 14-aminon acid central hydrophobic region of NS4A (amino acids 1678-1691 of the polyprotein or amino acids 21-34 of the NS4A), which has been shown to be sufficient for activation of the NS3 protease activity.

Functionally, the NS2/3 protease is also quite unique among viral proteases. Its sole role in viral maturation is to separate the NS2 from the rest of nonstructural proteins. As describe above, the functional HCV subgenomic RNAs (replicons) replicate in the absence of the structural proteins and NS2 in cells, indicating that the NS2/3 protease activity is not essential for RNA replication (Blight *et al* 2000; Lohmann et al 2001) although the NS2/3 protease activity is essential in vivo (Kolykhalov *et al* 2000). Based on these characteristics, the NS2/3 protease might be viewed as a positive-stranded RNA virus accessory protease, which is defined as a protease not involved directly in the proteolytic processing of key replicative proteins. Accessory proteases fall predominantly within the papain family, are found mostly in the N-terminal region of positive-stranded RNA virus polyproteins, and are wide spread among positive-stranded RNA viruses. Accessory proteases often are indispensable for virus reproduction although not directly involved in genome replication, (Gorbalenya *et al* 1996; Tijms *et al* 2001; Ziebuhr *et al* 2000).

Besides, the NS2/3 protease shares some features with proteases encoded by other positive-stranded RNA viruses. The rubella virus protease is perhaps the most functionally related to the NS2/3 protease. The rubella virus protease: (i) mediates a single *cis*-cleavage at its C terminus, (ii) has a Cys/His catalytic dyad, and (iii) requires divalent cations for its catalytic activity (Liu *et al* 1998). Recently, the rubella virus protease was proposed as a novel virus metalloprotease rather than a papain-like cysteine protease as originally thought (Liu *et al* 2000). It remains to be seen whether the NS2/3 protease and the rubella virus protease define a new class of viral metalloproteases.

Whereas the HCV NS3/4A protease has been characterized in great detail and is at present the focus of drug development efforts, the characterization of the NS2/3 protease and development of inhibitors of the NS2/3 protease has been severely hampered so far due to its autocatalytic nature and to the presence of a large, hydrophobic region that is an impediment to efficient heterologous expression and purification. The initial characterizations of processing at the NS2-NS3 junction were based on expression of the NS2-NS3 region in cell-free translation systems or various cellular systems. Usually, the systems involve detection of cleavage products with sodium dodecyl sulfate-polyacrylamide gel electrophoresis (SDS/PAGE) analysis and are not suitable for drug discovery. In order to utilize the systems in drug discovery, modifications have been sought, resulting in development of cell-based assays with high throughput (Wenzel *et al* 1999; Whitney *et al* 2002). The principle behind the assays lies in the dependence of the activity of a reporter on the cleavage between NS2 and 3. For example, Whitney *et al* reported an assay wherein the NS2/3 protease sequences were inserted between the beta-lactamase (BLA) reporter and an ubiquitin-based destabilization domain. In stable cells, NS2-3 mediated cis cleavage of NS2-3-BLA fusion protein resulted in differential stability of cleaved versus uncleaved BLA reporter, with the further much more stable due to devoid of ubiquitin-based destabilization domain and the later highly unstable due to the presence of ubiquitin-based destabilization domain, providing a robust readout for protease activity. The assay was adapted into a 384-well format on a fully automated platform. Screen effort using the assay, unfortunately, has not yielded drug-like small molecule inhibitors (Whitney *et al* 2002).

Not long ago, two groups have successfully reconstituted autoprocessing of a purified recombinant NS2/3 protease (Thibeault *et al* 2001; Pallaoro *et al* 2001). By deletion of a membrane-anchoring domain located at the N-terminus of NS2, NS2-3 precursor could be purified to homogeneity from inclusion bodies of *E. Coli*. Following refolding, the precursor is auto-cleaved under proper conditions. The advance will facilitate the detailed biochemical characterization of the enzyme and, hence, the discovery of inhibitors against the enzyme although no active compound with reasonable potency and drug like features has been disclosed so far.

4. NS3/4A PROTEASE

In contrast to the NS2/3 protease, our understandings on the NS3/4A protease is much more comprehensive. Consequently, inhibitors based different mechanism have been reported and some of them have advanced to clinic. It is expected that a drug specific for HCV NS3/4A protease will be added to the current regimens for HCV therapy in near future.

4.1 Role of NS3/4A protease in viral replication

Following release from NS2, NS3-NS5B polyprotein is further cleaved by the NS3/4A protease. A distinct temporal hierarchy of cleavage events was observed that is initiated by an intramolecular cut between the NS3-NS4A juncture, giving rise to NS3/4A, a heterodimeric protease. The protease in turn cleaves intermolecularly at the junction of NS5A-5B, releasing the mature NS5B, at the junction of NS4A-4B, releasing the mature NS4A, finally at the junction of NS4B and NS5A, giving rise to the mature NS4B and NS5A. The importance of the temporal order of the processing is not understood. Nevertheless, the NS3/4A protease is absolutely required for viral replication. Genetically disabling the activity of the protease renders an otherwise viable HCV cDNA non-infectious in chimpanzees (Kolykhalov *et al* 2000), thus validating the viral enzyme as a target for drug discovery.

In addition to its role in HCV polyprotein processing and thereby its indispensable role in HCV replication, the NS3/4A protease is proposed to be involved in regulation of cellular innate immune response.

Cellular control of virus infection is mediated through a variety of processes impacting different stages of the viral life cycle (Katze *et al* 2002). Interferon regulatory factors (IRFs) are key transcription factors that initiate this cellular antiviral state (Barnes *et al* 2002). IRF-3 is a latent cytoplasmic factor that is activated through phosphorylation upon viral infection. Phosphorylated IRF-3 translocates to the nucleus, where it induces transcription of type I IFNs and other antiviral genes. Foy *et al* (2003) first reported that the HCV NS3/4A serine protease blocks the phosphorylation and effector action of IRF-3. Disruption of the NS3/4A protease function by mutation or a ketoamide peptidomimetic inhibitor relieved this blockade and restored IRF-3 phosphorylation after cellular challenge with an unrelated virus. Thus, the NS3/4A protease represents a dual therapeutic target, the inhibition of which may block viral replication and restore IRF-3 control of HCV infection as well.

Recent work suggests that viral infections activate IRF-3 as well as NF-κB, another factor which also induces transcription of type I IFNs and other antiviral genes, through two independent signaling pathways. One pathway involves engagement of Toll-like receptor (TLR) 3 by its specific ligand, double-stranded RNA (dsRNA) (Alexopoulou *et al* 2001). TLRs are a family of innate immune-recognition receptors that recognize molecular patterns associated with microbial pathogens, and induce antimicrobial immune responses. The dsRNA is a molecular pattern associated with viral infection, because it is produced by most viruses at some point during their replication. The mammalian TLR3 recognizes dsRNA and that activation of the receptor induces the activation of NF-kappaB and IRF-3. The second pathway involves retinoic acid inducible gene I (RIG-I) (Yoneyama *et al* 2004). RIG-I encodes a DExD/H box RNA helicase that contains a helicase domain and a caspase recruitment domain. The helicase domain is responsible for the dsRNA-mediated signaling and the caspase recruitment domain transmits 'downstream' signals, resulting in the activation of transcription factors NF-kappaB and IRF-3. Towards the end, the activation of either pathway leads to expression of multiple protective cellular genes, including type I IFNs (Yoneyama *et al* 2004; Beutler 2004; Peters *et al* 2002; Grandvaux *et al* 2002).

Many viruses have evolved strategies that block the effector mechanisms induced through these pathways (Katze *et al* 2002). For HCV, it appears that both pathways are inhibited by the NS3/4A protease. Li *et al* (2005) showed that the NS3/4A protease caused specific proteolysis of Toll-IL-1 receptor domain-containing adaptor inducing IFN- (TRIF or TICAM-1), an adaptor protein linking TLR3 to kinases responsible for activating IRF-3 as well as NF-B. The NS3/4A expression from replicating HCV RNA was associated with reduced intracellular abundance of TRIF and inhibition of dsRNA-activated signaling through the TLR3 pathway. Foy *et al* (2005) reported that RIG-I signaling was suppressed by the protease activity of NS3/4A and treatment of cells with an active site inhibitor of the NS3/4A protease relieved this suppression and restored intracellular antiviral defenses.

4.2 Characteristics of NS3/4A protease

The mature form of NS3 protein extends from amino acids 1027 to 1657 of the polyprotein. The NS3 minimal protease domain has been mapped by deletion mutagenesis to the N-terminal 180 amino acids of NS3, namely, from 1027 to 1206 (Failla *et al* 1995; Bartenschlager *et al* 1994; Tanji *et al* 1994; Han *et al* 1995; Kolykhalov *et al* 1994). Within the region, the conserved residues that form the enzyme catalytic triad, namely, His-1083, Asp-1107 and Ser-1165, are found. The reminder of the NS3, i.e., from 1207 to 1657 (~450 amino acids) contains a helicase activity. The activity of both domains is retained when they are artificially separated (Figure 3).

In transfected cells, NS3 and NS4A form a stable complex on the membranes of ER (Failla *et al* 1995; Bartenschlager *et al* 1995). The domain on NS3 to interact with NS4A for complex formation has been mapped to about 30 amino acids at the N terminus (Failla *et al* 1995; Satoh 1995). The role of NS4A in the complex is dual. First, it enhances the proteolytic activity of NS3 (Failla *et al* 1995; Satoh 1995; Koch *et al* 1996). A 14-aminon acid central hydrophobic region of NS4A (amino acids 1678-1691) has been shown to be sufficient for the function by deletion mutagenesis (Koch *et al* 1996; Lin *et al* 1995; Tomei 1996; Shimizu 1996). This function of NS4A is recapitulated biochemically with purified proteins: the proteolytic activity of either full-length of NS3 or NS3 protease domain is enhanced in the presence of NS4A or just a synthetic peptides encompassing the 14-amino acid central region of NS4A (Lin *et al* 1995; Tomei 1996; Shimizu 1996). Second, NS4A targets the NS3 protein to the membrane of ER. In the transfected cells, NS3 becomes membrane-associated only when the NS4A is coexpressed. It is believed that a very hydrophobic segment proceeding to the 14-amino acid central region of NS4A forms a trans-membrane α-helix mediating the membrane targeting.

Both X-ray crystallography and NMR spectroscope have been used to determine the three dimensional structure of the NS3 protease, either in its free form or in complex with one or more of the following, helicase domain, cofactor, the zinc ion and inhibitors (Love 1995; Kim 1996; Barbato 1999; Yan 1998; Yao 1999; Marco 2000; Barbato 2000; Andrews 2003; Liu 2004). These studies revealed that structurally, the NS3 protease is part of the trypsin superfamily, but features such as a structural non-catalytic zinc moiety, a shallow active site and dependence on a second viral co-factor (NS4A), make it unique.

In the absence of a NS4A cofactor, the NS3 protease domain folds into two structural sub-domains, each containing a six-stranded β barrel, similar to the trypsin-like serine proteases. The catalytic triad is located in the crevice between two sub-domains, with the N-terminal sub-domain (residues 1-93) contributing the His-57 and Asp-81 for the catalytic triad and the C-terminal sub-domain (residues 94-180) contributing the Ser-139 of the catalytic triad. As a note, since these studies were preformed with NS3, NS4A or their subdomains, the numbering for the amino acid position starts from the 1st amino acid of NS3 and NS4A, not from the 1st amino acid of the polyprotein from now on. For comparison between two numberings, see Figure 3.

Binding of the NS4A peptide induces conformational changes in the NS3 protease (Figure 4). The most significant change happens around the N-terminal 28 residues of the protease which are unfolded in the unbound form. These residues fold a β-sheet when the NS4A peptide is bound. With the NS4A forming an additional β-strand sandwiched between two β-strands from the N-terminal subdomain, the N terminal subdomain of the NS3 protease now is an eight-stranded stranded β-barrel, structurally similar to the N-terminal domain of chymotrypsin. These structural observations are in agreement with the results by deletion mutagenesis which mapped the interaction domain of NS4A to the N-terminus of NS3 (see above). In addition, the structure explains the biochemical and mutational data that the central region (residues 21 to 34) of NS4A is sufficient for NS3 protease activation as described above. All the contacts observed between NS3 and NS4A involves only residues 21 to 32 of NS4A. The NS4A peptide binds in the extended conformation except for a kink at Ile-25 and Val-26. It forms hydrogen bonds with the first two β-strands of the N-terminal domain in an anti-parallel fashion. Gly-21 NH and Leu-31 CO are the only two backbone polar atoms of the NS4A central region (residue 21-32) that do not hydrogen bond with the NS3 protease domain. All the hydrophobic residues of NS4A are buried with non-polar atoms of the NS3 protease domain.

The commonly accepted mechanistic model of action of the serine proteases involves hydrogen bonds between carboxylate group of the Asp and the δ NH of the His, and the ε N of the His and the γ OH of the Ser residues. This hydrogen-binding network activates the γ O of the Ser which carries out nucleophilic attack on the C atom of the scissile bond (Fersht 1984; Polgar 1989; Lesk *et al* 1996). The side chain of Asp-81 is swung away from His-57 in the free-NS3 protease while Asp-81 carboxyl group points to the imidazole ring of His-57 in the NS4A- bound form of the NS3 protease. In addition, Ser-139 interacts with His-57 only in the NS4A-bound form of the NS3 protease. Thus, intercalation of NS4A into the N-terminal domain of the NS3 protease results in a spatial rearrangement of the active site towards the classical catalytic triad configuration. The observation is again consistent with the biochemical phenomenon that the catalytic efficiency of the NS3 protease is enhanced in the presence of the NS4A (see above).

The presence of a zinc-binding site in the NS3 protease was initially predicted by homology modeling (De Francesco *et al* 1996). It was later confirmed by biochemical analyses that a tightly-bound zinc ion is presence in an equimolar ratio with the NS3 protease (De Francesco *et al* 1996;

Stempniak *et al* 1997). In addition, the activity of NS3 protease required zinc ion (De Francesco *et al* 1998) and the addition of a metal ion chelator EDTA (Lin and Rice, 1995; Kakiuchi *et al* 1997) or a cupric ion in the proteolytic reaction (Hahm *et al* 1995; Han *et al* 1995; Kakiuchi *et al* 1997) caused some weak inhibition. The three dimensional structure studies revealed that the zinc ion is located opposite to the active site and is coordinated by three cysteine residues, Cys -97, 99 and 145, and through a water molecule to His 149 (Kim *et al* 1996; Love *et al* 1996; Yan *et al* 1998) (Figure 4). These metal ligating residues are situated in a long loop connecting two β-barrels and a short loop in the C-terminal subdomain. Hence, the metal binding may affect the relative position two β-barrels which in turn may affect the orientation of the catalytic residues since the catalytic triad residues are also distributed between these two β-barrels.

At last, although similar in geometry to other serine proteases, the catalytic triad (His57, Asp81 and Ser139) and oxy-anion hole reside in a shallow cleft that binds the substrate peptide, all of the customary substrate recognition loops around the cleft are missing in the NS3/4A protease, leaving the substrate-binding site remarkably undefined and exposed to solvent. This suggests that substrate recognition is based on subtle electrostatic interactions centered on the conserved sequences of the substrates along the extended protease contact surface. This feature has imposed a great challenge in developing small and potent inhibitors of the NS3/4A protease as will be discussed later.

4.3 *In vitro* system for evaluation of inhibitors of NS3/4A protease

Biochemical assays with purified proteins have been well established (for details, see review Kwong *et al* 1998). The proteins used in the assays mostly are a truncated form of NS3, namely, the protease domain of NS3, and a 14 amino acid synthetic peptide derived from NS4A central region or a truncated form of NS3 fused either at its N-terminus or C-terminus with 14 amino acids derived from NS4A central region simply because the production of the truncated form of NS3 in *E. coli* is easier, relative to the full length of NS3. It is in the form that the NS3/4 protease has been extensively characterized both biochemically and structurally. Nevertheless, NS3 and NS4A is, naturally, a membrane-bound multifunctional enzyme. It has been speculated that the membrane association might affect the specificity and catalysis of the NS3-4A protease as well as protein folding and interacting. Recently, Pamela *et al* (2005) established an assay to detect, using a unique internally quenched fluorogenic substrate (IQFS), NS3-4A protease activity within membrane fractions isolated from human cells expressing NS3-4A. With the assay, the

A)

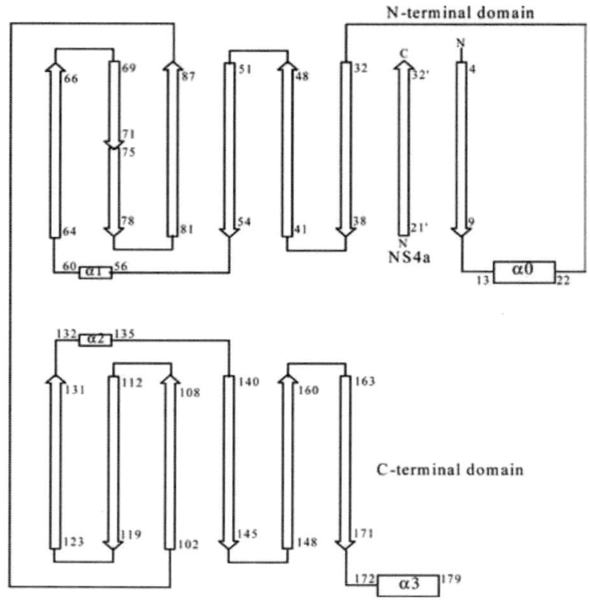

B)

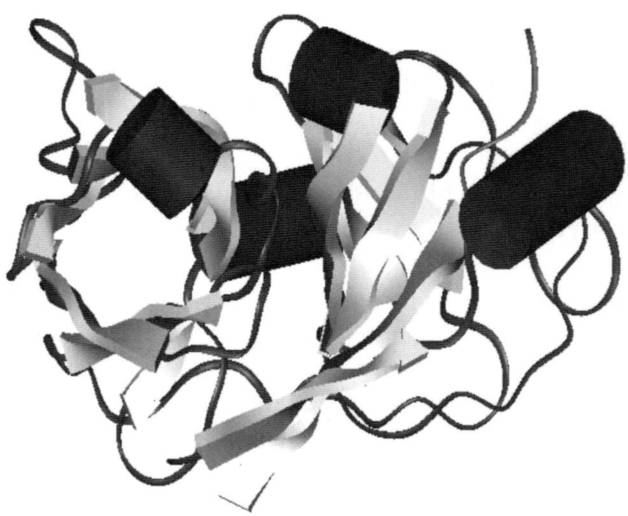

Figure 4: A) A schematic of the protein secondary structures in NS3 protease domain/NS4A complex. Helices are shown as cylinders and β-strands as arrows. **B)** The 3D structure of NS3 protease domain/NS4A complex. Helices are shown as red cylinders and β-strands as yellow arrows. NS4A is shown in orange color and the β-strand of NS4A is represented as yellow arrow. Figure 4a is modified and printed with permission from Yan Y. *et al* 1998.

authors found that steady-state kinetic parameters, such as *K*m and *k*cat, are quite similar to those determined with the traditional assays. The result indicate that that membrane association does not alter the enzymatic properties of the NS3-4A protease, but, it remain to be determined whether it affects the folding of NS3 and NS4A as well as the interaction between NS3 and NS4A.

As complement to the biochemical assays with purified enzymes, cell-based assays have also been developed because they can determine whether potential inhibitors are able to penetrate the cell, act in an appropriate cellular environment and act on the NS3/4A complex in an natural context. A number of these systems with the potential to identify inhibitors of the NS3/4A protease have been described (Kwong *et al* 1998). Some include the use of chimeras of either Sindbis virus or poliovirus containing the HCV NS3 protease, in which the production of infectious virus is dependent on the activity of the NS3 protease (Cho *et al* 1997; Hahm *et al* 1996). Other systems utilize reporter genes such as secreted alkaline phosphatase, the secretion of which is dependent on cleavage by NS3 (Lee *et al* 2003; Pacini *et al* 2004). The system could be used for confirmation of compounds identified with purified proteins and might be more valuable for discovery of hits targeting at the sites for protein-protein interaction.

4.4 Strategies for developing inhibitors of NS3/4A protease

Based on characteristics of the NS3/4A protease described above, three alternative approaches for development of HCV NS3/4A protease inhibitors were initially envisioned: (i) interference with the activation of the enzyme by its NS4A cofactor; (ii) binding to the structural zinc site; and (iii) binding to the active site. However, only the last approach has extensively been explored because the interaction between NS3 and NS4A involves a very large surface area, a feature not fitting to the traditional concept about an ideal target and because there is a great concern about likelihood to develop any zinc-ejector with an acceptable specificity.

To develop a potent inhibitor binding to the NS3/4A active site has initially been hindered by the structure of the active site: remarkably shallow, featureless and solvent-exposed. Nevertheless, a number of active site inhibitors have thus been described and at least 2 of them have been investigated in HCV infected patients. In the following paragraphs, we will discuss these inhibitors with a focus on the product based- analogs since they are representing the most promising classes.

As described above, the NS3/4A protease cleaves the viral polyprotein at four sites: NS3-4A, NS4A-NS4B, NS4B-NS5A and NS5A-NS5B. Cleavage at the first site is an intermolecular event (cis-cleavage) and the others are intramolecular (trans). According to Schechter and Berger nomenclature (Schechter *et al* 1967), the cleavage sites are designated as P6-P5-P4-P3-P2-P1—P1'-P2'-P3'-P4', with the scissile bond between P1 and P1', while the relative binding pockets of the enzyme are termed S6-S5-S4-S3-S2-S1—S1'-S2'-S3'-S4', with cleavage occurring after cysteine or threonine (Grakoui, *et al* 1993; Pizzi *et al* 1994).

An important class of peptidomimetic inhibitors is discovered based on the finding that the NS3/4A protease is susceptible to feedback inhibition by its N-terminal cleavage products, 1, 2 (Llinas-Brunet *et al* 1998; Steinkuhler *et al* 1998).

–P6–P5–P4—P3–P2–P1—
Asp-Glu-Met-Glu-Glu-Cys-OH 1
NS4A/NS4B product Ki = 0.6 uM

–P6–P5—P4—P3–P2–P1—
Asp–Asp–Ile–Val–Pro–Cys-OH 2
NS5A/NS5B product Ki = 71 uM

Capitalizing on this observation two groups have modified the natural amino acids in these hexapeptides to afford very potent hexapeptides inhibitors of the NS3/4A protease. (De Francesco *et al* 2000; Steinkuhler *et al* 2001). Based on these hexapeptides it was shown that they require two anchors, a P1 anchor and a P5-P6 acidic anchor for optimal active site binding as in example 3 and 4 (Ingallinella *et al* 1998; Beaulieu *et al* 2002).

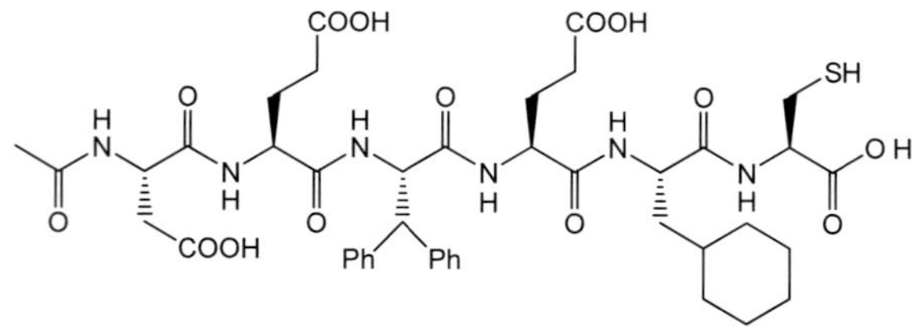

3 Ki = 0.040∝M µm

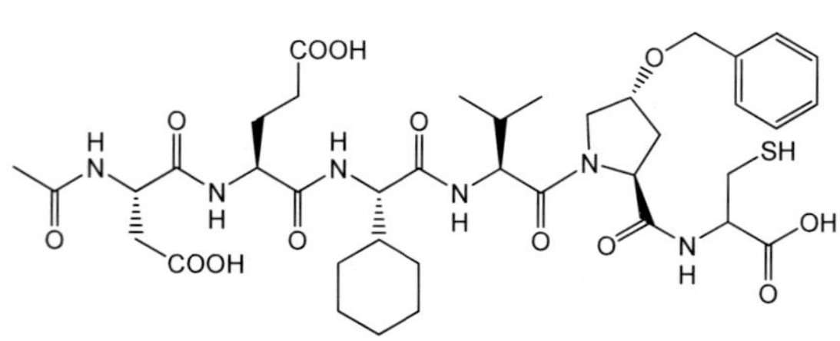

4 IC50 = 0.033 ∝M µm

The S1 pocket, is a small lipophilic pocket lined by hydrophobic residues of Val132, Leu135 and Phe154, is complimentary to the small and lipophilic cysteine side chain. In addition, the sulfhydryl group can interact with the aromatic ring of Phe154. The second anchor P5-P6 acid interacts with the basic amino acids Lys165, Arg161 and Arg123 of the protein. (Di Marco *et al* 2000; Koch *et al* 2001). The sulfhydryl group was a detriment for the development of effective therapeutics so major effort was devoted to find a suitable replacement for the P1 sulfhydryl group. Amino acids with small hydrophobic side chain like alanine, alpha-aminobutyric acid were tolerated but resulted in loss of potency. Amino acids with larger side chains also resulted in loss in potency due to steric incompatibilities (Steinkuhler *et al* 2001). An analysis of steric and electrostatic properties of the thiol group suggested a difluoromethyl group as a replacement for the thiol (Narjes *et al* 2002). Thus, introduction of (S)-4,4-difluoro-2-aminobutyric acid as cysteine replacement produced a hexapeptide 5 as potent as the initial hexapeptide 1.

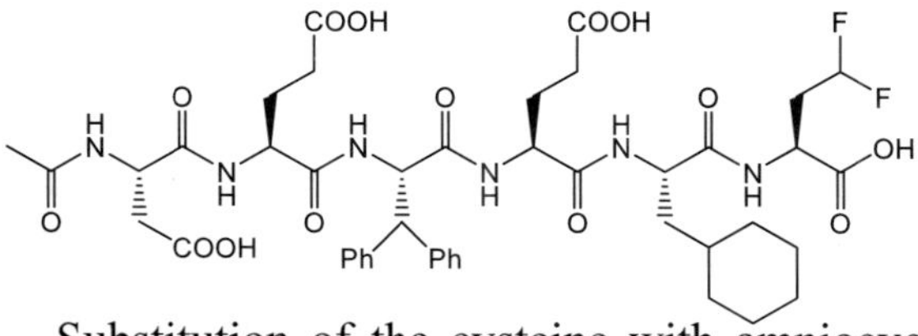

5 Ki = 0.02 μM

Substitution of the cysteine with amniocyclopropyl carboxylic acids at the P1 position also proved to be very effective giving hexapeptide 6, which was as potent as the parent (Llinas-Brunet *et al* 2000).

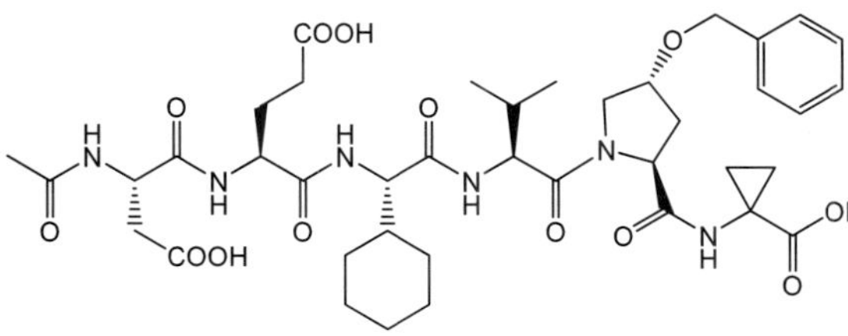

6 IC_{50} = 0.051 μM

Further optimization of the product-based inhibitors has produced potent inhibitors with smaller size. This demonstrated that the P5-P6 acid residues are not critical for activity. Several Boc of Cbz- protected tripeptides, e.g. 7, 8, have shown excellent potency against the NS3/4A protease (Pizzi *et al* 1994; Koch *et al* 2001).

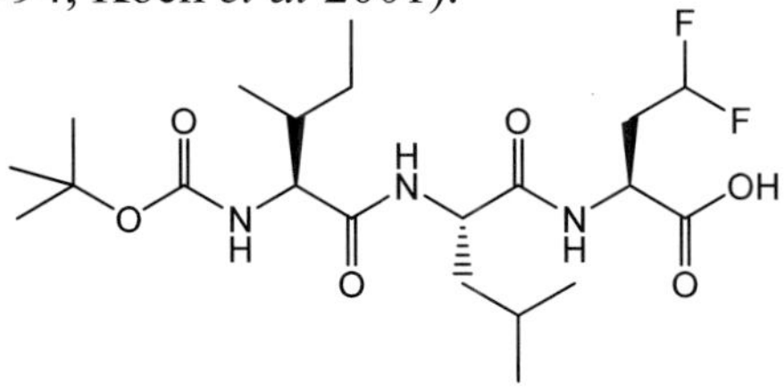

7 IC_{50} = 1.0μM

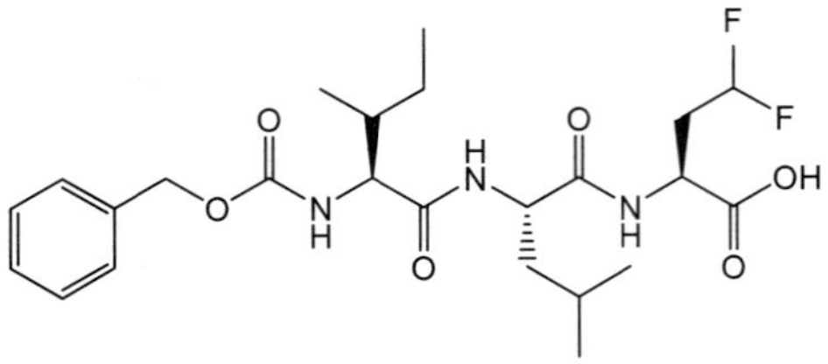

8 $IC_{50} = 1.7\ \mu M$

Alterations at P1-P4 positions were further explored, with particular focus on the P2 proline (Goudreau *et al* 2004). These modifications led to potent tetrapeptide with IC_{50} values in the low nanomolar range, compound 9 (Barbato *et al* 1999; Barbato *et al* 2001).

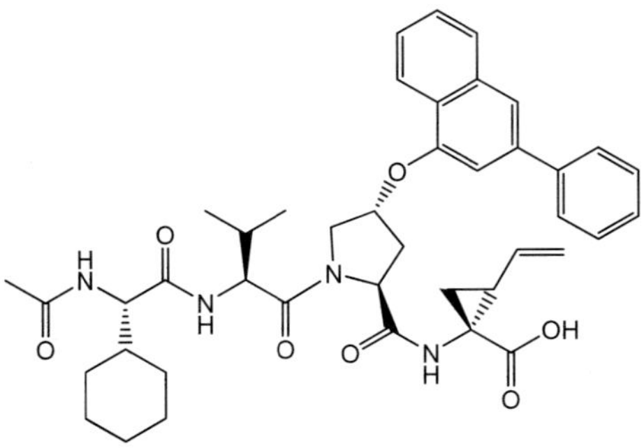

9 $IC_{50} = 0.013\ \mu M$

The limitations of peptide as drug candidates are well documented (Lipinski *et al* 2001). Therefore, a significant amount of work has been directed towards reducing the peptidic nature of these compounds. Very potent tripeptides have been synthesized by designing a macrocycle by connecting the P1 side chain with the P3 side chain. One such compound is BILN-2061 (Llinas-Brunet *et al* 2004).

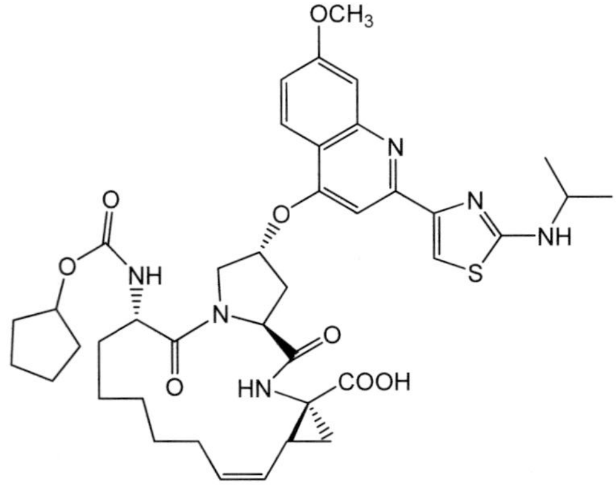

BILN-2061 $IC_{50} = 3.0$ nM

The potency of the BILN-2061 was determined using HCV subtype 1a and 1b replicons with an EC50 of 3 and 4 nM, respectively (Lamarre *et al* 2003). A proof-of-concept trial was conduced to determine the efficacy and tolerability of the inhibitor (Table 1). Thirty-one patients with HCV genotype 1 and minimal liver fibrosis received BILN 2061 for two days at

25 mg (Group A), 200 mg (Group B) or 500 mg (Group C), bid. All arms were placebo controlled-4 active drug to 1 placebo with 10 patients per arm. Viral load reduction by at least 100-fold were seen in seven out of nine, eight out of eight, and eight out of eight patients treated with 25, 200 and 500 mg, respectively. After the end of treatment, the viral load returned to baseline levels with 1-7 days. The drug was well tolerated (Lamarre *et al* 2003; Hinrichsen *et al* 2004).

Following the success of the first trial, several other 2-day monotherapy studies were conducted to evaluate the efficacy and tolerability in various patient groups. As summarized in Table 1, ten genotype 1 individuals with advanced fibrosis received the drug at 200mg bid (Group D) and ten genotype 1 patients with cirrhosis received the drug at a similar dose (Group E). Non-genotype 1 individuals with minimal fibrosis received 500mg bid (Group F). All arms were placebo controlled-4 active drug to 1 placebo with 10 patients per arm. Although the similar tolerability was observed among all groups, similar efficacy was only achieved in Group D and E genotype 1 patients. In comparison, in individuals with non-genotype 1 (Group F) there is clearly a reduction in response to BILN 2061 (Hinrichsen *et al* 2004; Reiser *et al* 2005). The results are actually in agreement with *in vitro* biochemical evaluation. BILN 2061 showed a decrease in affinity for the NS3/4A proteases of genotypes 2 and 3 (K(i), 80 to 90 nM) compared to genotype 1 enzymes (K(i), 1.5 nM) (Thibeault *et al* 2004).

Table 1: Summary of the HCV Viral Load Reduction from BILN 2061 Phase I//IIa.

Group		A	B	C	D	E	F
Total number of patients		9	8	8	8	8	8
Viral load reduction	Log	>1 >2 >3	>1 >2 >3	>1 >2 >3	>1 >2 >3	>1 >2 >3	>1 >2 >3
	Number of patients	9 7 3	8 8 3	8 8 7	8 8 4	8 8 6	4 3 0

Obviously, larger trails of prolonged BILN 2016 treatment are required to confirm efficacy and safety. Unfortunately, some cardiac toxicity was observed during 4-week high dosing in monkeys. There have been no reports of cardiac toxicity in humans receiving BILN 2061 at the doses studied, and further animal toxicity data is anxiously awaited (Benhamou Yves 2003).

Another strategy for the design of the NS3/4A protease inhibitors involves the introduction of electrophilic groups acting as classical serine traps. These include groups like boronic acids, alpha-diketones, ketoacids, alpha-ketoamides and ketoesters, compound 10 (Steinkuhler *et al* 2001; Fischmenn *et al* 2002). The serine hydroxyl group forms a reversible covalent bond to these electrophilic inhibitors of the NS3/4A protease.

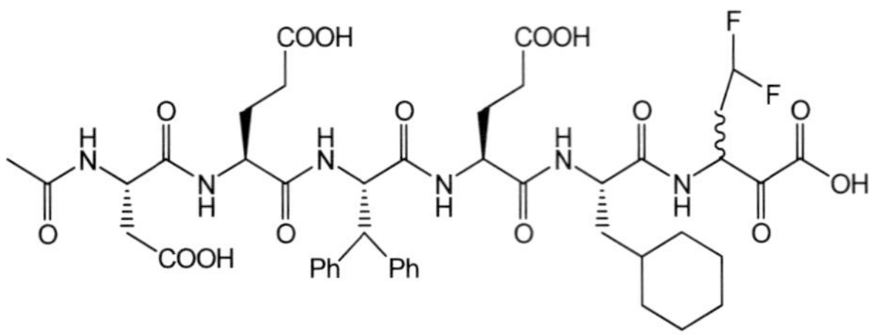

10 IC_{50} = 4 nM

Vertex Pharmaceuticals presently has a compound, VX-950 (Perni 2003; Perni *et al* 2004), based on this strategy, in the clinic that has showed promising results. The inhibitor demonstrates a potency of 0.4 μM (EC50) in HCV replicon assay (Lin *et al* 2004). Preclinical studies showed it to be orally bioavailable with favorable pharmacokinetic profile.

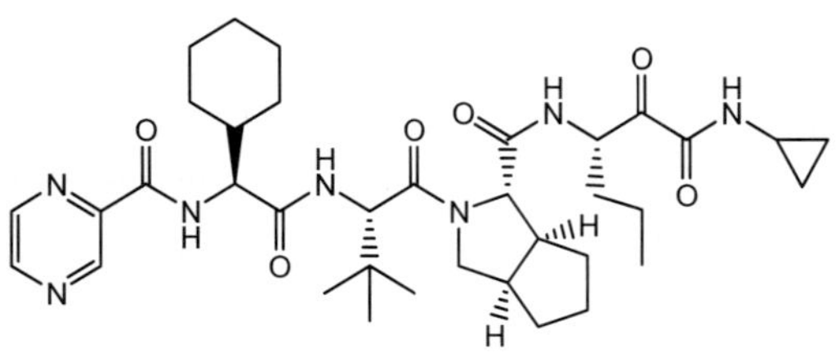

VX-950 Ki = 0.047 μM

Recently, the results of a Phase Ib clinical trial were disclosed (Reesink *et al* 2005). Patients with chronic hepatitis C (genotype 1) were dosed for 14 days at doses of 450 mg (n = 10), 750 mg (n = 8), and 1,250 mg (n =10), or placebo (n = 6). The safety of VX-950 was confirmed in this study, with no serious adverse events reported, and no discontinuations due to side effects. The most common adverse event reported was headache (28%). Regarding efficacy at inhibiting HCV replication, from a median of plasma HCV RNA at baseline of around 6 $\log_{10}$ IU/mL, no changes were seen in subjects receiving placebo, while those allocated to the 450 mg and 1,250 mg experienced a decrease of about 2 $\log_{10}$ IU/mL, and those receiving 750 mg had the maximum decline (median > 4 $\log_{10}$ IU/mL) at day 14. Table 2 below summarizes the number of subjects with undetectable HCV RNA at day 14 in each arm of the study. VX-950 might be further explored as monotherapy and studies of VX-950 in combination therapy are awaited as well.

Table 2: Patients with undetectable HCV RNA at day 14 of treatment with VX-950.

Dose of VX-950	Cut-off 30 IU/mL *	Cut-off 10 IU/mL #
450 mg (n = 10)	1	0
750 mg (n = 8)	4	2
1,250 mg (n = 10)	0	0

* viral RNA quantified with quantitative Roche COBAS TaqMan assay (detection limit < 30 IU/mL)

\# viral RNA quantified with qualitative Roche COBAS TaqMan assay (detection limit 10 IU/mL)

Other small molecules that have shown activity against HCV include murayaquinone (compound 11, Sch68631) (Chu *et al* 1996) isolated from Streptomyces and compound 12 (Sch351633) (Chu *et al* 1999) isolated from Penicillium griseofulvum.

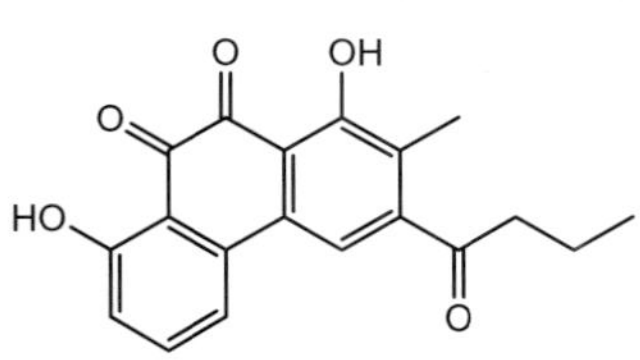

11 $IC_{50} = 7\ \mu M$

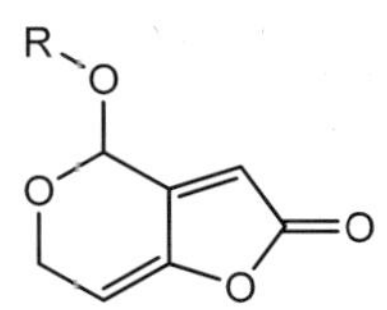

12 R = H, $IC_{50} = 3.8\ \mu g/ml$
R = Ac, $IC_{50} = 7.2\ \mu g/ml$
R = m-BrC_6H_4CO, $IC_{50} = 12.6\ \mu g/ml$

A few other compounds that have claimed HCV protease inhibitory activity are shown below. Compound 13 and its analogs showed activity against HCV protease but also showed inhibitory activity against human serine protease like chymotrypsin and elastase (Sudo *et al* 1997a). The following thiazolidone compounds 14, 15, 16, along with 17 and 18, identified through screening, have also claimed to possess HCV protease inhibitory activity (Sudo *et al* 1997b, Kakiuchi *et al* 1998).

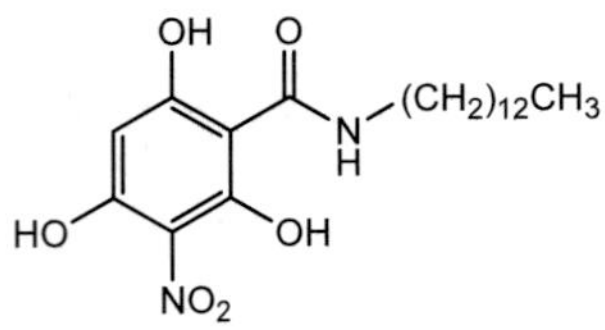

13

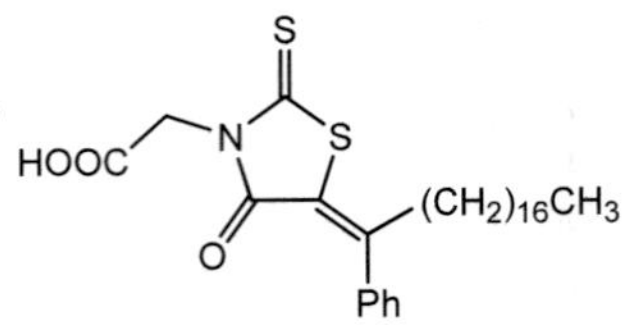

14

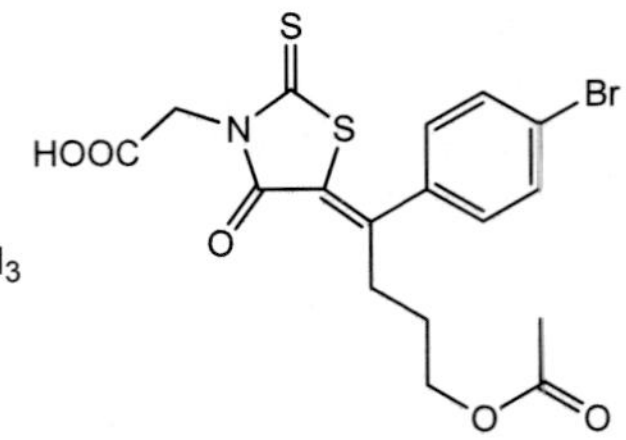

15

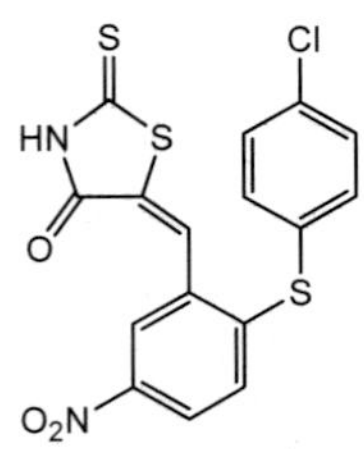

18

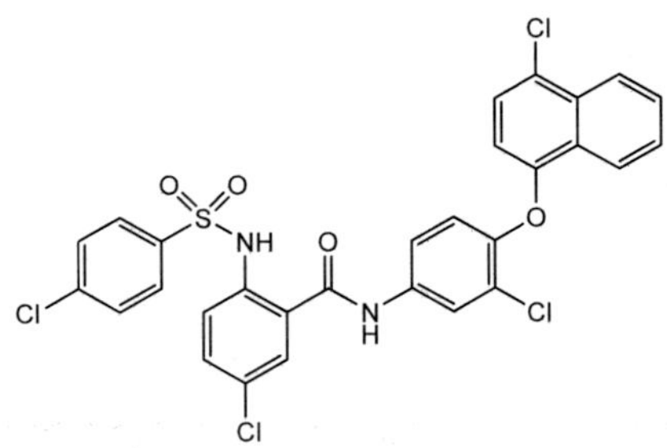

17

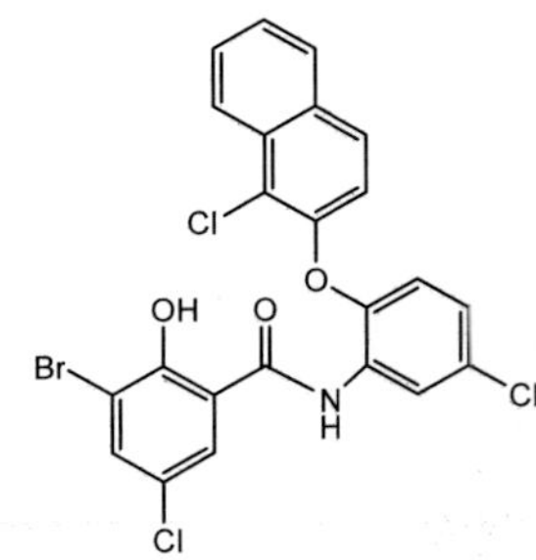

16

5. SUMMARY

HCV encodes two proteases: NS2/3 and NS3/4A. Although much is unknown about the NS2/3 protease, the NS3/4A protease has been well characterized both functionally and structurally. The NS3/4A is responsible fro the cleavage of all the non-structural proteins defined as essential components of the replication complexes. In addition, the N3/4A protease is proposed to be involved in regulation of cellular innate immune response. Structurally, the NS3 protease is part of the trypsin superfamily but with unique features such as a structural non-catalytic zinc moiety, a shallow active site and dependence on a second viral co-factor (NS4A). A potent class of peptidomimetic inhibitors is discovered based on the finding that the NS3/4A protease is susceptible to feedback inhibition by its N-terminal cleavage products. Two of such inhibitors have moved to early clinical development and both exhibit impressive antiviral efficacy. It is predicated that the inhibitors of the NS3/4A will soon be added to the current regime for treatment of chronic hepatitis C infected patients.

REFERENCES

Ahn J, Flamm S, 2004, Peginterferon-a2b and ribavirin. *Exp Rev Anti-infect Ther.* **2:** 17-25.

Alexopoulou L, Holt AC, Medzhitov R, Flavell RA, 2001, Recognition of double-stranded RNA and activation of NF-kappaB by Toll-like receptor 3. *Nature* **413:** 732-738.

Alter MJ, Kruszon-Moran D, Nainan OV, McQuillan GM, Gao F, Moyer LA, Kaslow RA, Margolis HS, 1999, The Prevalence of Hepatitis C Infection in the United States, 1998-1994. *N Engl J Med.* **341:** 556-562.

Andrew DM, Chaignot JM, Coomber BA, Dowle MD, Hind SL, Johnson MR, Jones PS, Mills G, Patikis A, Pateman TJ, Ed Robinson J, Slater MJ, Trivedi N, 2003, The design of potent, non-peptidic inhibitors of hepatitis C protease. *Eur J Med Chem.* **38:** 339-343.

Barbato G, Cicero DO, Nardi MC, Steinkuhler C, Cortese R, De Francesco R, Bazzo R, 1999, The solution structure of the N-terminal proteinase domain of the hepatitis C virus (HCV) NS3 protein provides new insights into its activation and catalytic mechanism. *J Mol Biol.* **289:** 371-384.

Barbato G, Cicero DO, Cordier F, Narjes F, Gerlach B, Sambucini S, Grzesiek S, Matassa V G, De Franscesco R, Bazzo R, 2000, Inhibitor binding induces active site stabilization of the HCV NS3 protein serine protease domain. *EMBO J.* **6:** 1195-1206.

Barnes B, Lubyova B, Pitha PM, 2002, On the role of IRF in host defense. *J Interferon Cytokine Res.* **22:** 59-71.

Bartenschlager R, Ahlborn-Laake L, Mous J, Jacobsen H, 1994, Kinetic and structural analyses of hepatitis C virus polyprotein processing. *J Virol.* **68:** 5045-5055.

Bartenschlager R, Lohmann V, Wilkinson T, Koch JO, 1995, Complex formation between the NS3 serine-type proteinase of the hepatitis C virus and NS4A and its importance for polyprotein maturation. *J Virol.* **69:** 7519-7528.

Beaulieu PL, Llinas-Brunet M, 2002, Therapies for hepatitis C infection: targeting the non-structural proteins of HCV. *Curr Med Chem.* **1:** 163-176.

Benhamou Yves, 2003, Short term anti-HCV activity and safety of BILN 2061 a novel oral HCV serine protease inhibitor. *HEP DART*. Kauai, Hawaii, USA.

Beutler B, 2004, Inferences, questions and possibilities in Toll-like receptor signalling. *Nature* **430:** 257-263.

Blight KJ, Kolykhalov AA, Rice CM, 2000, Efficient Initiation of HCV RNA Replication in Cell Culture. *Science.* **290:** 1972–1974.

Centers for Disease Control and Prevention, 2004, HIV/AIDS Surveillance Report, 2003. **15:** 1-46.

Cho YG, Moon HS, Sung YC, 1997, Construction of hepatitis C-SIN virus recombinants with replicative dependency on hepatitis C virus serine protease activity. *J Virol Methods.* **65:** 201-207.

Chu M, Mierzwa R, He L, King A, Patel M, Pichardo J, Hart A, Butkiewicz N, Puar MS, 1999, Isolation and structure of SCH 351633: a novel hepatitis C virus (HCV) NS3 protease inhibitor from the fungus Penicillium griseofulvum. *Bioorg Med Chem Lett.* **9:** 1949-1952.

Chu M, Mierzwa R, Truumees I, King A, Patel M, Berrie R, Hart A, Butkiewicz N, DasMahapatra B, 1996, Structure of Sch 68631: a new hepatitis C virus proteinase inhibitor from Streptomyces sp. *Tetrahedron Lett.* **37:** 7229-7232.

Cohen J. 1999, The scientific challenge of hepatitis C. *Science.* **285:** 26-30.

De Francesco RA, Urbani MC, Nardi MC, Tomei L, Steinkühler C, Tramontano A, 1996. A zinc binding site in viral serine proteinases. *Biochemistry.* **35:** 13282-13287.

De Francesco R, Pessi A, Steinkuhler C, 1998, The hepatitis C virus NS3 proteinase: structure and function of a zinc-containing serine proteinase. *Antivir Ther.* **3(Suppl 3):** 99-109.

De Francesco R, Steinkuhler C, 2000, Structure and function of the hepatitis C virus NS3-NS4A serine proteinase. *Curr Top Microbiol Immunol.* **242:** 149-169.

Di Marco S, Rizzi M, Volpari C, Walsh M, Narjes F, Colarusso S, De Francesco R, Matassa VG, Sollazzo M, 2000, Inhibition of the hepatitis C virus Colarusso NS3/4A protease thecrystal structures of two protease-inhibitor complexes. *J Biol Chem.* **275:** 7152-7157.

Einav S, Elazar M, Danieli T, Glenn JS, 2004, A nucleotide binding motif in hepatitis C virus (HCV) NS4B mediates HCV RNA replication. *J Virol.* **78:** 11288-11295.

Failla C, Tomei L, De Francesco R, 1995, An amino-terminal domain of the hepatitis C virus NS3 protease is essential for interaction with NS4A. *J Virol.* **69:** 1769-1777.

Fersht A, 1984, Enzyme structure and mechanism, 2nd. Edit. W.H. Freeman, San Francisco, CA.

Fischmenn TO, Weber PC, 2002, Peptide inhibitors of the hepatitis C virus serine protease within non-structural protein 3. *Curr Pharm Des.* **8:** 2533-2540.

Foy E, Li K, Wang C, Sumpter R Jr, Ikeda M, Lemon SM, Gale M Jr, 2003, Regulation of interferon regulatory factor-3 by the hepatitis C virus serine protease. *Science.* **300:** 1145-1148.

Foy E, Li K, Sumpter R Jr, Loo YM, Johnson CL, Wang C, Fish PM, Yoneyama M, Fujita T, Lemon SM, Gale M Jr, 2005, Control of antiviral defenses through hepatitis C virus disruption of retinoic acid-inducible gene-I signaling. *Proc Natl Acad Sci USA.* **102:** 2986-2991.

Fried MW, Shiffman ML, Reddy KR, Smith C, Marinos G, Goncales FL Jr, Haussinger D, Diago M, Carosi G, Dhumeaux D, Craxi A, Lin A, Hoffman J, Yu J, 2002, Peginterferon alfa-2a plus ribavirin for chronic hepatitis C virus infection. *N Engl J Med.* **347:** 975-982.

Gorbalenya AE, Snijder EJ, 1996, Viral cysteine proteases. *Perspect Drug Discov Des.* **6:** 64-86.

Goudreau N, Cameron DR, Bonneau P, Gorys V, Plouffe C, Poirier M, Lamarre D, Llinas-Brunet M, 2004, NMR Structural Characterization of Peptide Inhibitors Bound to the Hepatitis C Virus NS3 Protease: Design of a New P2 Substituent. *J Med Chem.* **47:** 123-132.

Grakoui A, McCourt DW, Wychowski C, Feinstone SM, Rice CM, 1993a, Characterization of the hepatitis C virus-encoded serine proteinase: Determination of proteinase-dependent polyprotein cleavage sites. *J Virol.* **67:** 2832-2843.

Grakoui A, McCourt DW, Wychowski C, Feinstone SM, Rice CM. 1993b, A second hepatitis C virus-encoded proteinase. *Proc Natl Acad Sci U S A.* **90:** 10583-10587.

Grandvaux N, tenOever BR, Servant MJ, Hiscott J, 2002, The interferon antiviral response: from viral invasion to evasion. *Curr Opin Infect Dis.* **15:** 259-267.

Griffin SD, Beales LP, Clarke DS Worsfold O, Evans SD, Jaeger J, Harris MP, Rowlands DJ, 2003, The p7 protein of hepatitis C virus forms an ion channel that is blocked by the antiviral drug, Amantadine. *FEBS Lett.* **535:** 34-38.

Hahm B, Han DS, Back SH, Song OK, Cho MJ, Kim CJ, Shimotohno K, Jang SK, 1995, NS3-4A of hepatitis C virus is a chymotrypsin-like protease. *J Virol.* **69:** 2534-2539.

Hahm BS, Back H, Lee TG, Wimmer E, Jang SK, 1996, Generation of a novel poliovirus with a requirement of hepatitis C virus protease activity. *Virology* **226:** 318-326.

Han DS, Hahm B, Rho HM, Jang SK, 1995, Identification of the protease domain in NS3 of hepatitis C virus. *J Gen Virol.* **76:** 985-993.

Hijikata M, Mizushima H, Akagi T, Mori S, Kakiuchi N, Kato N, Tanaka T, Kimura K, Shimotohno K, 1993, Two distinct proteinase activities required for the processing of a putative nonstructural precursor protein of hepatitis C virus. *J Virol.* **67:** 4665-4675.

Hinrichsen H, Benhamou Y, Wedemeyer H, Reiser M, Sentjens RE, Calleja JL, Forns X, Erhardt A, Cronlein J, Chaves RL, Yong CL, Nehmiz G, Steinmann GG, 2004, Short-term antiviral efficacy of BILN 2061, a hepatitis C virus serine protease inhibitor, in hepatitis C genotype 1 patients. *Gastroenterol.* **127:** 1347-1355.

Hirowatari Y, Hijikata M, Tanji Y, Nyunoya H, Mizushima H, Kimura K, Tanaka T, Kato N, Shimotohno K, 1993, Two proteinase activities in HCV polypeptide expressed in insect cells using baculovirus vector. *Arch Virol.* **133:** 349-356.

Hoofnagle JH, Mullen KD, Jones DB, Rustgi V, Di Bisceglie A, Peters M, Waggoner JG, Park Y, Jones EA, 1986, Treatment of chronic non-A,non-B hepatitis with recombinant human alpha interferon. A preliminary report. *N Engl J Med.* **315:** 1575-1578.

Huang M, Deshpande M, 2004, Hepatitis C drug discovery: in vitro and in vivo systems and drugs in the pipeline. *Exp Rev Anti-infect Ther.* **2:** 375-388.

Ingallinella P, Altamura S, Bianchi E, Taliani M, Ingenito R, Cortese R, De Francesco R, Steinkuehler C, Pessi A, 1998, Potent Peptide Inhibitors of Human Hepatitis C Virus NS3 Protease Are Obtained by Optimizing the Cleavage Products. *Biochemistry.* **37:** 8906-8914.

Kakiuchi N, Komoda Y, Hijikata M, Shimotohno K, 1997, Cleavage activity of hepatitis C virus serine proteinase. *J Biochem (Tokyo).* **122:** 749-755.

Kakiuchi N, Komoda Y, Komoda K, Takeshita N, Okada S, Tani T, Shimotohno K, 1998, Non-peptide inhibitors of HCV serine proteinase. *FEBS Lett.* **421:** 217-220.

Katze MG, He Y, Gale Jr M, 2002, Viruses and interferon: a fight for supremacy. *Nat. Rev. Immunol.* **2:** 675-677.

Kim JL, Morgenstern KA, Lin C, Fox T, Dwyer MD, Landro JA, Chambers SP, Markland W, Lepre CA, O'Malley ET, *et al* 1996, Crystal Structure of the Hepatitis C Virus NS3 Protease Domain Complexed with a Synthetic NS4A Cofactor Peptide. *Cell.* **87:** 343-355.

Koch JO, Lohmann V, Herian U, Bartenschlager R, 1996, In vitro studies on the activation of the hepatitis C virus NS3 proteinase by the NS4A cofactor. *Virology.* **221:** 54-66.

Koch U, Biasiol G, Brunetti M, Fattori D, Pallaoro M, Steinkuhler C, 2001, Role of charged residues in the catalytic mechanism of hepatitis C virus NS3 protease: electrostatic precollision guidance and transition-state stabilization. *Biochemistry.* **40:** 631-640.

Kolykhalov AA, Agapov EV, Rice CM, 1994, Specificity of the hepatitis C virus NS3 serine protease: effects of substitutions at the 3/4A, 4A/4B, 4B/5A, and 5A/5B cleavage sites on polyprotein processing. *J Virol.* **68:** 7525-33.

Kolykhalov AA, Mihalik K, Feinstone SM, Rice CM, 2000, Hepatitis C Virus-Encoded Enzymatic Activities and Conserved RNA Elements in the 3' Nontranslated Region Are Essential for Virus Replication In Vivo. *J Virol.* **74:** 2046-2051.

Kwong AD, Kim JL, Rao G, Lipovsek D, Raybuck SA, 1998, Hepatitis C virus NS3/4A protease. *Antivir Res.* **40:** 1-18.

Lamarre D, Anderson PC, Bailey M, Beaulieu P, Bolger G, Bonneau P, Bos M, Cameron DR, Cartier M, Cordingley MG, Faucher AM, Goudreau N, Kawai SH, Kukolj G, Lagace L, LaPlante SR, Narjes H, Poupart MA, Rancourt J, Sentjens RE, St George R, Simoneau B, Steinmann G, Thibeault D, Tsantrizos YS, Weldon SM, Yong CL, Llinas-Brunet M, 2003, An NS3 protease inhibitor with antiviral effects in humans infected with hepatitis C virus. *Nature.* **426:** 186-189.

Lauer GM, Walker BD, 2001, Hepatitis C Virus Infection. *N Engl J Med.* **345:** 41-52.

Lee JC, Shih YF, Hsu SP, Chang TY, Chen LH, Hsu JTA, 2003, Development of a cell-based assay for monitoring specific hepatitis C virus NS3/4A protease activity in mammalian cells. *Anal Biochem.* **316:** 152-170.

Lesk A, Fordham WD, 1996, Conservation and variability in the structure of serine proteinases of chymotrypsin family. *J Mol Biol.* **258:** 501-537.

Li K, Foy E, Ferreon JC, Nakamura M, Ferreon AC, Ikeda M, Ray SC, Gale M Jr, Lemon SM, 2005, Immune evasion by hepatitis C virus NS3/4A protease-mediated cleavage of the Toll-like receptor 3 adaptor protein TRIF. *Proc Natl Acad Sci USA.* **102:** 2992-2997.

Lin C, Rice CM, 1995, The hepatitis C virus NS3 serine proteinase and NS4A cofactor: establishment of a cell-free trans-processing assay. *Proc Natl Acad Sci USA.* **192:** 7622-7626.

Lin C, Lin K, Luong YP, Rao BG, Wei YY, Brennan DL, Fulghum JR, Hsiao HM, Ma S, Maxwell JP, Cottrell KM, Perni RB, Gates CA, Kwong AD, 2004, In vitro resistance studies of hepatitis C virus serine protease inhibitors, VX-950 and BILN 2061: structural analysis indicates different resistance mechanisms. *J Biol Chem.* **279:** 17508-17514.

Lindenbach BD, Rice CM, 2001, in *Fields Virology* (Knipe DM, and Howley PM, eds) Vol. 1, Fourth Ed., pp. 991–1041, Lippincott-Raven Publishers, Philadelphia.

Lipinski CA, Lombardo F, Dominy BW, Feeney PJ, 2001, Experimental and computational approaches to estimate solubility and permeability in drug discovery and development settings. *Adv Drug Delivery Rev.* **46:** 3-26.

Liu X, Ropp SL, Jackson RJ, Frey TK, 1998, The Rubella Virus Nonstructural Protease Requires Divalent Cations for Activity and Functions in trans. *J Virol.* **72:** 4463-4466.

Liu X, Yang J, Mohamad Ghazi A.M, Frey TK, 2000, Characterization of the Zinc Binding Activity of the Rubella Virus Nonstructural Protease. *J Virol.* **74:** 5949-5956.

Liu Y, Stoll VS, Richardson PL, Saldivar A, Klaus JL, Molla A, Kohlbrenner W, Kati WM, 2004, Hepatitis C NS3 protease inhibition by peptidyl-alpha-ketoamide inhibitors: kinetic mechanism and structure. *Arch Biochem Biophys.* **421:** 207-216.

Llinas-Brunet M., Bailey M, Fazal G, Goulet S, Halmos T, Laplante S, Maurice R, Poirier M, Poupart MA, Thibeault D, Wernic D, Lamarre D, 1998, Peptide-based inhibitors of the hepatitis C virus serine protease. *Bioorg Med Chem Lett.* **8:** 1713-1718.

Llinas-Brunet M, Bailey M, Fazal G, Ghiro E, Gorys V, Goulet S, Halmos T, Maurice R, Poirier M, Poupart MA, Rancourt J, Thibeault D, Wernic D, Lamarre D, 2000, Highly potent and selective peptide-based inhibitors of the hepatitis C virus serine protease: towards smaller inhibitors. *Bioorg Med Chem Lett.* **10:** 2267-2270.

Llinas-Brunet M, Bailey MD, Bolger G, Brochu C, Faucher A.-M, Ferland JM, Garneau M, Ghiro E, Gorys V, Grand-Maitre C, *et al* 2004, Structure-Activity Study on a Novel Series of Macrocyclic Inhibitors of the Hepatitis C Virus NS3 Protease Leading to the Discovery of BILN 2061. *J Med Chem.* **47:** 1605-1608.

Lohmann V, Korner F, Koch J, Herian U, Theilmann L, Bartenschlager R, 1999, Replication of subgenomic hepatitis C virus RNAs in a hepatoma cell line. *Science.* **285:** 110-113.

Lohmann V, Korner F, Dobierzewska A, Bartenschlager R, 2001, Mutations in Hepatitis C Virus RNAs Conferring Cell Culture Adaptation. *J Virol.* **75:**1437-1449.

Love RA, Parge HE, Wickersham JA, Hostomsky Z, Habuka N, Moomaw EW, Adachi T, Hostomska Z, 1996, The crystal structure of hepatitis C virus NS3 proteinase reveals a trypsin-like fold and a structural zinc binding site. *Cell.* **87:** 331-42.

Macdonald A, Harris M, 2004, Hepatitis C virus NS5A: tales of a promiscuous protein. *J Gen Virol.* **85:** 2485-502.

Manns MP, McHutchison JG, Gordon SC Rustgi VK, Shiffman M, Reindollar R, Goodman ZD, Koury K, Ling M, Albrecht JK,2001, Peginterferon alfa-2b plus ribavirin compared with interferon alfa-2b plus ribavirin for initial treatment of chronic hepatitis C: a randomised trial. *Lancet.* **358:** 958-965.

McHutchison JG, Gordon SC, Schiff ER Shiffman ML, Lee WM, Rustgi VK, Goodman ZD, Ling MH, Cort S, Albrecht JK,1998, Interferon alfa-2b alone or in combination with ribavirin as initial treatment for chronic hepatitis C. Hepatitis Interventional Therapy Group. *N Engl J Med.* **339:** 1485-1492.

Narjes F, Brunetti M, Colarusso S, Gerlach B, Koch U, Biasiol G, Fattori D, De Francesco R, Matassa VG, Steinkuehler CR, 2000, Ketoacids Are Potent Slow Binding Inhibitors of the Hepatitis C Virus NS3 Protease. *Biochemistry.* **39:** 1849-1861.

Pacini L, Bartholomew L, Vitelli A, Migliaccio G, 2004, Reporter substrates for assessing the activity of the hepatitis C virus NS3-4A serine protease in living cells. *Anal Biochem.* **331:** 46-59.

Pallaoro M, Lahm A, Biasiol G Brunetti M, Nardella C, Orsatti L, Bonelli F, Orru S, Narjes F, Steinkuhler C, 2001, Characterization of the hepatitis C virus NS2/3 processing reaction by using a purified precursor protein. *J Virol.* **75:** 9939-9946.

Perni RB, Byrn R, Chandorkar G, Chen SH, Colacino J, Chaturvedi P, Lin LF, Munroe J, Luong YP, Murko MA, *et al* 2003, VX-950: The discovery of an inhibitor of hepatitis C NS3-4A protease and a potential hepatitis C virus therapeutic. *54th annual Meeting of the American Association for the Study of Liver Diseases*, Boston, MA, USA 2003: Abstract 972.

Perni RB, Pitlik J, Britt SD, Court JJ, Courtney LF, Deininger DD, Farmer LJ, Gates CA, Harbeson SL, Levin RB, Lin C, Lin K, Moon YC, Luong YP, O'Malley ET, Rao BG, Thomson JA, Tung RD, Van Drie JH, Wei Y, 2004, Inhibitors of hepatitis C virus NS3.4A protease 2. Warhead SAR and optimization. *Bioorg Med Chem Lett.* **14:** 1441-1446.

Peters KL, Smith HL, Stark GR, Sen GC, 2002, IRF-3-dependent, NFB- and JNK-independent activation of the 561 and IFN- genes in response to double-stranded RNA. *Proc Natl Acad Sci USA.* **99:** 6322-6327.

Pieroni L, Santolini E, Fipaldini C, Pacini L, Migliaccio G, La Monica N, 1997, In vitro study of the NS2-3 protease of hepatitis C virus. *J Virol.* **71:** 6373-6380.

Pizzi E, Tramontano A, Tomei L, La Monica N, Failla C, Sardana M, Wood T, De Francesco R, 1994, Molecular model of the specificity pocket of the hepatitis C virus protease: implications for substrate recognition. *Proc Natl Acad Sci USA.* **91:** 888-892.

Polgar L, 1989, Mechanisms of Proteinase Action, CRC Press, Boca Raton, FA.

Poynard T, Marcellin P, Lee SS, Niederau C, Minuk GS, Ideo G, Bain V, Heathcote J, Zeuzem S, Trepo C, Albrecht J, 1998, Randomised trial of interferon alpha2b plus ribavirin for 48 weeks or for 24 weeks versus interferon alpha2b plus placebo for 48 weeks for treatment of chronic infection with hepatitis C virus. International Hepatitis Interventional Therapy Group (IHIT). *Lancet* **352:** 1426-1432.

Reed KE, Grakoui A, Rice CM, 1995, Hepatitis C virus-encoded NS2-3 protease: cleavage-site mutagenesis and requirements for bimolecular cleavage. *J Virol.* **69:** 4127-4136.

Reesink H, *et al* 2005, Initial results of a Phase 1 B, multiple-dose study of VX-950, a hepatitis C virus protease inhibitor. *Digestive Disease Week.* Chicago, IL. USA 2005: Abstract 527.

Reiser M, Hinrichsen H, Benhamou Y, Reesink HW, Wedemeyer H, Avendano C, Riba N, Yong CL, Nehmiz G, Steinmann GG, 2005, Antiviral efficacy of NS3-serine protease inhibitor BILN-2061 in patients with chronic genotype 2 and 3 hepatitis C. *Hepatology.* **41:** 832-835.

Santolini E, Pacini L, Fipaldini C, Migliaccio G, La Monica N, 1995, The NS2 protein of hepatitis C virus is a transmembrane polypeptide. *J Virol.* **69:** 7461-7471.

Satoh S, Tanji Y, Hijikata M, Kimura K, Shimotohno K, 1995, The N-terminal region of hepatitis C virus nonstructural protein 3 (NS3) is essential for stable complex formation with NS4A. *J Virol.* **69:** 4255-4260.

Schechter I, Berger A, 1967, On the size of the active site in proteases. I. Papain. *Biochem Biophys Res Commun.* **27:** 157-162.

Shimizu Y, Yamaji K, Masuho Y, Yokota T, Inoue H, Sudo K, Satoh S, Shimotohno K, 1996, Identification of the sequence on NS4A required for enhanced cleavage of the NS5A/5B site by hepatitis C virus NS3 protease. *J Virol.* **70:** 127-132.

Steinkuhler C, Biasiol G, Brunetti M, Urbani A, Koch U, Cortese R, Pessi A, De Francesco R, 1998, Product inhibition of the hepatitis C virus NS3 protease. *Biochemistry.* **37:** 8899-8905.

Steinkuhler C, Koch U, Narjes F, Matassa VG, 2001, Hepatitis C virus protease inhibitors: current progress and future challenges. *Curr Med Chem.* **8:** 919-932.

Stempniak M, Hostomska Z, Nodes BR, Hostomsky Z, 1997, The NS3 proteinase domain of hepatitis C virus is a zinc-containing enzyme. *J Virol.* **71:** 2881-2886.

Sudo K, Matsumoto Y, Matsushima M, Konno K, Shimotohno K, Shigeta S, Yokota T, 1997a, Novel hepatitis C virus protease inhibitors: 2,4,6-trihydroxy, 3-nitro-benzamide derivatives. *Antiviral Chem Chemother.* **8:** 541-544.

Sudo K, Matsumoto Y, Matsushima M, Konno K, Shimotohno K, Shigeta S, Yokota T, 1997b, Novel hepatitis C virus protease inhibitors: thiazolidine derivatives. *Biochem Biophys Res Commun.* **238:** 643-647.

Tanji Y, Hijikata M, Hirowatari Y, Shimotohno K, 1994, Hepatitis C virus polyprotein processing: kinetics and mutagenic analysis of serine proteinase-dependent cleavage. *J Virol.* **68:** 8418-8422.

Tellinghuisen TL, Marcotrigiano J, Rice CM, 2005, Structure of the zinc-binding domain of an essential component of the hepatitis C virus replicase. *Nature.* **435:** 374-379.

Thibeault D, Maurice R, Pilote L, amarre D, Pause A, 2001, In vitro characterization of a purified NS2/3 protease variant of hepatitis C virus. *J Biol Chem.* **276:** 46678-46684.

Thibeault D, Bousquet C, Gingras R, Lagace L, Maurice R, White PW, Lamarre D, 2004, Sensitivity of NS3 serine proteases from hepatitis C virus genotypes 2 and 3 to the inhibitor BILN 2061. *J Virol.* **78:** 7352-7359.

Tijms MA, van Dinten LC, Gorbalenya AE, Snijder EJ, 2001, A zinc finger-containing papain-like protease couples subgenomic mRNA synthesis to genome translation in a positive-stranded RNA virus *Proc Natl Acad Sci USA.* **98:** 1889-1894.

Tomei L, Failla C, Vitale RL, Bianchi E, De Francesco R, 1996, A central hydrophobic domain of the hepatitis C virus NS4A protein is necessary and sufficient for the activation of the NS3 protease. *J Gen Virol.* **77:** 1065-1070.

Varaklioti A, Vassilaki N, Georgopoulou U, Mavromara P, 2002, Alternate translation occurs within the core coding region of the hepatitis C viral genome. *J Biol Chem.* **277:** 17713-17721.

Walewski JL, Keller TR, Stump DD, Branch AD, 2001, Evidence for a new hepatitis C virus antigen encoded in an overlapping reading frame. *RNA* **7:** 710-21.

Wenzel M, Troxell J, Buckheit R, Huang M, 1999, Establishment of a cell based assay for evaluation of compounds against HCV NS2-3 protease activity. *Antivir Ther.* **4(Supplement):** A95.

Whitney M, Stack JH, Darke PL, Zheng W, Terzo J, Inglese J, Strulovici B, Kuo LC, Pollock BA, 2002, A collaborative screening program for the discovery of inhibitors of HCV NS2/3 cis-cleaving protease activity. *J Biomol Screen* **7:** 149-154.

WHO, 1997, Hepatitis C: Global prevalence. *Wkly Epidemiol Rec.* **72:** 341-344.

Wu Z, Yao N, Le VH, Weber P, 1998, Mechanism of autoproteolysis at the NS2-NS3 junction of the hepatitis C virus polyprotein. *Trends Biochem Sci.* **23:** 92-94.

Yan Y, Li Y, Munshi S, Sardana V, Cole JL, Sardana M, Steinkuehler C, Tomei L, De Francesco R, Kuo LC, Chen Z, 1998, Complex of NS3 protease and NS4a peptixe of BK strain hepatitis C virus: A 2.2 A resolution structure in a hexagonal crystal form. *Prot Sci.* **7:** 837-847.

Yao N, Reichert P, Taremi SS, Prosise WW, Weber PC, 1999, Molecular views of viral polyprotein processing revealed by the crystal structure of the hepatitis C virus bifunctional protease-helicase. *Structure.* **7:** 1353.

Yoneyama M, Kikuchi M, Natsukawa T, Shinobu N, Imaizumi T, Miyagishi M, Taira K, Akira S, Fujita T, 2004, The RNA helicase RIG-I has an essential function in double-stranded RNA-induced innate antiviral responses. *Nat Immunol.* **5:** 730-737.

Xu Z, Choi J, Yen TS, Lu W, Strohecker A, Govindarajan S, Chien D, Selby MJ, Ou J, 2001, Synthesis of a novel hepatitis C virus protein by ribosomal frameshift. *EMBO J.* **20:** 3840-3848.

Ziebuhr J, Snijder EJ, Gorbalenya AE, 2000, Virus-encoded proteinases and proteolytic processing in the Nidovirales. *J Gen Virol.* **81:** 853-879.

Chapter 8

Angiotensin Converting Enzyme in the Pathophysiology of Liver Fibrosis

Yao Hong Wei
Department of Pharmacology, School of Medicine, Zhejiang University, 353 Yan'an Road, Hangzhou 310031, the People's Republic of China.

1. INTRODUCTION

Hepatic fibrosis is a dynamic process caused by chronic liver injury due to various etiologies (hepatotropic viruses infection, alcohol abuse, and metal overload), eventually leading to cirrhosis. It is predominantly characterized by excessive accumulation of extracellular matrix (ECM) caused by both an increased synthesis and decreased or unbalanced degradation of ECM. In advanced stages, the liver contains approximately 6 times more ECM than normal, including collagens (I, III, and IV), fibronectin, undulin, elastin, laminin, hyaluronan, and proteoglycans. Decreased activity of ECM-removing MMPs is mainly due to an overexpression of their specific inhibitors (TIMPs). The accumulation of ECM proteins distorts the hepatic architecture by forming a fibrous scar, and the subsequent development of nodules of regenerating hepatocytes defines cirrhosis. Cirrhosis produces hepatocellular dysfunction and increased intrahepatic resistance to blood flow, which result in hepatic insufficiency and portal hypertension, respectively (Bhaskar 2004). However, the molecular bases for the development of liver fibrosis and subsequent portal hypertension are not entirely elucidated.

Molecular changes in liver tissue and their relation to liver fibrosis have been of particular interest in recent years. Because of the high incidence of liver cirrhosis in the general population (Karsan *et al* 2004) and the risk of portal hypertension/hepatocellular carcinoma, the investigation of the underlying basic pathophysiology is of great clinical importance. Studies have shown that activation of the renin-angiotensin system (RAS)

U. Lendeckel and Nigel M. Hooper (eds.), Proteases in Gastrointestinal Tissue, 183-207.

contributes to fibrotic changes in liver tissue. Angiotensin II (Ang II, or Ang 1-8) is thought to be responsible for most of the physiological and pathophysiological effects of the RAS, and angiotensin converting enzyme inhibitor (ACEI) that reduces the formation of Ang II has been highly successful in the management of hypertension, is standard therapy following myocardial infarction to delay the development of heart failure, and reduces the rate of progression of renal disease (Johnston 1994; Dzau 2001). Ang II has been also considered a potential mediator of liver fibrosis development, which is attenuated by ACEI or Ang II receptor blocker (Jonsson *et al* 2001; Paizis *et al* 2002; Tuncer *et al* 2003). Furthermore, Ang II could induce intrahepatic portal hypertension (Garcia-Pagan *et al* 1995). Enhancement of the adrenergic vasoconstrictor influence on the portal system (Goodfriend *et al* 1996), direct contractile influence on activated stellate cells, and sodium and fluid retention induced by stimulation of aldosterone secretion are possible mechanisms that contribute to the portal hypertensive effect of Ang II. Bradykinin, one of the substrates of angiotensin converting enzyme (ACE), may contribute to the protective effect of tissue fibrosis (Pawluczyk *et al* 2004). Therefore, blockade of the RAS by ACEI/Ang II receptor antagonists should be beneficial for prevention of hepatic fibrosis, and subsequent liver cirrhosis.

2. STUCTURE AND FUNCTION OF ACE

ACE (also known as peptidyl dipeptidase A, EC 3.4.15.1), which was first isolated in 1956, is a type-I membrane-anchored dipeptidyl carboxypeptidase that is essential for blood pressure regulation and electrolyte homeostasis through the RAS system. There are two isoforms of ACE that are transcribed from the same gene in a tissue-specific manner. In somatic tissues it exists as a glycoprotein composed of a single, large polypeptide chain of 1,277 amino acids, whereas in sperm cells it is a lower-molecular-mass glycoform of 701 amino acids.

ACE is present in many different cell types such as neuronal cells and renal proximal tubular cells. It is mostly found in endothelial cells. It is attached to the endothelial surface membrane by an anchor peptide and it can be cleaved and released into the blood circulation as soluble enzyme. In liver, ACE is also produced by cells of macrophage lineage, proliferating bile duct epithelial cells, and detected at the gene level in activated human hepatic stellate cells (HSCs) (Bataller *et al* 2001; Paizis *et al* 2002; Bataller *et al* 2003; Leung *et al* 2003). In bile duct ligation liver fibrosis, the levels of both ACE gene expression and activity were markedly up-regulated (Paizis *et al* 2002). Furthermore, increased hepatic ACE is mainly distributed in areas of bile ductular proliferation and active fibrogenesis following bile duct ligation.

As enzyme, ACE basically converts the decapeptide angiotensin I (Ang I or angiotensin 1-10) into the octapeptide Ang II through cleavage of the carboxyl terminal dipeptide histidyl-leucine. Furthermore, it also can inactivate bradykinin by proteolytic cleavage of a dipeptide moiety, and increase bradykinin level.

However the classical view of the RAS has been challenged by the discovery of the enzyme ACE2 (Donoghue *et al* 2000; Tipnis *et al* 2000), in addition to the increasing awareness that many angiotensin peptides other than Ang II have biological activity and physiological importance. ACE2 is described originally for its ability to generate angiotensin 1-9 (Ang 1-9) from Ang I (Donoghue *et al* 2000), it also degrades Ang II to the biologically active peptide, angiotensin 1-7 (Ang 1-7) (Oudit *et al* 2003). Indeed, the catalytic efficiency of ACE2 for Ang II is 400-fold greater than for Ang I (Vickers *et al* 2002), indicating that the major role for ACE2 is the conversion of Ang II to Ang 1-7. The potential role of Ang 1-7 as a cardioprotective peptide with vasodilator, anti-growth and anti-proliferative actions has been recognized (Ferrario *et al* 1997; Ferrario *et al* 2002). The data suggest that ACE2 might function to limit the vasoconstrictor action of Ang II through its inactivation, in addition to counteracting the actions of Ang II through the formation of the agonist, Ang 1-7. Interestingly, the in vitro enzymatic activity of ACE2 is unaffected by ACEI (Donoghue *et al* 2000; Tipnis *et al* 2000), but there are no data as to the effect of angiotensin receptor blockers on ACE2 activity.

The regulation of ACE2 on heart and kidney function is mediated by its Mas receptor, a G-protein-coupled receptor encoded by the MAS1 protooncogene (Santos *et al* 2003; Kostenis *et al* 2005). Recent study revealed that Mas could act as a physiological antagonist of the Ang II type 1 (AT1) receptor; mice lacking the Mas gene show enhanced Ang II-mediated vasoconstriction in mesenteric micro-vessels (Kostenis *et al* 2005). Therefore, the AT1-Mas complex could be of great importance as a target for pharmacological intervention in cardiovascular and renal diseases. Although an absence of cardiac fibrosis in ACE2-deficient hypertensive mice, a role of ACE2 in tissue fibrosis is not clear (Crackower *et al* 2002). Further investigation into function of ACE2 in tissue repair and remodeling of wild type animal is intriguing.

3. PATHOGENESIS OF LIVER FIBROSIS

Hepatic fibrosis is the result of the wound-healing response of the liver to repeated injury. After an acute liver injury, parenchymal cells regenerate and replace the necrotic or apoptotic cells. This process is associated with an inflammatory response and a limited deposition of ECM. If the hepatic injury persists, then eventually the liver regeneration fails, and hepatocytes are substituted with abundant ECM, including fibrillar collagen. As fibrotic liver diseases advance, disease progression from collagen bands to bridging fibrosis to frank cirrhosis occurs.

3.1 HSCs activation in liver fibrosis

HSCs are the main ECM-producing cells in the injured liver (Gabele *et al* 2003). In the normal liver, HSCs reside in the space of Disse and are the major storage sites of vitamin A. Following chronic injury, HSCs activate or transdifferentiate into myofibroblast-like cells, acquiring contractile, proinflammatory, and fibrogenic properties (Milani *et al* 1990; Marra 1999). Activated HSCs migrate and accumulate at the sites of tissue repair, secreting large amounts of ECM and regulating ECM degradation. Collagen synthesis in HSCs is regulated at the transcriptional and posttranscriptional levels (Lindquist *et al* 2000).

Interestingly, HSCs express a number of neuroendocrine markers (e.g., reelin, nestin, neurotrophins, synaptophysin, and glial-fibrillary acidic protein) and bear receptors for neurotransmitters (Geerts 2001; Oben *et al* 2003; Sato *et al* 2003). For example, HSCs contain catecholamine biosynthetic enzymes, release norepinephrine, and are growth-inhibited by adrenoceptor antagonists. In addition, HSCs from mice with reduced levels of norepinephrine grow poorly in culture and exhibit inhibited activation during liver injury. Finally, growth and injury-related fibrogenic responses are rescued by adrenoceptor agonists (Oben *et al* 2004). Thus, the development of liver fibrosis is regulated by neurotransmitters (i.e., sympathetic nervous system inhibitors may be novel therapies to improve the repair of damaged livers).

Hepatic cell types other than HSCs may also have fibrogenic potential. Myofibroblasts derived from small portal vessels proliferate around biliary tracts in cholestasis-induced liver fibrosis to initiate collagen deposition (Kinnman *et al* 2002; Magness *et al* 2004). HSCs and portal myofibroblasts differ in specific cell markers and response to apoptotic stimuli (Knittel *et al* 1999). The relative importance of each cell type in liver fibrogenesis may depend on the origin of the liver injury. While HSCs are the main fibrogenic cell type in pericentral areas, portal myofibroblasts may predominate when liver injury occurs around portal tracts. Culture of $CD34^{+}CD38^{-}$ hematopoietic stem cells with various growth factors has been shown to generate HSCs and myofibroblasts of bone marrow origin that infiltrate human livers undergoing tissue remodeling (Forbes *et al* 2004; Suskind *et al* 2004). These data indicate that cells originating in bone marrow can be a source of fibrogenic cells in the injured liver. Other potential sources of fibrogenic cells (i.e., epithelial-mesenchymal transition and circulating fibrocytes) have not been demonstrated in the liver (Kalluri *et al* 2003; Phillips *et al* 2004; Yao *et al* 2004).

A complex interplay among different hepatic cell types takes place during hepatic fibrogenesis. Hepatocytes are targets for most hepatotoxic agents, including hepatitis viruses, alcohol metabolites, and bile acids. Damaged hepatocytes release reactive oxygen species (ROS) and fibrogenic mediators, and induce the recruitment of white blood cells by inflammatory cells. Apoptosis of damaged hepatocytes stimulates the fibrogenic actions of liver myofibroblasts. Inflammatory cells, either lymphocytes or polymorphonuclear cells, activate HSCs to secrete collagen. HSCs activation is also influenced by paracrine cytokines (TNF-α, TGF-β, PDGF, etc) produced by Kupffer cells (KCs) in the initiation and perpetuation of its activation (Yao *et al* 2004). In the experimental liver injury, KCs infiltration precedes HSCs activation (Friedman 1995; Toda *et al* 2000). In vitro, exposure of HSCs soon after culture to conditioned medium from cultures of KCs accelerates the process of its activation, and enhances its proliferation and fibrogenesis (Yao *et al* 2004; Zhang *et al* 2004). Epithelial cells stimulate the accumulated portal myofibroblasts to initiate collagen deposition around damaged bile ducts in primary biliary cirrhosis and primary sclerosis cholangitis (Kinnman *et al* 2002). Moreover, activated HSCs secrete inflammatory chemokines, express cell adhesion molecules, and modulate the activation of inflammatory cells, which in turn facilitate its activation (Vinas *et al* 2003). Therefore, a vicious circle in which inflammatory and fibrogenic cells stimulate each other is likely to occur in liver fibrosis (Maher 2001).

In addition, the composition of the ECM can directly modulate HSCs proliferation and collagen synthesis. When cultured on plastic, HSCs activate (Yao *et al* 2004) similar to those activated in vivo following a fibrogenic stimulus. HSCs activation can be inhibited (at least delayed) and even partially reversed when the cells are cultured on a basement membrane-like substrate, namely Matrigel (Sohara *et al* 2002). Type IV collagen, fibrinogen, and urokinase type plasminogen activator stimulate resident HSCs by activating latent cytokines such as TGF-β1 (Gressner *et al* 2002). Fibrillar collagens can bind and stimulate HSCs via discoidin domain receptor DDR2 and integrins. Moreover, the altered ECM can serve as a reservoir for growth factors and MMPs (Olaso *et al* 2001).

3.2 Cytokines and chemokines involved in liver fibrosis

Cytokines regulating the inflammatory response to injury regulate hepatic fibrogenesis in vivo and in vitro (Marra 2002). Among pro-fibrotic growth factors, TGF-β1 appears to be a key mediator in liver fibrogenesis (Gressner *et al* 2002). In HSCs, TGF-β favors the transition to myofibroblast-like cells, stimulates the synthesis of ECM proteins, and inhibits their degradation. Strategies aimed at disrupting TGF-β1 synthesis and/or signaling pathways markedly decrease fibrosis in experimental models (Shek *et al* 2004). PDGF is also the most potent mitogen for HSCs and is upregulated in the fibrotic liver; its inhibition attenuates experimental liver fibrogenesis (Borkham-Kamphorst *et al* 2004). In addition to TGF-β1 and PDGF, other cytokines such as TNF-α, IL-1β, IL-6, and IL-13 are also important profibrotic mediators, inhibition and/or gene knockout of those cytokines attenuate the progress of liver fibrosis (Natsume *et al* 1999; Schwabe *et al* 2003; Kaviratne *et al* 2004; Sudo *et al* 2005).

In contrast to above-mentioned profibrotic cytokine, IL-10, IFN-γ, and IFN-α, which is anti-inflammatory cytokines, possess antifibrogenic properties by inhibiting HSCs activation, down-regulating profibrogenic cytokines and their intracellular signaling, and TIMP expression (Mallat *et al* 1995; Louis *et al* 1998; Song *et al* 2002; Inagaki *et al* 2003; Zhang *et al* 2004). However, a high production of IL-10 is observed in mice liver fibrosis chronically injected with Con A (Louis *et al* 2000). This may be viewed as a negative-feedback response of the immune system to avoid cell activation, proinflammatory cytokine production and tissue destruction.

Cytokines with vasoactive properties also regulate liver fibrogenesis. Vasodilator substances (e.g., nitric oxide, relaxin) exert antifibrotic effects while vasoconstrictors (e.g., norepinephrine, Ang II) have opposite effects (Williams *et al* 2001; Oben *et al* 2004). Endothelin-1, a powerful vasoconstrictor, stimulates fibrogenesis through its type A receptor (Cho *et al* 2000). Among vasoactive cytokines, Ang II seems to play a major role in liver fibrogenesis. Ang II is the effector peptide of the RAS, which is a major regulator of arterial pressure homeostasis in humans. In addition, Ang II induces hepatic inflammation and stimulates an array of fibrogenic actions in activated HSCs, including cell proliferation, cell migration, secretion of proinflammatory cytokines, and collagen synthesis (Bataller *et al* 2003; Bataller *et al* 2003) (see 4.2 section). Key components of RAS system are locally expressed in chronically injured livers, and activated HSCs de novo generate Ang II (Yoshiji *et al* 2001; Yoshiji *et al* 2002). Pharmacological and/or genetic ablation of Ang II markedly attenuates experimental liver fibrosis (Yoshiji *et al* 2001; Kanno *et al* 2003; Yao *et al* 2004).

Adipokines, which are cytokines mainly derived from the adipose tissue, regulate liver fibrogenesis. Leptin is required for HSCs activation and fibrosis development (Ikejima *et al* 2002; Marra 2002). In contrast, adiponectin markedly inhibits liver fibrogenesis in vitro and in vivo (Kamada *et al* 2003). The actions of these cytokines may explain why obesity influences fibrosis development (Ortiz *et al* 2002).

Chemokines stimulate key biological processes in HSCs such as activation, proliferation, and migration (Marra *et al* 1999; Schwabe *et al* 2003). These responses are required for the accumulation of activated HSCs at the sites of hepatic injury, a key feature in the hepatic wound healing response. HSCs are not only a target, they also can amplify inflammation through the release of chemokines including monocyte chemoattractant protein-1 (MCP-1), macrophage inflammatory protein-2 (MIP-2), cytokine-induced neutrophil chemoattractant/IL-8, and RANTES (Regulated upon Activation, Normal T-cell Expressed and Secreted), and are believed to contribute to the attraction of inflammatory cells into the injured liver (Maher *et al* 1998; Marra *et al* 1998; Friedman 2000; Schwabe *et al* 2003). Therefore, the chemokine system appears to affect fibrogenesis by regulating the cross-talk between HSCs and cells of the immune system to achieve a concerted cellular response during the hepatic wound healing process. However, it is unclear how chemokines expression by HSCs affects liver injury and whether inhibition of chemokines may be beneficial or can be compensated for by other chemokines.

3.3 Intracellular signaling of HSCs activation

Data on intracellular pathways regulating liver fibrogenesis are mainly derived from studies using cultured HSCs, while understanding of their role in vivo is progressing through experimental fibrogenesis studies using knockout mice. The classical model system to study HSCs activation is culturing quiescent HSCs on a plastic substrate following their isolation. However, molecular mechanism to initiate and perpetuate HSCs activation is not entirely understood. It is believed that the induction of transcription factors plays a pivotal role in this process. The expression of gene involving in fibrogenesis is characteristically controlled by transcription factors.

HSCs activation is associated with an unusual persistent activation of NF-κB. In most cells NF-κB is transiently activated; however following HSCs activation, NF-κB is persistently activated with a reduction in IκBα expression (Elsharkawy *et al* 1999). As a result, many NF-κB responsive genes including IL-6 and intercellular adhesion molecule 1 (ICAM-1) are constitutively expressed in the activated, but not in quiescent HSCs. The expression of NF-κB in liver tissue significantly increases in CCl_4-induced rats hepatic fibrosis (Yao *et al* 2004), and NF-κB plays an important role in the activated HSCs by protecting these cells against TNF-α-induced apoptosis (Lang *et al* 2000). However, studies have shown that NF-κB is not a key regulatory factor for HSCs activation since inhibiting NF-κB activation does not alter activated HSCs cellular morphology, α-SMA or collagen gene expression (Lang *et al* 2000). Furthermore, hepatic mRNA values of RelA, the main element of active NF-κB, correlate inversely with fibrosis progression ($r = 0.51$; $P < 0.04$), and NF-κB p65 inhibits transcription of the endogenous α1(I) collagen gene in HSCs (Rippe *et al* 1999; Boya *et al* 2001). Thus, a role of NF-κB in liver fibrogenesis needs further investigation.

AP-1 represents another family of transcription factors that shows increased and persistent activity in the activated HSCs. In addition to regulating MMP gene expression, AP-1 is also important in regulating other genes involved in matrix remodeling in the activated HSCs. JunD is the most important of the AP-1 proteins in the activated HSCs as it is required for both TIMP-1 and IL-6 gene expression (Smart *et al* 2001). Interestingly, a shift occurs during cellular activation in the expression patter of AP-1 proteins. Initially c-Fos, Fra1, c-Jun, and JunB are induced; however, these are replaced by persistent AP-1 activation involving Fra2, FosB, and JunD (Bahr *et al* 1999). This suggests that although AP-1 is important in controlling gene expression in the activated HSC, it probably is not a 'master controller' for HSCs activation.

Myocyte enhancer factor-2 (MEF-2) activation is critical for HSCs activation and maintenance of the activated HSCs phenotype (Wang *et al* 2004). MEF-2 expression closely parallels HSCs activation and when HSCs are induced to revert to the quiescent state by culture on Matrigel substrate, MEF-2 expression decreases. Using RNAi to induce sequence-specific RNA degradation resulting in a posttranscriptional inhibition of gene expression, the results showed that inhibiting MEF-2 expression reduced expression of genes associated with activated HSCs, including α-SMA and α1(I) collagen, and inhibits HSCs proliferation. Therefore, MEF-2, as a key nuclear mediator, may participate in the pathologic process of liver fibrogenesis in vivo.

HSCs activation is also associated with induction of the Kruppel-like transcription factor family, which includes Sp1, BTEB1, and KLF6. Each of these transcription factors increases expression of α1(I) collagen and TGF-β (Kim *et al* 1998; Ratziu *et al* 1998; Chen *et al* 2000). Members of the CCAAT/enhancer binding protein (C/EBP) family of transcription factors are also induced following HSCs activation and appear to be important in controlling gene expression of the α1(I) collagen gene (Greenwel *et al* 2000).

Although transcription factor activation plays a critical role at initiating and maintaining the activated state of HSCs, this event is probably not the primary event responsible for HSCs activation. Transcription factors are often activated following the stimulation of intracellular signaling cascades resulting in posttranslational modifications to existing proteins. Following HSCs activation stimulation of several intracellular signaling cascades have been described.

Extracellular-regulated kinase (ERK), which is stimulated in experimentally induced liver injury, mediates proliferation and migration of HSCs (Marra *et al* 1999). PDGF, a potent proliferative cytokine for HSCs, has been shown to activate MAPK signaling, specifically JNK, ERK, p38

MAPK. Both JNK and ERK activation induces HSCs proliferation. JNK regulates apoptosis of hepatocytes as well as the secretion of inflammatory cytokines by cultured HSCs (Schwabe *et al* 2001; Schwabe *et al* 2004). However, activation of p38 MAPK activity inhibits the proliferative response (Gabele *et al* 2003). Activation of JNK and ERK has been shown to stimulate binding activities of both AP-1 and STAT1 transcription factors to their cognate recognition sites (Marra *et al* 1995; Marra *et al* 1996). As described (Rippe *et al* 2004), MEF-2 activation is dependent on both ERK and p38 activity, thus demonstrating that further upstream events are necessary for transcription factor activation and subsequent transcriptional activities.

The TGF-β1-activated Smad signaling pathway stimulates experimental hepatic fibrosis and is a potential target for therapy (Schnabl *et al* 2001; Dooley *et al* 2003). Smad7 overexpression totally blocked TGF-β signal transduction, shown by inhibiting Smad2/3 phosphorylation and nuclear translocation of activated Smad complexes, resulting in decreased collagen I expression (Dooley *et al* 2003). Smad7 also abrogated TGF-β-dependent proliferation inhibition of HSCs. Gene transfer of Smad7 inhibits experimental liver fibrogenesis in vivo (Dooley *et al* 2003). Meanwhile, TGF-β also simulates MAPK signaling in HSCs, and eventually induces α1(I) collagen gene expression (Dooley *et al* 2001; Cao *et al* 2002). However, Smad and p38 MAPK signaling independently and additively regulate α1(I) collagen gene expression by transcriptional activation, whereas p38 MAPK and not Smad signaling increases alpha1(I) collagen mRNA stability (Tsukada *et al* 2005).

The focal adhesion kinase (FAK)-phosphatidylinositol 3-kinase (PI3K)-Akt-signaling pathway mediates agonist-induced fibrogenic actions in HSCs (Marra *et al* 1999). The expressions of FAK protein and mRNA are greatly increased in fibrotic rat livers (Jiang *et al* 2004). Inhibition of FAK activity blocks PDGF-induced activation of PI3K and Akt, HSCs migration, and cell attachment. Expression of type I collagen protein and α1(I) collagen mRNA in HSCs is increased by Akt activation and inhibited when PI3K activity is blocked (Reif *et al* 2003). The PI3K signaling pathway, stimulated following PDGF treatment in activated HSCs, leads to Akt and $p70^{S6}$ kinase activation resulting with increased HSCs proliferation and chemotaxis (Marra *et al* 1997; Reif *et al* 2003). Therefore, FAK-PI3K-Akt signaling pathway plays an important role in HSCs adhesion, migration, and collagen synthesis.

FAK is regulated by the Rho family of GTPases in response to adhesion in HSC. Because FAK is tyrosine phosphorylated in response to plating of HSCs on fibronectin, while a specific Rho-associated coiled-coil forming protein kinase (p160ROCK) inhibitor, Y-27632, treatment inhibits the tyrosine phosphorylation of FAK (Iwamoto *et al* 2000). Indeed, the small GTPase, Rho, is present in activated HSCs and that Rho and one of its targets, p160ROCK, signaling pathways play an important role in the activation of HSCs (Yee 1998; Kato *et al* 1999). A p160ROCK inhibitor influences activated HSCs behavior such as morphological alterations, proliferation, contraction, migration and Type 1 collagen production, and prevents the progress of liver fibrosis (Yee 1998; Iwamoto *et al* 2000; Murata *et al* 2001; Tada *et al* 2001). Thus, inhibition of the RhoA-p160ROCK pathway may be beneficial for the treatment of liver fibrogenesis by abolishing cell proliferation and collagen gene expression in HSCs.

Activation of NADPH oxidase by Ang II induces ROS in the activated HSCs with subsequent stimulation of HSCs genes (Bataller *et al* 2003). These actions are largely mediated by ROS generated by a nonphagocytic form of NADPH oxidase. Disruption of an active NADPH oxidase prevents HSCs activation by Ang II and protects mice from developing severe liver injury following prolonged alcohol intake and/or bile duct ligation (Kono *et al* 2000; Bataller *et al* 2003).

Peroxisome proliferator-activated receptor-γ (PPAR-γ) is a member of the steroid/thyroid hormone nuclear receptor superfamily. The PPAR pathway regulates HSCs activation and experimental liver fibrosis. Expression of PPAR-γ protein is dramatically reduced in HSCs activated both in vitro (Marra *et al* 2000; Miyahara *et al* 2000; Galli *et al* 2002). PPAR-γ agonists dose-dependently inhibit HSCs proliferation and MCP-1 at the gene and protein levels induced by PDGF and TGF-β, and attenuate liver fibrosis in vivo (Marra *et al* 2000; Galli *et al* 2002).

Recent studies suggest a role for intracellular pathways signaled by Toll-like receptors (TLR) and β-cathepsin in HSCs (Canbay *et al* 2003; Paik *et al* 2003). LPS directly acts through TLR4 and then activates NF-κB and JNK to induce proinflammatory chemokines (IL-8 and MCP-1) and adhesion molecules (ICAM-1 and VCAM-1) in activated human HSCs. Therefore, HSCs in addition to KCs may be a target for LPS-induced liver injury and provide a direct link between inflammatory and fibrotic liver injury.

In summary, a great deal of intracellular signals takes part in HSCs activation and subsequent liver fibrogenesis. Future studies will require careful and directed regulation of each signaling pathway in order to accurately assess its role in the HSCs activation process.

4. ACE IN THE PATHOPHYSIOLOGY OF LIVER FIBROSIS

As forementioned description, ACE mainly converts the decapeptide Ang I into the octapeptide Ang II, and inactivates circulating bradykinin. Therefore, the effect of ACE in liver fibrosis chiefly got involved in actions of Ang II and bradykinin.

A growing number of studies have suggested that Ang II plays an important role in liver fibrosis development, and treatment with Ang II inhibitor and/or receptor blocker dramatically attenuated liver fibrosis (Bataller *et al* 2000, 2003; Kono *et al* 2000; Wei *et al* 2001; Paizis *et al* 2002; Kanno *et al* 2003; Tuncer *et al* 2003; Rippe *et al* 2004; Yao *et al* 2004). Likewise, the kallikrein-kinin system is also involved in the development of tissue fibrosis and liver cirrhosis (Stewart *et al* 1972; Wong *et al* 1977; Wirth *et al* 1997; Cugno *et al* 2001).

4.1 ACE's changes and its inhibitor in liver fibrosis

ACE is known to be produced by cells of macrophage lineage and has been detected at the gene level in activated human HSCs (Bataller *et al* 2001; Bataller *et al* 2003). Hepatic inflammatory cells, activated stellate cells, or proliferating bile duct epithelial cells may be the possible sources of ACE in bile duct ligation liver fibrosis (Paizis *et al* 2002). The low baseline levels of both ACE gene expression and activity in the normal liver (Leung *et al* 2003) are markedly up-regulated in bile duct ligation rat liver (Paizis *et al* 2002). Increased hepatic ACE is mainly distributed in areas of bile ductular proliferation and active fibrogenesis following bile duct ligation. Clinical study revealed that approximately 30.0% of 151 patients with chronic alcoholism and alcoholic liver disease have elevated ACE levels (Borowsky *et al* 1982). The mean serum ACE level of those patients is elevated to (30.8 ± 13) U/mL compared with (22.8 ± 6) U/mL in control subjects. Abstinence from alcohol for 6 to 27 months by 11 patients is associated with persistently normal serum ACE levels. Likewise, the serum activity of ACE significantly increases in patients with cirrhosis compared with the activity of the same enzyme in healthy subjects (Huskic *et al* 1999). Therefore, ACE plays an important role in liver fibrosis. Inhibition of ACE results in regression or prevents the development of hepatic fibrosis in animal models (Jonsson *et al* 2001; Yoshiji *et al* 2001; Tuncer *et al* 2003; Yao *et al* 2004; Yoshiji *et al* 2005). As a result of ACE inhibition, the level of Ang II decreases, while bradykinin level increases (see 4.2, and 4.3 sections).

Besides increased bradykinin level, ACEI may potentiate the effects of bradykinin using mechanisms that are independent of their ability to inhibit ACE activity, per se. For example, ACEI can potentiate bradykinin activity in the presence of ACE-resistant bradykinin B2 receptor agonists (Hecker *et al* 1994). Furthermore, the bradykinin-potentiating effects of ACEI are not mimicked by the synthetic ACE substrate hippuryl-L-histidyl-L-leucine, which is as equally effective at blocking bradykinin catabolism as ACEI

(Bossaller *et al* 1992; Hecker *et al* 1994). Moreover, when B2 receptors are desensitized and no longer responsive to extra agonist, ACEI can reactivate B2 receptor-mediated signaling (Benzing *et al* 1999). Several possibilities may explain these phenomena. There is evidence to suggest that ACEI may exert their effect directly on the bradykinin-B2 receptor (Bossaller *et al* 1992; Hecker *et al* 1994), although ACEI binding to receptor is yet to be demonstrated. It has also been suggested that binding of ACEI to ACE results in a conformational change, which is transduced directly to the B2 receptor in a sort of ACE : B2 receptor "cross-talk" (Benzing *et al* 1999). It has been suggested that the variability in ACEI efficacy, as seen with different molecules of the same class, may be dependent on the ACEI's unique structural properties, which are able to facilitate bradykinin B2 receptor signaling (Hecker *et al* 1997).

4.2 Ang II in the pathophysiology of liver fibrosis

Blockade of Ang II can attenuate the development of hepatic fibrosis in animal models. In a rat model of pig serum-induced fibrosis, administration of perindopril and candesartan blocks hepatic fibrosis and decreases the expression of α-SMA, a maker of activated HSCs (Yoshiji *et al* 2001). In a rat bile duct ligation model, administration of captopril causes a decrease of TGF-β1 and collagen gene expression and delayes the progression of hepatic fibrosis (Jonsson *et al* 2001). Our in vivo experiments (Yao *et al* 2004) also demonstrated that captopril (100 $mg{\cdot}kg^{-1}$, ig) and losartan (2.5, 5, 10 $mg{\cdot}kg^{-1}$, ig) significantly attenuate the progress of liver fibrosis induced by CCl_4. However, irbesartan does not cause a significant reduction of matrix deposition in the liver, although it suppresses the overexpression of TGF-β1 and type I collagen gene (Paizis *et al* 2001). These conflicting findings can be attributed to differences in the method of fibrogenesis or in the drugs tested.

Activated human (Bataller *et al* 2000) and rat (Wei *et al* 2000) HSCs express AT1 receptors. Ang II can induce contraction and proliferation of HSCs, but not quiescent HSCs (Bataller *et al* 2000); the interaction of Ang II with its AT1 receptor plays a pivotal role in the development of liver fibrosis through the activation of HSCs (Yoshiji *et al* 2001). The exact reason why Ang II acts only on activated HSCs, but not on quiescent HSCs is not clear. It may be a result of either the machinery required for cell contraction or the absence of AT1 receptor in quiescent HSCs. Ang II could induce a marked dose-dependent increase in intracellular calcium concentration ($[Ca^{2+}]_i$) and cell contraction of activated HSCs (Bataller *et al* 2000). The increase in $[Ca^{2+}]_i$ is largely dependent on the entrance of Ca^{2+} through L-type Ca^{2+} channels (Bataller *et al* 1998). It has been shown that there is a lack of these L-type Ca^{2+} channels in quiescent HSCs and their up-regulation after HSCs activation (Itatsu *et al* 1998). The results suggest that activated HSCs are targets of the action of Ang II in the intrahepatic circulation.

TIMP-1 level is markedly up-regulated both in humans and murine fibrosis models (Iredale 1997). TIMP-1 significantly promotes the development of liver fibrosis in a transgenic mouse model (Yoshiji *et al* 2000). In a rat model of reversible liver fibrosis, matrix remodeling and resolution of liver fibrosis are closely associated with a marked decrease in TIMP-1 expression (Iredale *et al* 1998). TIMP-1 expression is significantly increased by Ang II in activated HSCs in a time- and dose-dependent manner. The suppression of Ang II by perindopril significantly attenuates liver fibrosis development in association with TIMP-1 inhibition and HSCs activation. TIMP-1 mRNA upregulation by Ang II is abolished by candesartan and the PKC inhibitor, LY333531 in a dose-dependent manner (Yoshiji *et al* 2003). Therefore, Ang II induces the TIMP-1 through PKC signaling pathway in rat liver fibrosis development.

NADPH oxidase mediates the actions of Ang II on HSCs and plays a critical role in liver fibrogenesis (Bataller *et al* 2003; Arteel 2004). Ang II phosphorylates $p47^{phox}$, a regulatory subunit of NADPH oxidase, and induces ROS formation via NADPH oxidase activity. An increase of DNA synthesis, cell migration, procollagen α1(I) mRNA expression, and secretion of TGF-β1 and inflammatory cytokines (IL-8 and MCP-1) in human HSCs stimulated with Ang II are attenuated by N-acetylcysteine and diphenylene iodonium, an NADPH oxidase inhibitor. HSCs isolated from $p47^{phox-/-}$ mice display a blunted response to Ang II compared with wild type cells. After bile duct ligation, $p47^{phox-/-}$ mice show attenuated liver injury and fibrosis compared with wild type counterparts. Moreover, the expression of α-SMA and TGF-beta1 is reduced in $p47^{phox-/-}$ mice.

Recent studies have reported that AT1 receptor is also expressed in hepatic KCs, and Ang II stimulates mRNA expression of TGF-β and fibronectin in hepatic KCs (Leung *et al* 2003). Losartan or saralasin markedly decrease the mRNA expression of fibronectin and TNF-α and TGF-β1 levels in culture supernatants of KCs stimulated with Ang II (Leung *et al* 2003; Yao *et al* 2004). Therefore, Ang II is involved in the liver fibrotic process because of its role as a pro-inflammatory cytokine, the interaction of Ang II and AT1 receptor in hepatic KCs is one of the important regulatory pathways in the development of liver fibrosis.

Except for HSCs and hepatic KCs, AT1 receptor is also expressed in hepatic mast cells in the bile duct-ligation model of rats hepatic fibrogenesis (Paizis *et al* 2002). Studies into the role of mast cells in hepatic fibrosis are limited, but mast cell infiltration and hyperplasia were obvious in a variety of experimental models of rat liver fibrosis (Armbrust *et al* 1997; Gaca *et al* 1999). Mast cells are themselves capable of secreting TGF-β1 and producing extracellular matrix components (Thompson *et al* 1991; Gordon *et al* 1994).

However, the action and downstream cascade of AT1 receptor in mast cells, particularly in the course of liver fibrosis, were unclear, and require further investigation.

Angiogenesis is an essential process in many pathological events, such as tumor growth, and even in liver fibrogenesis (Yoshiji *et al* 2002; Vogten *et al* 2004). In experimental liver fibrogenesis, VEGF receptor expression increases in the liver. VEGF receptor-1 neutralizing monoclonal antibody (mAb) and VEGF receptor-2 mAb treatment significantly attenuate the development of fibrosis associated with the suppression of neovascularization in the liver (Yoshiji *et al* 2002). In addition, the progression of fibrosis can be inhibited by anti-angiogenic agents (TNP-470 and angiostatin) (Wang *et al* 2000; Vogten *et al* 2004). Ang II, a peptide hormone, has been shown to induce neovascularization and enhance vessel density in experimental systems. Pro-angiogenesis of Ang II is partially mediated by potentiating the expression of VEGF in endothelial cells (Rizkalla *et al* 2003; Imanishi *et al* 2004). Therefore, inhibition of Ang II, such as ACEI and AT1 receptor blocker, would be an alternative new strategy for the treatment of liver fibrosis through inhibiting neovascularization.

The progression of hepatic fibrosis often leads to cirrhosis and is associated with liver cancer. Classically, it has been considered the vasoconstrictor action of Ang II on the postsinusoidal venules that leads to an increase in hepatic portal pressure (Arroyo *et al* 1981). Administration of Ang II increases intrahepatic pressure in experimental and human cirrhosis while AT1 receptor blocker abrogates the effect of Ang II (Rockey *et al* 1996; Schneider *et al* 1999; Yang *et al* 2002). The effect of Ang II receptor blockade in cirrhotic patients is controversial. In cirrhotic patients receiving Ang II receptor blocker showed a decrease in portal pressure associated with a fall in arterial pressure (Gonzalez-Abraldes *et al* 2001; Schepke *et al* 2001; Debernardi-Venon *et al* 2002). In contrast, losartan induces a significant reduction in portal pressure without affecting the arterial pressure (Schneider *et al* 1999). The discrepant results of losartan remained to be elucidated. Therefore, the clinical use of ACEI or Ang II receptor blockers in cirrhotic patients must be very cautious.

4.3 Bradykinin in the pathophysiology of liver fibrosis

ACE also catalyzes the degradation of bradykinin (Regoli *et al* 1980) except inhibits Ang II production, it is thought that ACEI may exert their beneficial actions by partially protecting endogenously produced bradykinin from degradation. In vitro studies (Pawluczyk *et al* 2004) showed addition of exogenous bradykinin to macrophage-conditioned medium-treated mesangial cells results in a (22.5 ± 1.4) % ($P < 0.02$) reduction in secreted fibronectin levels. However, bradykinin levels are significantly reduced in culture supernatants of mesangial cells treated with perindoprilat, results which are contrary to what might have been expected following inhibition of bradykinin catabolism. These paradoxical observations may be explained when increased ligation to an increased number of bradykinin B2 receptors is taken into account, because bradykinin B2 receptor expression is up regulated by (71 ± 30)% in response to perindoprilat treatment (P = 0.032). Moreover, the bradykinin B2 receptor antagonist HOE 140 reverses the perindoprilat-mediated reduction in mesangial cell fibronectin levels. The results indicated that ACEI -induced renoprotection is mediated, at least in part, via the actions of bradykinin. Transgenic rats overexpressing increased endogenous bradykinin exhibited reduced interstitial fibrosis in the unilateral ureteral obstruction model of renal injury. Furthermore, genetic manipulation or pharmacologic blockade of the bradykinin B2 receptor increases interstitial fibrosis. The increased interstitial fibrosis in bradykinin B2 receptor genetic ablation mice is accompanied by reduced activity of plasminogen activators and MMP-2 (Schanstra *et al* 2002), suggesting that the protective effects of bradykinin involve activation of a B2 receptor/PA/MMP-2 cascade. These results indicate bradykinin would be beneficial to preventing the development of renal fibrosis. However, bradykinin plays a positive role in vascular smooth muscle cells fibrosis (Douillet *et al* 2000). It increases α2 chain of type I collagen mRNA levels, α2 chain of type I collagen promoter activity, and TIMP-1 production via autocrine activation of TGF-β1 in vascular smooth muscle cells. In addition, the MAPK pathway may be responsible for bradykinin signals mediating the production of α2 chain of type I collagen and TIMP-1. The different results of bradykinin on tissue fibrosis remained to be clarified.

The action of bradykinin on liver fibrosis is unclear at the present time. Further understanding of the cellular and molecular mechanisms by which bradykinin might modulate liver fibrosis could lead to the development of new strategies for intervention and treatment of this diseases.

5. CONCLUSION

The pathophysiological mechanisms of liver fibrosis are very complex. Among these, the activation of ACE seems to play an important role in the development of hepatic fibrosis. Inhibition of ACE promotes regression or prevents the development of hepatic fibrosis though lowering Ang II and elevating bradykinin. Aside from those, ACEI may strengthen the effects of bradykinin, which are independent of their ability to inhibit ACE activity. Therefore, ACEI is a promising new agent for the treatment of liver fibrosis.

Blockade of the RAS system by ACEI should be beneficial for improvement of fluid and salt secretion and reduce portal pressure in cirrhotic patients. However, concerns have been raised about their safety because of arterial hypotension and deterioration of renal function. Evaluation of the above studies is difficult because most were neither placebo controlled nor randomized (Vlachogiannakos *et al* 2001). Furthermore, as patient characteristics differed considerably between studies (for example, Child-Pugh class, presence of ascites, salt restriction, use of diuretics, and renal function impairment) it is difficult to make comparisons. Further investigation along these lines may prove to be very exciting.

REFERENCES

Armbrust T, Batusic D, Ringe B, Ramadori G, 1997, Mast cells distribution in human liver disease and experimental rat liver fibrosis. Indications for mast cell participation in development of liver fibrosis. *J Hepatol.* **26:** 1042-1054.

Arroyo V, Bosch J, Mauri M, Ribera F, Navarro-Lopez F, Rodes J, 1981, Effect of angiotensin-II blockade on systemic and hepatic haemodynamics and on the renin-angiotensin-aldosterone system in cirrhosis with ascites. *Eur J Clin Invest.* **11:** 221-229.

Arteel GE, 2004, "HOPE" for the liver? Mechanistic insight into the role of the renin-angiotensin system in hepatic fibrosis. *Hepatology.* **40:** 263-265.

Bahr MJ, Vincent KJ, Arthur MJ, Fowler AV, Smart DE, Wright MC, Clark IM, Benyon RC, Iredale JP, Mann DA, 1999, Control of the tissue inhibitor of metalloproteinases-1 promoter in culture-activated rat hepatic stellate cells: regulation by activator protein-1 DNA binding proteins. *Hepatology.* **29:** 839-848.

Bataller R, Nicolas JM, Ginees P, Gorbig MN, Garcia-Ramallo E, Lario S, Tobias E, Pinzani M, Thomas AP, Arroyo V, Rodes J, 1998, Contraction of human hepatic stellate cells activated in culture: a role for voltage-operated calcium channels. *J Hepatol.* **29:** 398-408.

Bataller R, Gines P, Nicolas JM, Gorbig MN, Garcia-Ramallo E, Gasull X, Bosch J, Arroyo V, Rodes J, 2000, Angiotensin II induces contraction and proliferation of human hepatic stellate cells. *Gastroenterology.* **118:** 1149-1156.

Bataller R, Gines P, Lora JM, Sole M, Nicolas JM, Jimenez W, Arroyo V, Rodes J, 2001, Evidence for a local renin-angiotensin systemin human liver: expression in activated hepatic stellate cells (abstr). *Hepatology.* **34:** 908.

Bataller R, Gabele E, Schoonhoven R, Morris T, Lehnert M, Yang L, Brenner DA, Rippe RA, 2003, Prolonged infusion of angiotensin II into normal rats induces stellate cell activation and proinflammatory events in liver. *Am J Physiol Gastrointest Liver Physiol.* **285:** G642-651.

Bataller R, Sancho-Bru P, Gines P, Lora JM, Al-Garawi A, Sole M, Colmenero J, Nicolas JM, Jimenez W, Weich N, Gutierrez-Ramos JC, Arroyo V, Rodes J, 2003, Activated human hepatic stellate cells express the renin-angiotensin system and synthesize angiotensin II. *Gastroenterology.* **125:** 117-125.

Bataller R, Schwabe RF, Choi YH, Yang L, Paik YH, Lindquist J, Qian T, Schoonhoven R, Hagedorn CH, Lemasters JJ, Brenner DA, 2003, NADPH oxidase signal transduces angiotensin II in hepatic stellate cells and is critical in hepatic fibrosis. *J Clin Invest.* **112:** 1383-1394.

Benzing T, Fleming I, Blaukat A, Muller-Esterl W, Busse R, 1999, Angiotensin-converting enzyme inhibitor ramiprilat interferes with the sequestration of the B2 kinin receptor within the plasma membrane of native endothelial cells. *Circulation.* **99:** 2034-2040.

Bhaskar ME, 2004, Management of cirrhosis and ascites. *N Engl J Med.* **351:** 300-301; author reply 300-301.

Borkham-Kamphorst E, Stoll D, Gressner AM, Weiskirchen R, 2004, Antisense strategy against PDGF B-chain proves effective in preventing experimental liver fibrogenesis. *Biochem Biophys Res Commun.* **321:** 413-423.

Borowsky SA, Lieberman J, Strome S, Sastre A, 1982, Elevation of serum angiotensin-converting enzyme level. Occurrence in alcoholic liver disease. *Arch Intern Med.* **142:** 893-895.

Bossaller C, Auch-Schwelk W, Grafe M, Graf K, Baumgarten C, Fleck E, 1992, Effects of converting enzyme inhibition on endothelial bradykinin metabolism and endothelium-dependent vascular relaxation. *Agents Actions Suppl.* **38 (Pt 3):** 171-177.

Boya P, Larrea E, Sola I, Majano PL, Jimenez C, Civeira MP, Prieto J, 2001, Nuclear factor-kappa B in the liver of patients with chronic hepatitis C: decreased RelA expression is associated with enhanced fibrosis progression. *Hepatology.* **34:** 1041-1048.

Canbay A, Guicciardi ME, Higuchi H, Feldstein A, Bronk SF, Rydzewski R, Taniai M, Gores GJ, 2003, Cathepsin B inactivation attenuates hepatic injury and fibrosis during cholestasis. *J Clin Invest.* **112:** 152-159.

Cao Q, Mak KM, Lieber CS, 2002, DLPC decreases TGF-beta1-induced collagen mRNA by inhibiting p38 MAPK in hepatic stellate cells. *Am J Physiol Gastrointest Liver Physiol.* **283:** G1051-1061.

Chen A, Davis BH, 2000, The DNA binding protein BTEB mediates acetaldehyde-induced, jun N-terminal kinase-dependent alphaI(I) collagen gene expression in rat hepatic stellate cells. *Mol Cell Biol.* **20:** 2818-2826.

Cho JJ, Hocher B, Herbst H, Jia JD, Ruehl M, Hahn EG, Riecken EO, Schuppan D, 2000, An oral endothelin-A receptor antagonist blocks collagen synthesis and deposition in advanced rat liver fibrosis. *Gastroenterology.* **118:** 1169-1178.

Crackower MA, Sarao R, Oudit GY, Yagil C, Kozieradzki I, Scanga SE, Oliveira-dos-Santos AJ, da Costa J, Zhang L, Pei Y, Scholey J, Ferrario CM, Manoukian AS, Chappell MC, Backx PH, Yagil Y, Penninger JM, 2002, Angiotensin-converting enzyme 2 is an essential regulator of heart function. *Nature.* **417:** 822-828.

Cugno M, Salerno F, Nussberger J, Bottasso B, Lorenzano E, Agostoni A, 2001, Bradykinin in the ascitic fluid of patients with liver cirrhosis. *Clin Sci (Lond).* **101:** 651-657.

Debernardi-Venon W, Barletti C, Alessandria C, Marzano A, Baronio M, Todros L, Saracco G, Repici A, Rizzetto M, 2002, Efficacy of irbesartan, a receptor selective antagonist of angiotensin II, in reducing portal hypertension. *Dig Dis Sci.* **47:** 401-404.

Donoghue M, Hsieh F, Baronas E, Godbout K, Gosselin M, Stagliano N, Donovan M, Woolf B, Robison K, Jeyaseelan R, Breitbart RE, Acton S, 2000, A novel angiotensin-converting enzyme-related carboxypeptidase (ACE2) converts angiotensin I to angiotensin 1-9. *Circ Res.* **87:** E1-9.

Dooley S, Streckert M, Delvoux B, Gressner AM, 2001, Expression of Smads during in vitro transdifferentiation of hepatic stellate cells to myofibroblasts. *Biochem Biophys Res Commun.* **283:** 554-562.

Dooley S, Hamzavi J, Breitkopf K, Wiercinska E, Said HM, Lorenzen J, Ten Dijke P, Gressner AM, 2003, Smad7 prevents activation of hepatic stellate cells and liver fibrosis in rats. *Gastroenterology.* **125:** 178-191.

Douillet CD, Velarde V, Christopher JT, Mayfield RK, Trojanowska ME, Jaffa AA, 2000, Mechanisms by which bradykinin promotes fibrosis in vascular smooth muscle cells: role of TGF-beta and MAPK. *Am J Physiol Heart Circ Physiol.* **279:** H2829-2837.

Dzau VJ, 2001, Theodore Cooper Lecture: Tissue angiotensin and pathobiology of vascular disease: a unifying hypothesis. *Hypertension.* **37:** 1047-1052.

Elsharkawy AM, Wright MC, Hay RT, Arthur MJ, Hughes T, Bahr MJ, Degitz K, Mann DA, 1999, Persistent activation of nuclear factor-kappaB in cultured rat hepatic stellate cells involves the induction of potentially novel Rel-like factors and prolonged changes in the expression of IkappaB family proteins. *Hepatology.* **30:** 761-769.

Ferrario CM, Chappell MC, Tallant EA, Brosnihan KB, Diz DI, 1997, Counterregulatory actions of angiotensin-(1-7). *Hypertension.* **30:** 535-541.

Ferrario CM, Averill DB, Brosnihan KB, Chappell MC, Iskandar SS, Dean RH, Diz DI, 2002, Vasopeptidase inhibition and Ang-(1-7) in the spontaneously hypertensive rat. *Kidney Int.* **62:** 1349-1357.

Forbes SJ, Russo FP, Rey V, Burra P, Rugge M, Wright NA, Alison MR, 2004, A significant proportion of myofibroblasts are of bone marrow origin in human liver fibrosis. *Gastroenterology.* **126:** 955-963.

Friedman SL, 1995, Parenchymal Fe and collagen gene expression: an iron-clad association? *Hepatology.* **21:** 1197-1199.

Friedman SL, 2000, Molecular regulation of hepatic fibrosis, an integrated cellular response to tissue injury. *J Biol Chem.* **275:** 2247-2250.

Gabele E, Brenner DA, Rippe RA, 2003, Liver fibrosis: signals leading to the amplification of the fibrogenic hepatic stellate cell. *Front Biosci.* **8:** d69-77.

Gaca MD, Pickering JA, Arthur MJ, Benyon RC, 1999, Human and rat hepatic stellate cells produce stem cell factor: a possible mechanism for mast cell recruitment in liver fibrosis. *J Hepatol.* **30:** 850-858.

Galli A, Crabb DW, Ceni E, Salzano R, Mello T, Svegliati-Baroni G, Ridolfi F, Trozzi L, Surrenti C, Casini A, 2002, Antidiabetic thiazolidinediones inhibit collagen synthesis and hepatic stellate cell activation in vivo and in vitro. *Gastroenterology.* **122:** 1924-1940.

Garcia-Pagan JC, Bosch J, Rodes J, 1995, The role of vasoactive mediators in portal hypertension. *Semin Gastrointest Dis.* **6:** 140-147.

Geerts A, 2001, History, heterogeneity, developmental biology, and functions of quiescent hepatic stellate cells. *Semin Liver Dis.* **21:** 311-335.

Gonzalez-Abraldes J, Albillos A, Banares R, Del Arbol LR, Moitinho E, Rodriguez C, Gonzalez M, Escorsell A, Garcia-Pagan JC, Bosch J, 2001, Randomized comparison of long-term losartan versus propranolol in lowering portal pressure in cirrhosis. *Gastroenterology.* **121:** 382-388.

Goodfriend TL, Elliott ME, Catt KJ, 1996, Angiotensin receptors and their antagonists. *N Engl J Med.* **334:** 1649-1654.

Gordon JR, Galli SJ, 1994, Promotion of mouse fibroblast collagen gene expression by mast cells stimulated via the Fc epsilon RI. Role for mast cell-derived transforming growth factor beta and tumor necrosis factor alpha. *J Exp Med.* **180:** 2027-2037.

Greenwel P, Dominguez-Rosales JA, Mavi G, Rivas-Estilla AM, Rojkind M, 2000, Hydrogen peroxide: a link between acetaldehyde-elicited alpha1(I) collagen gene up-regulation and oxidative stress in mouse hepatic stellate cells. *Hepatology.* **31:** 109-116.

Gressner AM, Weiskirchen R, Breitkopf K, Dooley S, 2002, Roles of TGF-beta in hepatic fibrosis. *Front Biosci.* **7:** d793-807.

Hecker M, Porsti I, Bara AT, Busse R, 1994, Potentiation by ACE inhibitors of the dilator response to bradykinin in the coronary microcirculation: interaction at the receptor level. *Br J Pharmacol.* **111:** 238-244.

Hecker M, Blaukat A, Bara AT, Muller-Esterl W, Busse R, 1997, ACE inhibitor potentiation of bradykinin-induced venoconstriction. *Br J Pharmacol.* **121:** 1475-1481.

Huskic J, Kulenovic H, Kardum D, Babic N, Knezevic Z, 1999, [Serum angiotensin converting enzyme in patients with primary liver carcinoma]. *Med Arh.* **53:** 61-63.

Ikejima K, Takei Y, Honda H, Hirose M, Yoshikawa M, Zhang YJ, Lang T, Fukuda T, Yamashina S, Kitamura T, Sato N, 2002, Leptin receptor-mediated signaling regulates hepatic fibrogenesis and remodeling of extracellular matrix in the rat. *Gastroenterology.* **122:** 1399-1410.

Imanishi T, Hano T, Nishio I, 2004, Angiotensin II potentiates vascular endothelial growth factor-induced proliferation and network formation of endothelial progenitor cells. *Hypertens Res.* **27:** 101-108.

Inagaki Y, Nemoto T, Kushida M, Sheng Y, Higashi K, Ikeda K, Kawada N, Shirasaki F, Takehara K, Sugiyama K, Fujii M, Yamauchi H, Nakao A, de Crombrugghe B, Watanabe T, Okazaki I, 2003, Interferon alfa down-regulates collagen gene transcription and suppresses experimental hepatic fibrosis in mice. *Hepatology.* **38:** 890-899.

Iredale JP, 1997, Tissue inhibitors of metalloproteinases in liver fibrosis. *Int J Biochem Cell Biol.* **29:** 43-54.

Iredale JP, Benyon RC, Pickering J, McCullen M, Northrop M, Pawley S, Hovell C, Arthur MJ, 1998, Mechanisms of spontaneous resolution of rat liver fibrosis. Hepatic stellate cell apoptosis and reduced hepatic expression of metalloproteinase inhibitors. *J Clin Invest.* **102:** 538-549.

Itatsu T, Oide H, Watanabe S, Tateyama M, Ochi R, Sato N, 1998, Alcohol stimulates the expression of L-type voltage-operated Ca2+ channels in hepatic stellate cells. *Biochem Biophys Res Commun.* **251:** 533-537.

Iwamoto H, Nakamuta M, Tada S, Sugimoto R, Enjoji M, Nawata H, 2000, A p160ROCK-specific inhibitor, Y-27632, attenuates rat hepatic stellate cell growth. *J Hepatol.* **32:** 762-770.

Jiang HQ, Zhang XL, Liu L, Yang CC, 2004, Relationship between focal adhesion kinase and hepatic stellate cell proliferation during rat hepatic fibrogenesis. *World J Gastroenterol.* **10:** 3001-3005.

Johnston CI, 1994, Tissue angiotensin converting enzyme in cardiac and vascular hypertrophy, repair, and remodeling. *Hypertension.* **23:** 258-268.

Jonsson JR, Clouston AD, Ando Y, Kelemen LI, Horn MJ, Adamson MD, Purdie DM, Powell EE, 2001, Angiotensin-converting enzyme inhibition attenuates the progression of rat hepatic fibrosis. *Gastroenterology.* **121:** 148-155.

Kalluri R, Neilson EG, 2003, Epithelial-mesenchymal transition and its implications for fibrosis. *J Clin Invest.* **112:** 1776-1784.

Kamada Y, Tamura S, Kiso S, Matsumoto H, Saji Y, Yoshida Y, Fukui K, Maeda N, Nishizawa H, Nagaretani H, Okamoto Y, Kihara S, Miyagawa J, Shinomura Y, Funahashi T,Matsuzawa Y, 2003, Enhanced carbon tetrachloride-induced liver fibrosis in mice lacking adiponectin. *Gastroenterology.* **125:** 1796-1807.

Kanno K, Tazuma S, Chayama K, 2003, AT1A-deficient mice show less severe progression of liver fibrosis induced by CCl(4). *Biochem Biophys Res Commun.* **308:** 177-183.

Karsan HA, Rojter SE, Saab S, 2004, Primary prevention of cirrhosis. Public health strategies that can make a difference. *Postgrad Med.* **115:** 25-30.

Kato M, Iwamoto H, Higashi N, Sugimoto R, Uchimura K, Tada S, Sakai H, Nakamuta M, Nawata H, 1999, Role of Rho small GTP binding protein in the regulation of actin cytoskeleton in hepatic stellate cells. *J Hepatol.* **31:** 91-99.

Kaviratne M, Hesse M, Leusink M, Cheever AW, Davies SJ, McKerrow JH, Wakefield LM, Letterio JJ, Wynn TA, 2004, IL-13 activates a mechanism of tissue fibrosis that is completely TGF-beta independent. *J Immunol.* **173:** 4020-4029.

Kim Y, Ratziu V, Choi SG, Lalazar A, Theiss G, Dang Q, Kim SJ, Friedman SL, 1998, Transcriptional activation of transforming growth factor beta1 and its receptors by the Kruppel-like factor Zf9/core promoter-binding protein and Sp1. Potential mechanisms for autocrine fibrogenesis in response to injury. *J Biol Chem.* **273:** 33750-33758.

Kinnman N, Housset C, 2002, Peribiliary myofibroblasts in biliary type liver fibrosis. *Front Biosci.* **7:** d496-503.

Knittel T, Kobold D, Piscaglia F, Saile B, Neubauer K, Mehde M, Timpl R, Ramadori G, 1999, Localization of liver myofibroblasts and hepatic stellate cells in normal and diseased rat livers: distinct roles of (myo-)fibroblast subpopulations in hepatic tissue repair. *Histochem Cell Biol.* **112:** 387-401.

Kono H, Rusyn I, Yin M, Gabele E, Yamashina S, Dikalova A, Kadiiska MB, Connor HD, Mason RP, Segal BH, Bradford BU, Holland SM, Thurman RG, 2000, NADPH oxidase-derived free radicals are key oxidants in alcohol-induced liver disease. *J Clin Invest.* **106:** 867-872.

Kostenis E, Milligan G, Christopoulos A, Sanchez-Ferrer CF, Heringer-Walther S, Sexton PM, Gembardt F, Kellett E, Martini L, Vanderheyden P, Schultheiss HP, Walther T, 2005, G-Protein-Coupled Receptor Mas Is a Physiological Antagonist of the Angiotensin II Type 1 Receptor. *Circulation.*

Lang A, Schoonhoven R, Tuvia S, Brenner DA, Rippe RA, 2000, Nuclear factor kappaB in proliferation, activation, and apoptosis in rat hepatic stellate cells. *J Hepatol.* **33:** 49-58.

Leung PS, Suen PM, Ip SP, Yip CK, Chen G, Lai PB, 2003, Expression and localization of AT1 receptors in hepatic Kupffer cells: its potential role in regulating a fibrogenic response. *Regul Pept.* **116:** 61-69.

Lindquist JN, Marzluff WF, Stefanovic B, 2000, Fibrogenesis. III. Posttranscriptional regulation of type I collagen. *Am J Physiol Gastrointest Liver Physiol.* **279:** G471-476.

Louis H, Van Laethem JL, Wu W, Quertinmont E, Degraef C, Van den Berg K, Demols A, Goldman M, Le Moine O, Geerts A, Deviere J, 1998, Interleukin-10 controls neutrophilic infiltration, hepatocyte proliferation, and liver fibrosis induced by carbon tetrachloride in mice. *Hepatology.* **28:** 1607-1615.

Louis H, Le Moine A, Quertinmont E, Peny MO, Geerts A, Goldman M, Le Moine O, Deviere J, 2000, Repeated concanavalin A challenge in mice induces an interleukin 10-producing phenotype and liver fibrosis. *Hepatology.* **31:** 381-390.

Magness ST, Bataller R, Yang L, Brenner DA, 2004, A dual reporter gene transgenic mouse demonstrates heterogeneity in hepatic fibrogenic cell populations. *Hepatology.* **40:** 1151-1159.

Maher JJ, Lozier JS, Scott MK, 1998, Rat hepatic stellate cells produce cytokine-induced neutrophil chemoattractant in culture and in vivo. *Am J Physiol.* **275:** G847-853.

Maher JJ, 2001, Interactions between hepatic stellate cells and the immune system. *Semin Liver Dis.* **21:** 417-426.

Mallat A, Preaux AM, Blazejewski S, Rosenbaum J, Dhumeaux D, Mavier P, 1995, Interferon alfa and gamma inhibit proliferation and collagen synthesis of human Ito cells in culture. *Hepatology.* **21:** 1003-1010.

Marra F, Pinzani M, DeFranco R, Laffi G, Gentilini P, 1995, Involvement of phosphatidylinositol 3-kinase in the activation of extracellular signal-regulated kinase by PDGF in hepatic stellate cells. *FEBS Lett.* **376:** 141-145.

Marra F, Choudhury GG, Abboud HE, 1996, Interferon-gamma-mediated activation of STAT1alpha regulates growth factor-induced mitogenesis. *J Clin Invest.* **98:** 1218-1230.

Marra F, Gentilini A, Pinzani M, Choudhury GG, Parola M, Herbst H, Dianzani MU, Laffi G, Abboud HE,Gentilini P, 1997, Phosphatidylinositol 3-kinase is required for platelet-derived growth factor's actions on hepatic stellate cells. *Gastroenterology*. **112:** 1297-1306.

Marra F, DeFranco R, Grappone C, Milani S, Pastacaldi S, Pinzani M, Romanelli RG, Laffi G,Gentilini P, 1998, Increased expression of monocyte chemotactic protein-1 during active hepatic fibrogenesis: correlation with monocyte infiltration. *Am J Pathol.* **152:** 423-430.

Marra F, 1999, Hepatic stellate cells and the regulation of liver inflammation. *J Hepatol.* **31:** 1120-1130.

Marra F, Arrighi MC, Fazi M, Caligiuri A, Pinzani M, Romanelli RG, Efsen E, Laffi G, Gentilini P, 1999, Extracellular signal-regulated kinase activation differentially regulates platelet-derived growth factor's actions in hepatic stellate cells, and is induced by in vivo liver injury in the rat. *Hepatology*. **30:** 951-958.

Marra F, Romanelli RG, Giannini C, Failli P, Pastacaldi S, Arrighi MC, Pinzani M, Laffi G, Montalto P, Gentilini P, 1999, Monocyte chemotactic protein-1 as a chemoattractant for human hepatic stellate cells. *Hepatology*. **29:** 140-148.

Marra F, Efsen E, Romanelli RG, Caligiuri A, Pastacaldi S, Batignani G, Bonacchi A, Caporale R, Laffi G, Pinzani M, Gentilini P, 2000, Ligands of peroxisome proliferator-activated receptor gamma modulate profibrogenic and proinflammatory actions in hepatic stellate cells. *Gastroenterology*. **119:** 466-478.

Marra F, 2002, Chemokines in liver inflammation and fibrosis. *Front Biosci.* **7:** d1899-1914.

Marra F, 2002, Leptin and liver fibrosis: a matter of fat. *Gastroenterology*. **122:** 1529-1532.

Milani S, Herbst H, Schuppan D, Kim KY, Riecken EO, Stein H, 1990, Procollagen expression by nonparenchymal rat liver cells in experimental biliary fibrosis. *Gastroenterology*. **98:** 175-184.

Miyahara T, Schrum L, Rippe R, Xiong S, Yee HF, Jr., Motomura K, Anania FA, Willson TM,Tsukamoto H, 2000, Peroxisome proliferator-activated receptors and hepatic stellate cell activation. *J Biol Chem*. **275:** 35715-35722.

Murata T, Arii S, Nakamura T, Mori A, Kaido T, Furuyama H, Furumoto K, Nakao T, Isobe N,Imamura M, 2001, Inhibitory effect of Y-27632, a ROCK inhibitor, on progression of rat liver fibrosis in association with inactivation of hepatic stellate cells. *J Hepatol*. **35:** 474-481.

Natsume M, Tsuji H, Harada A, Akiyama M, Yano T, Ishikura H, Nakanishi I, Matsushima K, Kaneko S, Mukaida N, 1999, Attenuated liver fibrosis and depressed serum albumin levels in carbon tetrachloride-treated IL-6-deficient mice. *J Leukoc Biol*. **66:** 601-608.

Oben JA, Yang S, Lin H, Ono M, Diehl AM, 2003, Norepinephrine and neuropeptide Y promote proliferation and collagen gene expression of hepatic myofibroblastic stellate cells. *Biochem Biophys Res Commun*. **302:** 685-690.

Oben JA, Diehl AM, 2004, Sympathetic nervous system regulation of liver repair. *Anat Rec A Discov Mol Cell Evol Biol*. **280:** 874-883.

Oben JA, Roskams T, Yang S, Lin H, Sinelli N, Torbenson M, Smedh U, Moran TH, Li Z, Huang J, Thomas SA, Diehl AM, 2004, Hepatic fibrogenesis requires sympathetic neurotransmitters. *Gut*. **53:** 438-445.

Olaso E, Ikeda K, Eng FJ, Xu L, Wang LH, Lin HC, Friedman SL, 2001, DDR2 receptor promotes MMP-2-mediated proliferation and invasion by hepatic stellate cells. *J Clin Invest*. **108:** 1369-1378.

Ortiz V, Berenguer M, Rayon JM, Carrasco D, Berenguer J, 2002, Contribution of obesity to hepatitis C-related fibrosis progression. *Am J Gastroenterol*. **97:** 2408-2414.

Oudit GY, Crackower MA, Backx PH, Penninger JM, 2003, The role of ACE2 in cardiovascular physiology. *Trends Cardiovasc Med.* **13:** 93-101.

Paik YH, Schwabe RF, Bataller R, Russo MP, Jobin C, Brenner DA, 2003, Toll-like receptor 4 mediates inflammatory signaling by bacterial lipopolysaccharide in human hepatic stellate cells. *Hepatology.* **37:** 1043-1055.

Paizis G, Gilbert RE, Cooper ME, Murthi P, Schembri JM, Wu LL, Rumble JR, Kelly DJ, Tikellis C, Cox A, Smallwood RA, Angus PW, 2001, Effect of angiotensin II type 1 receptor blockade on experimental hepatic fibrogenesis. *J Hepatol.* **35:** 376-385.

Paizis G, Cooper ME, Schembri JM, Tikellis C, Burrell LM, Angus PW, 2002, Up-regulation of components of the renin-angiotensin system in the bile duct-ligated rat liver. *Gastroenterology.* **123:** 1667-1676.

Pawluczyk IZ, Patel SR, Harris KP, 2004, The role of bradykinin in the antifibrotic actions of perindoprilat on human mesangial cells. *Kidney Int.* **65:** 1240-1251.

Phillips RJ, Burdick MD, Hong K, Lutz MA, Murray LA, Xue YY, Belperio JA, Keane MP, Strieter RM, 2004, Circulating fibrocytes traffic to the lungs in response to CXCL12 and mediate fibrosis. *J Clin Invest.* **114:** 438-446.

Ratziu V, Lalazar A, Wong L, Dang Q, Collins C, Shaulian E, Jensen S, Friedman SL, 1998, Zf9, a Kruppel-like transcription factor up-regulated in vivo during early hepatic fibrosis. *Proc Natl Acad Sci USA.* **95:** 9500-9505.

Regoli D, Barabe J, 1980, Pharmacology of bradykinin and related kinins. *Pharmacol Rev.* **32:** 1-46.

Reif S, Lang A, Lindquist JN, Yata Y, Gabele E, Scanga A, Brenner DA, Rippe RA, 2003, The role of focal adhesion kinase-phosphatidylinositol 3-kinase-akt signaling in hepatic stellate cell proliferation and type I collagen expression. *J Biol Chem.* **278:** 8083-8090.

Rippe RA, Schrum LW, Stefanovic B, Solis-Herruzo JA, Brenner DA, 1999, NF-kappaB inhibits expression of the alpha1(I) collagen gene. *DNA Cell Biol.* **18:** 751-761.

Rippe RA, Brenner DA, 2004, From quiescence to activation: Gene regulation in hepatic stellate cells. *Gastroenterology.* **127:** 1260-1262.

Rizkalla B, Forbes JM, Cooper ME, Cao Z, 2003, Increased renal vascular endothelial growth factor and angiopoietins by angiotensin II infusion is mediated by both AT1 and AT2 receptors. *J Am Soc Nephrol.* **14:** 3061-3071.

Rockey DC, Weisiger RA, 1996, Endothelin induced contractility of stellate cells from normal and cirrhotic rat liver: implications for regulation of portal pressure and resistance. *Hepatology.* **24:** 233-240.

Santos RA, Simoes e Silva AC, Maric C, Silva DM, Machado RP, de Buhr I, Heringer-Walther S, Pinheiro SV, Lopes MT, Bader M, Mendes EP, Lemos VS, Campagnole-Santos MJ, Schultheiss HP, Speth R, Walther T, 2003, Angiotensin-(1-7) is an endogenous ligand for the G protein-coupled receptor Mas. *Proc Natl Acad Sci USA.* **100:** 8258-8263.

Sato M, Suzuki S, Senoo H, 2003, Hepatic stellate cells: unique characteristics in cell biology and phenotype. *Cell Struct Funct.* **28:** 105-112.

Schanstra JP, Neau E, Drogoz P, Arevalo Gomez MA, Lopez Novoa JM, Calise D, Pecher C, Bader M, Girolami JP, Bascands JL, 2002, In vivo bradykinin B2 receptor activation reduces renal fibrosis. *J Clin Invest.* **110:** 371-379.

Schepke M, Werner E, Biecker E, Schiedermaier P, Heller J, Neef M, Stoffel-Wagner B, Hofer U, Caselmann WH, Sauerbruch T, 2001, Hemodynamic effects of the angiotensin II receptor antagonist irbesartan in patients with cirrhosis and portal hypertension. *Gastroenterology.* **121:** 389-395.

Schnabl B, Kweon YO, Frederick JP, Wang XF, Rippe RA, Brenner DA, 2001, The role of Smad3 in mediating mouse hepatic stellate cell activation. *Hepatology.* **34:** 89-100.

Schneider AW, Kalk JF, Klein CP, 1999, Effect of losartan, an angiotensin II receptor antagonist, on portal pressure in cirrhosis. *Hepatology*. **29:** 334-339.

Schwabe RF, Schnabl B, Kweon YO, Brenner DA, 2001, CD40 activates NF-kappa B and c-Jun N-terminal kinase and enhances chemokine secretion on activated human hepatic stellate cells. *J Immunol.* **166:** 6812-6819.

Schwabe RF, Bataller R, Brenner DA, 2003, Human hepatic stellate cells express CCR5 and RANTES to induce proliferation and migration. *Am J Physiol Gastrointest Liver Physiol.* **285:** G949-958.

Schwabe RF, Uchinami H, Qian T, Bennett BL, Lemasters JJ, Brenner DA, 2004, Differential requirement for c-Jun NH2-terminal kinase in TNFalpha- and Fas-mediated apoptosis in hepatocytes. *Faseb J.* **18:** 720-722.

Shek FW, Benyon RC, 2004, How can transforming growth factor beta be targeted usefully to combat liver fibrosis? *Eur J Gastroenterol Hepatol.* **16:** 123-126.

Smart DE, Vincent KJ, Arthur MJ, Eickelberg O, Castellazzi M, Mann J, Mann DA, 2001, JunD regulates transcription of the tissue inhibitor of metalloproteinases-1 and interleukin-6 genes in activated hepatic stellate cells. *J Biol Chem.* **276:** 24414-24421.

Sohara N, Znoyko I, Levy MT, Trojanowska M, Reuben A, 2002, Reversal of activation of human myofibroblast-like cells by culture on a basement membrane-like substrate. *J Hepatol.* **37:** 214-221.

Song E, Chen J, Wang K, Zhang H, Su F, Wang M, Heemann U, 2002, Intrasplenic transplantation of syngenic hepatocytes modified by IFN-gamma gene ameliorates hepatic fibrosis in rats. *Transpl Int.* **15:** 472-478.

Stewart D, Blendis LM, Williams R, 1972, Studies on the prekallikrein-bradykininogen system in liver disease. *J Clin Pathol.* **25:** 410-414.

Sudo K, Yamada Y, Moriwaki H, Saito K, Seishima M, 2005, Lack of tumor necrosis factor receptor type 1 inhibits liver fibrosis induced by carbon tetrachloride in mice. *Cytokine.* **29:** 236-244.

Suskind DL, Muench MO, 2004, Searching for common stem cells of the hepatic and hematopoietic systems in the human fetal liver: CD34+ cytokeratin 7/8+ cells express markers for stellate cells. *J Hepatol.* **40:** 261-268.

Tada S, Iwamoto H, Nakamuta M, Sugimoto R, Enjoji M, Nakashima Y, Nawata H, 2001, A selective ROCK inhibitor, Y27632, prevents dimethylnitrosamine-induced hepatic fibrosis in rats. *J Hepatol.* **34:** 529-536.

Thompson HL, Burbelo PD, Gabriel G, Yamada Y, Metcalfe DD, 1991, Murine mast cells synthesize basement membrane components. A potential role in early fibrosis. *J Clin Invest.* **87:** 619-623.

Tipnis SR, Hooper NM, Hyde R, Karran E, Christie G, Turner AJ, 2000, A human homolog of angiotensin-converting enzyme. Cloning and functional expression as a captopril-insensitive carboxypeptidase. *J Biol Chem.* **275:** 33238-33243.

Toda K, Kumagai N, Tsuchimoto K, Inagaki H, Suzuki T, Oishi T, Atsukawa K, Saito H, Morizane T, Hibi T, Ishii H, 2000, Induction of hepatic stellate cell proliferation by LPS-stimulated peripheral blood mononuclear cells from patients with liver cirrhosis. *J Gastroenterol.* **35:** 214-220.

Tsukada S, Westwick JK, Ikejima K, Sato N, Rippe RA, 2005, SMAD and p38 MAPK signaling pathways independently regulate alpha1(I) collagen gene expression in unstimulated and transforming growth factor-beta-stimulated hepatic stellate cells. *J Biol Chem.* **280:** 10055-10064.

Tuncer I, Ozbek H, Ugras S, Bayram I, 2003, Anti-fibrogenic effects of captopril and candesartan cilexetil on the hepatic fibrosis development in rat. The effect of AT1-R blocker on the hepatic fibrosis. *Exp Toxicol Pathol.* **55:** 159-166.

Vickers C, Hales P, Kaushik V, Dick L, Gavin J, Tang J, Godbout K, Parsons T, Baronas E, Hsieh F, Acton S, Patane M, Nichols A, Tummino P, 2002, Hydrolysis of biological peptides by human angiotensin-converting enzyme-related carboxypeptidase. *J Biol Chem.* **277:** 14838-14843.

Vinas O, Bataller R, Sancho-Bru P, Gines P, Berenguer C, Enrich C, Nicolas JM, Ercilla G, Gallart T, Vives J, Arroyo V, Rodes J, 2003, Human hepatic stellate cells show features of antigen-presenting cells and stimulate lymphocyte proliferation. *Hepatology.* **38:** 919-929.

Vlachogiannakos J, Tang AK, Patch D, Burroughs AK, 2001, Angiotensin converting enzyme inhibitors and angiotensin II antagonists as therapy in chronic liver disease. *Gut.* **49:** 303-308.

Vogten JM, Drixler TA, te Velde EA, Schipper ME, van Vroonhoven TJ, Voest EE, Borel Rinkes IH, 2004, Angiostatin inhibits experimental liver fibrosis in mice. *Int J Colorectal Dis.* **19:** 387-394.

Wang X, Tang X, Gong X, Albanis E, Friedman SL, Mao Z, 2004, Regulation of hepatic stellate cell activation and growth by transcription factor myocyte enhancer factor 2. *Gastroenterology.* **127:** 1174-1188.

Wang YQ, Ikeda K, Ikebe T, Hirakawa K, Sowa M, Nakatani K, Kawada N, Kaneda K, 2000, Inhibition of hepatic stellate cell proliferation and activation by the semisynthetic analogue of fumagillin TNP-470 in rats. *Hepatology.* **32:** 980-989.

Wei H, Lu H, Li D, Zhan Y, Wang Z, Huang X, 2001, The expression of AT1 receptor on hepatic stellate cells in rat fibrosis induced by CCl4. *Chin Med J (Engl).* **114:** 583-587.

Wei HS, Li DG, Lu HM, Zhan YT, Wang ZR, Huang X, Zhang J, Cheng JL, Xu QF, 2000, Effects of AT1 receptor antagonist, losartan, on rat hepatic fibrosis induced by CCl(4). *World J Gastroenterol.* **6:** 540-545.

Williams EJ, Benyon RC, Trim N, Hadwin R, Grove BH, Arthur MJ, Unemori EN, Iredale JP, 2001, Relaxin inhibits effective collagen deposition by cultured hepatic stellate cells and decreases rat liver fibrosis in vivo. *Gut.* **49:** 577-583.

Wirth KJ, Bickel M, Hropot M, Gunzler V, Heitsch H, Ruppert D, Scholkens BA, 1997, The bradykinin B2 receptor antagonist Icatibant (HOE 140) corrects avid Na+ retention in rats with CCl4-induced liver cirrhosis: possible role of enhanced microvascular leakage. *Eur J Pharmacol.* **337:** 45-53.

Wong PY, Talamo RC, Williams GH, 1977, Kallikrein-kinin and renin-angiotensin systems in functional renal failure of cirrhosis of the liver. *Gastroenterology.* **73:** 1114-1118.

Yang YY, Lin HC, Huang YT, Lee TY, Hou MC, Lee FY, Liu RS, Chang FY, Lee SD, 2002, Effect of 1-week losartan administration on bile duct-ligated cirrhotic rats with portal hypertension. *J Hepatol.* **36:** 600-606.

Yao HW, LI J, Chen JQ, 2004, Effect of losartan, an angiotensin II antagonist, on hepatic fibrosis induced by CCl4 in rats. *Dig Dis Sci.* **49:** 1589-1594.

Yao HW, Li J, Chen JQ, Xu SY, 2004, [The active metabolite of leflunomide A771726 inhibits proliferation and collagen synthesis of hepatic stellate cell]. *Zhejiang Da Xue Xue Bao Yi Xue Ban.* **33:** 515-518, 528.

Yao HW, Li J, Chen JQ, Xu SY, 2004, Inhibitory effect of leflunomide on hepatic fibrosis induced by CCl4 in rats. *Acta Pharmacol Sin.* **25:** 915-920.

Yao HW, Xie QM, Chen JQ, Deng YM, Tang HF, 2004, TGF-beta1 induces alveolar epithelial to mesenchymal transition in vitro. *Life Sci.* **76:** 29-37.

Yee HF, Jr., 1998, Rho directs activation-associated changes in rat hepatic stellate cell morphology via regulation of the actin cytoskeleton. *Hepatology.* **28:** 843-850.

Yoshiji H, Kuriyama S, Miyamoto Y, Thorgeirsson UP, Gomez DE, Kawata M, Yoshii J, Ikenaka Y, Noguchi R, Tsujinoue H, Nakatani T, Thorgeirsson SS, Fukui H, 2000, Tissue inhibitor of metalloproteinases-1 promotes liver fibrosis development in a transgenic mouse model. *Hepatology*. **32:** 1248-1254.

Yoshiji H, Kuriyama S, Yoshii J, Ikenaka Y, Noguchi R, Nakatani T, Tsujinoue H, Fukui H, 2001, Angiotensin-II type 1 receptor interaction is a major regulator for liver fibrosis development in rats. *Hepatology*. **34:** 745-750.

Yoshiji H, Kuriyama S, Fukui H, 2002, Angiotensin-I-converting enzyme inhibitors may be an alternative anti-angiogenic strategy in the treatment of liver fibrosis and hepatocellular carcinoma. Possible role of vascular endothelial growth factor. *Tumour Biol*. **23:** 348-356.

Yoshiji H, Kuriyama S, Yoshii J, Ikenaka Y, Noguchi R, Yanase K, Namisaki T, Yamazaki M, Tsujinoue H, Imazu H, Fukui H, 2003, Angiotensin-II induces the tissue inhibitor of metalloproteinases-1 through the protein kinase-C signaling pathway in rat liver fibrosis development. *Hepatol Res*. **27:** 51-56.

Yoshiji H, Kuriyama S, Noguchi R, Yoshii J, Ikenaka Y, Yanase K, Namisaki T, Kitade M, Yamazaki M, Tsujinoue H, Fukui H, 2005, Combination of interferon-beta and angiotensin-converting enzyme inhibitor, perindopril, attenuates the murine liver fibrosis development. *Liver Int*. **25:** 153-161.

Zhang LJ, Chen YX, Chen ZX, Huang YH, Yu JP, Wang XZ, 2004, Effect of interleukin-10 and platelet-derived growth factor on expressions of matrix metalloproteinases-2 and tissue inhibitor of metalloproteinases-1 in rat fibrotic liver and cultured hepatic stellate cells. *World J Gastroenterol*. **10:** 2574-2579.

Zhang X, Yu WP, Gao L, Wei KB, Ju JL, Xu JZ, 2004, Effects of lipopolysaccharides stimulated Kupffer cells on activation of rat hepatic stellate cells. *World J Gastroenterol*. **10:** 610-613.

Chapter 9

Matrix Metalloproteinases in Chronic Liver Disease and Liver Transplantation

Hein W. Verspaget, Johan P. Kuyvenhoven, Cornelis F.M. Sier, Bart van Hoek
Leiden University Medical Center, Department of Gastroenterology and Hepatology, PO Box 9600, 2300 RC Leiden, The Netherlands

1. INTRODUCTION

Matrix metalloproteinases (MMPs) are the main degrading enzymes of extracellular matrix proteins and basement membranes, and they play an important role in the processes of tissue remodeling and repair in many physiological and pathological processes. A subgroup of the MMP family, the gelatinases MMP-2 and MMP-9, is thought to be particularly involved in the degradation of matrix in the liver. MMP-2 can be expressed by many cell types in the liver, however, the hepatic stellate cell is suggested to be the main cellular source. The principal source of MMP-9 in the liver is the Kupffer cell, but MMP-9 can also be released from inflammatory cells, e.g. neutrophils. The potential contribution to and role of (circulating) MMP-2 and MMP-9 in liver fibrosis, hepatocellular carcinoma (HCC), ischemia/reperfusion (I/R) injury and acute rejection after orthotopic liver transplantation (OLT) is described.

2. MATRIX METALLOPROTEINASES

MMPs encompass a family of enzymes whose main function is degradation of the extracellular matrix. MMPs are important for many normal processes requiring matrix turnover, e.g., embryonic development, wound healing and angiogenesis. In addition to matrix degradation for normal tissue remodeling and repair, MMPs have also been implicated in a variety of pathological

U. Lendeckel and Nigel M. Hooper (eds.), Proteases in Gastrointestinal Tissue, 209-234.

processes, including tumour metastasis, periodontal disease, atherosclerosis, and pulmonary emphysema (Nagase and Woessner 1999).

The family of MMPs can be loosely divided into four subgroups, identified by their structure and substrate preference, i.e., interstitial collagenases, gelatinases, stromelysins and membrane-type MMPs. Currently, more than 25 different MMPs have been described in the mammalian systems (Table 1). All MMPs have been assigned an MMP number and most also have a common name.

Table 1. List of major MMP-subgroups with some of their main substrates (Benyon and Arthur 2001; Hoekstra *et al* 2001).

Group	Descriptive name	Number	Principal substrate
Collagenases	Interstitial collagenase	MMP-1	All: fibrillar collagens I, II and III
	Neutrophil collagenase	MMP-8	
	Collagenase-3	MMP-13	
	Collagenase-4	MMP-18	Collagen I, not known
Stromelysins	Stromelysin-1	MMP-3	All: proteolycans, ECM glycoproteins
	Stromelysin-2	MMP-10	and nonfibrillar collagens IV and V
	Stromelysin-3	MMP-11	Serine protease inhibitor
Gelatinases	Gelatinase A (72 kDa)	MMP-2	Both: collagens IV and V, gelatin,
	Gelatinase B (92 kDa)	MMP-9	elastin, laminin
Membrane-type	MT1-MMP	MMP-14	ProMMP-2 and proMMP-13, collagens I, II and III
	MT2-MMP	MMP-15	ProMMP-2, laminin
	MT3-MMP	MMP-16	Collagen III, fibronectin
	MT4-MMP	MMP-17	Fibrinogen, fibrin, activates TNF-α
	MT5-MMP	MMP-24	ProMMP-2, proteoglycans
	MT6-MMP	MMP-25	Collagen IV, fibronectin, fibrin
Others	Matrilysin-1	MMP-7	All: elastin, nonfibrillar collagen
	Matrilysin-2	MMP-26	
	Metalloelastase	MMP-12	

The main characteristics of these MMPs are (Woessner 1991; Parsons *et al* 1997; Duffy and McCarthy 1998):

1. the catalytic activity depends on a metal ion (i.e., Zn^{2+} at the active site);
2. most are secreted in a latent form;
3. the zymogen forms can be activated by other proteinases or organomercurials;
4. they are inhibited by tissue inhibitors of metalloproteinases (TIMPs);
5. they share common amino-acid sequences;
6. the enzymes cleave at least one component of the extracellular matrix (ECM).

MMPs contain at least three domains: a signal peptide that directs the translational product to the endoplasmic reticulum for secretion; a propeptide domain that is removed when the enzyme is activated and a catalytic domain.

Most MMPs also possess a C-terminal domain with sequence homology to hemopexin. The gelatinases differ from the other MMPs in that, the catalytic domain is separated from the hemopexin-like domain by a fibronectin-like domain. The latter is required to bind and cleave collagen and elastin (Woessner 1991; Murphy and Docherty 1992; Nguyen *et al* 2001; Sternlicht and Werb 2001).

The regulation of MMPs is stringent and occurs at several levels (Parsons *et al* 1997).

(1) Gene expression. Normal gene expression of MMPs is characterized by tightly controlled regulation to maintain normal tissue function. The expression is transcriptionally regulated by numerous stimulatory and suppressive factors such as growth factors (e.g., transforming growth factor-beta), hormones, cytokines [e.g., tumor necrosis factor-alpha (TNF-α) and interleukin (IL)-1], and cellular transformation. Not only soluble factors but also cell-matrix and cell-cell interactions play a role in the expression of MMPs (Nagase and Woessner 1999).

Single nucleotide polymorphisms in gene promoters of MMPs have been shown to affect transcriptional activity. The –1306 C/T transition in the MMP-2 promoter sequence disrupts an Sp1 site and thus results in strikingly lower promoter activity (Price *et al* 2001). In contrast, the –1562 C/T transition in the promoter of MMP-9 results in higher promoter activity, which appeared to be due to preferential binding of a putative transcription repressor protein to the C allelic promoter (Zhang *et al* 1999).

(2) Secretion in latent form. MMPs are produced and secreted in a latent proenzyme form so they require activation in order to have any effect on the extracellular matrix. Several enzyme activators, which include the plasminogen activator (PA)/plasmin system, plasma kallikrein, neutrophil elastase, and trypsin have been implicated in the activation of MMPs (Murphy and Docherty 1992). Unlike other MMPs, proMMP-2 is constitutively expressed by many cell types and activation occurs at the cell surface (Corcoran *et al* 1996). Since the activation occurs in the immediate pericellular milieu, the local degradation of the matrix can be closely regulated, e.g., by an invasive cell. The major proMMP-2 activation pathway appears to be through MT1-MMP and is regulated by TIMP-2 in a trimolecular interaction (Sternlicht and Werb 2001). The involvement of the PA/plasmin system in the activation of proMMP-2 is controversial (Lijnen *et al* 1998; Sternlicht and Werb 2001). Yet, activation of proMMP-2 involves cleavage by MT1-MMP, yielding an intermediate form that may be activated by plasmin (Baramova *et al* 1997).

In contrast, proMMP-9 is not constitutively expressed but the secretion can be induced and is controlled by other factors. For example, proMMP-9 is synthesized by differentiating neutrophils in the bone marrow, stored in specific granules of circulating neutrophils, and released following neutrophil activation by inflammatory cytokines (Opdenakker *et al* 2001; Sternlicht and Werb 2001). ProMMP-9 activation can occur directly via plasmin dependent mechanisms (Corcoran *et al* 1996; Lijnen *et al* 1998). Plasmin is a proteinase which is generated by the activation of the proenzyme plasminogen by the action of tissue-type plasminogen activator (tPA) and urokinase-type PA. tPA is active upon secretion and can also directly interact with ECM components. Activation of proMMP-9 can also be plasmin-independent, e.g. mediated by a second MMP (MMP-2 or matrilysin) (Corcoran *et al* 1996; Opdenakker *et al* 2001).

(3) Inhibition by TIMPs. Four naturally occurring specific inhibitors of MMPs have been described, namely tissue inhibitors of matrix metalloproteinases (TIMP)-1,-2,-3, and -4. The TIMPs reversibly inhibit active MMPs by forming a strong 1:1 stoichiometric non-covalent complex, resulting in loss of proteolytic activity. In addition to binding to the active enzyme, TIMP-1 forms preferentially complexes with proMMP-9, while TIMP-2 binds to proMMP-2 (Duffy and McCarthy 1998). TIMPs may also exert direct growth-promoting activity independent of their metalloproteinase inhibitory activity (Corcoran *et al* 1996; Sternlicht and Werb 2001).

(4) MMP catabolism and clearance. Little is known about autoproteolysis of active MMPs but some cleavages seem to inactivate MMPs (Sternlicht and Werb 2001). The degradation and excretion pathways of MMPs and TIMPs in the body have not been examined to date (Zucker *et al* 1998). Therefore, it is not known whether hepatic or renal dysfunction influences the clearance of MMPs.

The gelatinases MMP-2 and MMP-9

The gelatinases, which are also known as type IV collagenases, degrade gelatin (denatured collagen) and type I, IV, V, VII, and X collagen. Type IV collagen is particularly abundant in basement membranes, which separate organ parenchyma from the underlying stroma. These enzymes also cleave the noncollagenous proteins elastin, fibronectin, and laminin. This subgroup of MMPs has 2 distinct members, known as gelatinase A (MMP-2) and gelatinase B (MMP-9). Generally, these 2 gelatinases are thought to have a similar substrate specificity (Duffy and McCarthy 1998). Some characteristics of these enzymes are shown in Table 2.

Table 2. Characteristics of the gelatinases (Nguyen *et al* 2001).

Common names	**Gelatinase A**	**Gelatinase B**
Nomenclature	**MMP-2**	**MMP-9**
Substrate specificity	Gelatin, collagen type IV and V, elastin, laminin	Gelatin, collagen type IV and V, elastin, laminin
Molecular mass	72 kD	92 kD
Molecular mass of active species	64 kD, 62 kD	82 kD, 67 kD
Physiological activators	MT1-MMP, type I collagen, hepatocyte growth factor	Serine proteases, MMP-2 and MMP-7
Latent form binds to TIMP	TIMP-2	TIMP-1
Synthesis by cells	Constitutive	Inducible

MMP-9 is released predominantly from neutrophils and macrophages, but the principal source in the liver is the Kupffer cell, the resident macrophage of the liver (Winwood *et al* 1995). In addition, one study demonstrated some MMP-9 labeling of hepatocytes close to the portal areas (Geisler *et al* 1997). Neutrophils do not produce MMP-2 or TIMP, whereas most other cell types do (Opdenakker *et al* 2001). Monocytes, lymphocytes, dendritic cells, fibroblasts, and tumor cell lines produce MMP-2 constitutively, albeit sometimes in small quantities. MMP-9 is an inducible enzyme in most of these cell types. In the liver, the hepatic stellate cell is suggested to be the main cellular source of MMP-2. Following liver injury, these cells become activated and can express a wide range of MMPs and TIMPs, but in particular MMP-2 (Benyon and Arthur 2001). From other nonparenchymal liver cells, MMP-2 and MMP-9 synthesis has only been demonstrated in sinusoidal endothelial cells (Upadhya *et al* 1997).

Methods of detection

MMPs can be detected by a variety of techniques, each with its own advantages and disadvantages. Immunohistochemistry, enzyme-linked immunosorbent assay (ELISA), mRNA detection, gelatin-zymography and Western blotting are the main techniques used. Immunohistochemistry and mRNA detection can be used to localize the MMPs, thus determining their site of production, but they do not detect enzyme activity. Gelatin-zymography has the advantage of measuring enzymatic activity quantitatively and of distinguishing the active from the inactive enzyme. However, only MMP-2 and MMP-9 can be measured easily with this technique (Parsons *et al* 1997). Our group applied highly specific ELISAs for determining MMP-2 and MMP-9, which measure the grand total of pro-enzyme, active- and inhibitor-complexed forms of the respective MMP (Hanemaaijer *et al* 1998; Sier *et al* 2000; Gveric *et al* 2001). MMP-2 and MMP-9 enzymatic activities can also be determined in blood samples by using specific biochemical immunosorbent activity assays (BIA) (Capper *et al* 1999; Sier *et al* 2000; Gveric *et al* 2001). Free, active MMPs, however, cannot be detected in most blood samples because of rapid complex formation with specific inhibitors in the circulation.

3. MATRIX METALLOPROTEINASES IN CHRONIC LIVER DISEASE

3.1 Liver fibrosis

Longstanding alcohol abuse, viral hepatitis (especially hepatitis B and hepatitis C), autoimmune hepatitis and cholestatic liver diseases, such as primary biliary cirrhosis, are important causes of chronic liver disease in Western countries. In chronic liver disease, a process of tissue remodeling develops, in which destruction of hepatic cells is followed by repair mechanisms characterized by increased collagen production, accumulation of ECM and progressive destruction of the organ architecture. Ultimately, hepatic fibrosis leads to cirrhosis, characterized by nodule formation and organ contraction, which can lead to life-threatening complications such as portal hypertension, hepatic failure and hepatocellular carcinoma. The pathological accumulation of ECM can be a result of an increase in synthesis or a decrease in degradation of ECM, or a combination of both, since hepatic fibrosis is a dynamic process (Arthur 2000; Okazaki *et al* 2000; Benyon and Arthur 2001; Schuppan *et al* 2001). Activated hepatic stellate cells are central to the process of fibrosis as the major source of fibrillar matrix components (Iredale *et al* 1998; Friedman 2000).

Like other parenchyma, the normal liver contains an epithelial component (hepatocytes), an endothelial lining (which in the liver is distinguished by fenestrae), tissue macrophages (Kupffer cells), and a perivascular mesenchymal cell called the stellate cell. The cellular elements of the liver are organized within sinusoids, with the subendothelial space of Disse separating the hepatocytes from the sinusoidal endothelium. The space of Disse contains a basement membrane-like matrix, allowing maximized passage of molecules from the fenestrated sinusoidal endothelium to hepatocytes and providing structural integrity of the liver parenchyma (Benyon and Arthur 1998; Friedman 2000). The main components of the ECM in normal liver are collagen type I, III, IV, V, and VI, although other types of collagen are present in smaller proportions. There are also many noncollagenous matrix components, including fibronectin, laminin, elastin and proteoglycans

(Schuppan 1990; Okazaki *et al* 2000). MMPs, e.g. synthesized by hepatic stellate cells within the space of Disse, are the main degrading enzymes of the ECM proteins, such as collagen, gelatin and laminin, and therefore play an important role in the process of tissue remodelling (Woessner 1991; Murphy and Docherty 1992).

In the liver, stellate cells express virtually all key components required for matrix degeneration (Iredale *et al* 1998; Okazaki *et al* 2000; Schuppan *et al* 2001). In particular, they are the key source of MMP-2, which is responsible for the degradation of type IV collagen, a major component of the basement membrane. Conversely, active MMP-2 has been shown to promote proliferation of activated stellate cells (Murawaki *et al* 1997). An increased mRNA expression of MMP-2, but also of TIMP-1 and TIMP-2, was reported in liver biopsy samples of patients with cirrhosis (Milani *et al* 1994; Benyon *et al* 1996; Murawaki *et al* 1997; Lichtinghagen *et al* 1998; Theret *et al* 1998). In patients with chronic hepatitis and cirrhosis there is evidence of an increased expression in hepatic stellate cells of MMP-2 and MT1-MMP mRNA, with the latter enzyme being able to activate proMMP-2 (Takahara *et al* 1997). The presence of MMP gene transcripts does not per se provide clues as to the presence of the corresponding enzymatic activity in the tissue. Albeit, as assessed by gelatin-zymography, MMP-2 could also be detected in human fibrotic liver but not in normal liver tissue (Preaux *et al* 1999; Murawaki *et al* 1999).

In accordance to increased production of MMPs in liver tissue samples, *serum* MMP-2, and also TIMP-1 and TIMP-2 concentrations, were markedly increased in patients with liver cirrhosis, and showed a good correlation with the degree of liver fibrosis (Ueno *et al* 1996; Ebata *et al* 1997; Kasahara *et al* 1997; Murawaki *et al* 1999; Boeker *et al* 2002). However, in one study no correlation was observed between plasma MMP-2 and both liver fibrosis and grade of inflammation in patients with chronic hepatitis C (Walsh *et al* 1999).

Kupffer cells can influence stellate cells through the secretion of MMP-9 (Winwood *et al* 1995). MMP-9 can activate latent transforming growth factor-beta, which is the dominant stimulus to ECM production by stellate cells (Yu and Stamenkovic 2000; Bissell *et al* 2001). In human liver, MMP-9 mRNA expression was increased in patients with chronic hepatitis and cirrhosis, as compared to controls, but there was no correlation with the grade of inflammation in liver biopsies or serum aspartate aminotransferase (AST) (Lichtinghagen *et al* 2001). In addition, both cirrhotic and normal liver samples displayed a 92-kDa gelatinolytic band corresponding to Kupffer cell-derived MMP-9 (Preaux *et al* 1999). Data on *serum* MMP-9 in patients with chronic liver disease are conflicting. Both lower (Kuo *et al* 2000; Lichtinghagen *et al* 2000) and similar (Hayasaka *et al* 1996) levels are reported compared to controls.

In summary, the available evidence suggests that stellate cells express a combination of MMPs and TIMPs that have the ability to degrade normal matrix, while inhibiting degradation of fibrillar collagens that accumulate in liver fibrosis. This pattern is characterized by MMP-2 and MT1-MMP expression (schematic presentation Figure 1), which seems to lead to localized pericellular degradation of normal matrix. In addition, there is a relative increase in expression of TIMPs leading to a more global inhibition of degradation of fibrillar liver collagens (Arthur 2000; Benyon and Arhur 2001). Kupffer cells, on the other hand, seem to be involved in the production of the inducible MMP-9.

3.2 Hepatocellular carcinoma

Hepatocellular carcinoma (HCC) is an epithelial cancer originating from hepatocytes and is one of the most common cancers worldwide, especially in Asia. The annual incidence in patients with cirrhosis ranges between 3-10% (Tran *et al* 2002). The most important etiologic factors implicated in HCC are the hepatitis B and C viruses, abuse of alcohol, and hemochromatosis (Bruix *et al* 2001). Although many improvements have been made in terms of diagnosis and treatment, the prognosis of HCC is still very poor (Kuyvenhoven *et al* 2001). HCC frequently shows early invasion to blood vessels as well as intra- and extrahepatic metastasis. In western countries HCC develops multifocally in the chronically injured liver in approximately 90% of the cases, where altered turn-over and increased deposition of extracellular matrix proteins has been reported. In malignancy, MMPs seem to be induced and used by invasive tumours to remodel the local environment, allowing tumour growth, neo-angiogenesis, and metastasis (Chambers and Matrisian 1997; Brown 1998). The source of MMPs in human cancer was originally assumed to be the carcinoma cells. However, it seems that the expression of several MMPs can also be induced in stromal tissue, with the highest levels of induction in the invasive tumour margins (Brown 1998).

The expression of MMPs in HCC is poorly understood and the evidence from various researches is contradictory. High levels of MMP-2 mRNA and MMP-2 activation have been reported in HCC (Musso 1997; Theret *et al* 1998; Ogata *et al* 1999). By contrast, another study reported a lower expression of MMP-2 in tumour tissue than in non-tumour tissue (Sakamoto *et al* 2000). In a study by Määttä *et al*, MMP-2 mRNA was expressed predominantly by cells of the tumour stroma (Määttä *et al* 2000), whereas others demonstrated that MMP-2 was preferentially located at the invading border of tumour tissue (Harada *et al* 1998). Increased amounts of MMP-2 were found by zymography in tissue samples of HCC, as compared with adjacent non-tumourous liver tissue (Määttä *et al* 2000). In addition, MMP-2 activity was significantly higher in tumours arising in cirrhotic livers than in those arising in non-cirrhotic livers, and it associated with the stage of fibrosis (Theret *et al* 2001). In contrast to tumour samples, *serum* MMP-2 levels were not significantly different between patients with liver cirrhosis and those with HCC (Ueno 1996; Murawaki *et al* 1999; Giannelli *et al* 2002). Moreover, these studies found no correlation between MMP-2 and alpha-fetoprotein, tumour size or tumour differentiation. In these studies, all patients with HCC had underlying cirrhosis (Murawaki *et al* 1999) or severe active hepatitis (Ueno *et al* 1996). Therefore, these studies suggest that the increased serum MMP-2 levels in patients with HCC is derived from the non-tumourous part of the liver rather than from the carcinoma (Figure 1).

In HCC, MMP-9 was also found to be increased and mRNA was found to be expressed mainly by neoplastic epithelial cells and to a lesser extent in stromal cells (Määttä *et al* 2000; Sakamoto 2000). Increased MMP-9 mRNA expression, as measured by Northern hybridization, was associated with capsular infiltration (Arii *et al* 1996). Zymography showed almost equal amounts of the latent form of MMP-9 in both tumour and adjacent liver tissue, while its active form was present only in HCC (Määttä *et al* 2000). Hayasaka *et al* (1996), even suggested that MMP-9 could be a diagnostic marker for HCC, because the mean plasma levels of MMP-9 in patients with HCC were significantly elevated compared to controls, patients with chronic hepatitis and patients with cirrhosis.

The important role of MMPs in the process of tumour growth and metastasis has led to the development of specific MMP inhibitors (e.g., batimastat), which have been used in the treatment of several malignancies (Brown 1998; Hoekstra *et al* 2001). Up to now MMP inhibitors have not been used, however, in clinical trials including patients with HCC.

3.3 Ischemia/reperfusion injury after liver transplantation

Orthotopic liver transplantation (OLT) has become an established therapy for patients with end-stage liver disease and acute liver failure. Interruption and subsequent restoration of the blood flow is unavoidable in transplantation of organs. Organ injury caused by this transient ischemia followed by reperfusion is one of the main causes of initial poor function after OLT (Maring *et al* 1997). The spectrum of clinical manifestations of ischemia and reperfusion (I/R) injury can range from asymptomatic elevation of liver enzymes to primary non-function of the liver. Hypothermia and specific preservation solutions are used to limit the injury to the graft during and immediately after preservation (Strasberg *et al* 1994; Farmer *et al* 2000).

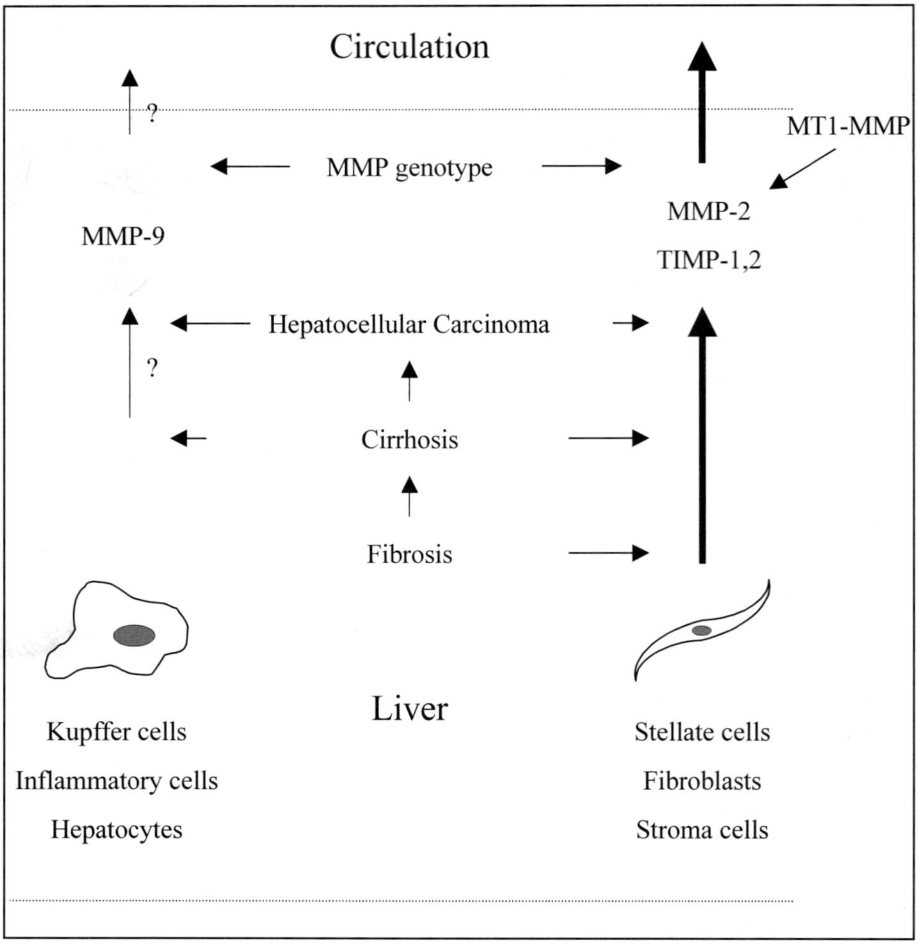

Figure 1: Changes in the expression of MMP-2 and MMP-9 in chronic liver diseases, with the sequence of events and the major contributors. The solid MMP-directed arrows indicate the strength of the changes observed.

Hepatic I/R injury is a complex, multifactorial pathophysiologic process that affects all types of hepatic cells, such as Kupffer cells, endothelial cells, hepatocytes and neutrophils (Clavien 1998; Lichtman and Lemasters 1999; Fan *et al* 1999; Farmer *et al* 2000; Kukan and Haddad 2001; Serracino-Inglott *et al* 2001; Selzner *et al* 2003). The histopathological characteristics of ischemic preservation include hepatic vacuolisation and swelling of endothelial cells. Within minutes after reperfusion with oxygenated blood, endothelial cells round up and eventually detach from the connective tissue matrix, consisting of cords of collagen linked to the cells through intermediate molecules such as fibronectin (Farmer *et al* 2000). This process of detachment appears to be mediated by proteases (Clavien 1998). Hepatocytes retain their viability and initially seem minimally affected (Farmer *et al* 2000). Soon thereafter, Kupffer cells become activated, as indicated by degranulation, increased phagocytosis, and release of oxygen free radicals and inflammatory mediators, such as TNF-α, IL-1, and platelet activating factor. Together, Kupffer cell activation and endothelial cell injury lead to profound microcirculatory disturbances and sinusoidal accumulation of leukocytes and platelets (Fan *et al* 1999; Farmer *et al* 2000). In the late phase of injury, neutrophils infiltrate the liver in response to chemoattractants released by activated Kupffer cells and expression of intercellular adhesion molecules on endothelial cells (Lichtman and Lemasters 1999). Accumulation of activated neutrophils within the hepatic parenchyma causes further hepatocyte damage several hours after reperfusion through the release of oxidants and proteases (Clavien 1998; Lentsch *et al* 2000). Microcirculatory changes appear to reach a maximum within 48 hours after reperfusion (Farmer *et al* 2000).

In the liver, MMPs-secreted by lipocytes, Kupffer cells, endothelial cells or neutrophils are capable of digesting connective tissue matrix that, for example, anchors sinusoidal lining cells to underlying cords of collagen in the space of Disse, and have an important role in exposing the matrix to neutrophils and platelets upon reperfusion (Arthur *et al* 1992; Goetzl *et al* 1996; Lichtman and Lemasters 1999; Lentsch *et al* 2000; Opdenakker *et al* 2001). Upadhya *et al* (1997; 1999; 2000) have shown that the gelatinases MMP-2 and MMP-9 may play an important role in hepatic I/R injury. Liver effluents, collected after various periods of preservation, contained MMP-2 and MMP-9, and their gelatinolytic activity increased with time of cold preservation. Furthermore, cultured endothelial cells produce these gelatinases when stored in the cold. In addition, several preservation solutions, e.g. University of Wisconsin solution with lactobionate and reduced glutathione, were found or even designed to inhibit MMP activity (Upadhya and Strasberg 2000). Hepatic MMP expression was also evaluated by Northern blot analysis using a model of normothermic partial liver I/R in rats (Cursio *et al* 2002). MMP and TIMP expression was induced in a specific time-dependent pattern following I/R. The transcripts of MMP-9 in liver lobes were rapidly induced after reperfusion, and returned to basal levels after 24 hours. A second phase was noted after 48 hours. MMP-2 and MT1-MMP expression was low after reperfusion and showed a peak 2-3 days after I/R, followed by a slow decline. Finally, TIMP-1 and TIMP-2 mRNA presented a similar pattern of induction with a peak at 48 hours. The gelatinolytic activity of MMP-9 in liver tissue increased rapidly after reperfusion with a biphasic profile, reflecting the accumulation of MMP-9 mRNA. Pre-treatment of the animals with the phosphinic MMP inhibitor RXPO3 significantly reduced markers of parenchyma injury and apoptosis (Cursio *et al* 2002).

MMPs are also involved in I/R injury in other organs and diseases. Increased MMP-9 activity and mRNA expression was found after reperfusion using a rat lung transplantation model (Yano *et al* 2001). In myocardial ischemia and reperfusion, increased levels of MMP-9 were reported as well (Danielsen *et al* 1998). Increased levels of MMP-9 were also found in rats after cardiac transplantation as compared to normal rat hearts and compared to rats who were treated with an MMP inhibitor after reperfusion (Falk *et al* 2002). Studies on the role of MMP-2 in I/R injury are conflicting. An acute release of MMP-2 was noted in coronary effluents of rats during reperfusion after ischemia of isolated, perfused hearts (Cheung *et al* 2000). However, MMP-2 activity and mRNA expression did not change during ischemia and after reperfusion in the rat lung transplantation model (Yano *et al* 2001). Also, in the kidney, MMPs did not seem to play a role during the early phase of experimental I/R injury in the rat (Ziswiler *et al* 2001).

3.4 Acute rejection after liver transplantation

Acute cellular rejection of the liver allograft remains an important problem following OLT and is the major reason that immunosuppressive therapy must be administered. Complications related to the administration of immunosuppressive therapy remain a predominant cause of mortality in the liver transplantation recipient (Asfar *et al* 1996). Most commonly, the onset of rejection occurs between the fourth and fourteenth postoperative day. There are few typical symptoms of hepatic rejection, although fever and malaise are not uncommon. The first signs of rejection are elevation of liver function tests. Leucocytosis and eosinophilia are also frequently present. The bile, if available for inspection, will be lighter and less viscous. In most cases acute rejection responds well to additional immunosuppression. The rejection incidence varies between 20-70%, depending on the immunosuppressive regimen and the diagnostic criteria used in the different studies (Wiesner *et al* 1998; Neuberger 1999). Other factors that influence the incidence of acute rejection include the indication for OLT, age, race of the recipient, and preservation injury (Neuberger 1999).

Many centers perform routine biopsy on approximately the seventh postoperative day because of the frequency of rejection at this time point. The typical histopathological findings include a mixed portal inflammation, containing activated lymphocytes, mononuclear cells, and frequently eosinophils. Polymorphonuclear leucocytes may also be present. Other critical findings include bile duct inflammation and venous endotheliitis (Batts 1999). Acute rejection is usually graded into three categories: mild, moderate and severe. A 0- to 9-point scale, the Rejection Activity Index, can be used as a numerical score with the option to further characterize rejection histologically (Wiesner *et al* 1998).

Acute rejection is characterized by an immunological attack on the allograft, which is mediated by cellular components of the immune system. T lymphocytes are the predominant cellular components. CD4+ cells appear to have a dominant role in initiating and amplifying the immune response, and CD8+ cells have a central effector role. The macrophages are pivotal in the immune response as the antigen-presenting cells. The other cells, identified in the portal tract, such as polymorphonuclear leukocytes and eosinophils, most likely reflect the influence of local cytokine production (Hall 1991; Millis 1999). The interaction between the donor antigen and recipient antigen-presenting cell provide the signals stimulating responder CD4+ cells. These cells then produce a number of cytokines, of which IL-2 seems to be the most important. These cytokines can change endothelial behaviour, causing an increase in vascular permeability and the upregulation of adhesion molecule expression on endothelial cells (Bumgardner and Orosz 1999). Adhesion molecules not only provide important cellular interactions of T cells with antigen presenting cells, but the integrins also promote leukocyte migration and extravasation, adhesion to endothelial cells and extracellular matrix (Vierling 1999). In addition to the effects of cytokines on adhesion molecule expression, cytokines such as TNF-α, IL-1 and IFN-γ have also been demonstrated to influence the secretion of MMPs by infiltrating lymphocytes (Johnatty *et al* 1997). MMP promote matrix degradation and facilitate lymphocyte trafficking through the gelatinous extracellular matrix of the allograft. Tissue injury and immune responses thus induce a complex of tissue repair and remodelling processes (Bumgardner and Orosz 1999).

Degradation of extracellular matrix, as evidenced by the increase of laminin, hyaluronic acid and fibronectin receptor, was found to be a prominent feature in acute hepatic allograft rejection (Mueller *et al* 1998; Demirci *et al* 1999). T-cells, that infiltrate the allograft, secrete predominantly the gelatinases MMP-2 and MMP-9, after β1-integrin and adhesion molecule dependent stimulation by cytokines and inflammatory mediators (Goetzl *et al* 1996). Also in a rat model of small bowel rejection, upregulated MMP-2 and MMP-9 expression was demonstrated in crypt epithelium and submucosal areas, as well as in T cell areas of the small bowel during rejection (Kimizuka *et al* 2002).

4. THE LEIDEN EXPERIENCE WITH MATRIX METALLOPROTEINASES IN LIVER DISEASE AND ORTHOTOPIC LIVER TRANSPLANTATION

The main focus of our studies was to assess the clinical impact of circulating gelatinase-type matrix metalloproteinases MMP-2 and MMP-9 in several chronic liver diseases, with emphasis on orthotopic liver transplantation (OLT). In addition to this, we have investigated the interaction between MMPs and the fibrinolytic system during OLT. Finally, the influence of functional gene promoter polymorphisms of these MMPs was investigated.

First the clinical significance of serum MMP-2 and MMP-9 was assessed in 91 patients with several chronic liver diseases and in 60 controls (Kuyvenhoven *et al* 2003a). Serum levels of MMP-2 were significantly higher in patients with chronic liver disease compared to controls, and increased according to the progression of liver disease in patients with cirrhosis. There was a strong correlation between MMP-2 and serum markers of liver dysfunction (bilirubin, albumin, and prothrombin time). Inversely, serum MMP-9 levels had an opposite correlation with these parameters, and were found to be decreased in patients with chronic liver disease as compared to controls. However, the MMP-2 and MMP-9 serum levels in an individual patient were not found to be useful markers for liver function because of a wide overlap in levels between the different Child-Pugh stages. In patients with HCC, MMP-2 levels were significantly higher than in controls, but comparable to patients with chronic liver disease. MMP-9 yielded no significant differences between patients with or without HCC and controls. Due to a considerable overlap of serum MMP-2 and MMP-9 levels in patients with chronic liver disease with or without HCC, these parameters can not be used as diagnostic markers for HCC in the context of chronic liver disease.

Next we assessed the evolution of plasma MMP-2 and MMP-9, and their inhibitors TIMP-1 and TIMP-2, in 24 patients during OLT (Kuyvenhoven *et al* 2004a). Plasma TIMP-1, TIMP-2 and MMP-2 levels gradually decreased during transplantation. Approximately two-third of total MMP-2 appeared to be in its activatable proMMP form. No release of MMP-2 from the graft could be detected. In contrast, plasma levels of MMP-9 increased sharply during OLT. Peak MMP-9 levels of about eight times above baseline were found at 30 minutes after reperfusion. This is probably due to a combination of absence of clearance by the donor liver during the anhepatic period and release from the ischemically injured liver graft after reperfusion. Most MMP-9 appeared to be in its active/inhibitor-complexed form. There was a significant correlation between plasma MMP-9 and tissue-type plasminogen activator (t-PA) levels, but not with TNF-α. In conclusion, OLT is associated with a sharp increase of MMP-9 during the anhepatic and postreperfusion periods, which coincided with the changes in t-PA, suggesting common underlying mechanisms of induction and regulation. It is known that OLT is associated with increased fibrinolytic activity due to elevated plasmin generation, which might activate some MMPs. Therefore the effect of serine-protease inhibition by aprotinin was investigated. No significant differences in MMP-2 and MMP-9 were observed between patients treated with aprotinin and placebo. Also, the composition of these MMPs was not altered by the use of aprotinin, suggesting that serine–protease/plasmin-independent pathways are responsible for MMP activation during OLT.

MMPs have been suggested to play an important role in I/R injury during OLT. In patients with more severe I/R injury the MMP-9 concentration, particularly of the active/inhibitor-complexed form, remained high at 120 minutes postreperfusion compared to patients with no or mild I/R injury (Figure 2). The decrease in MMP-2 (Figure 3), TIMP-1 and TIMP-2 during OLT occurred irrespective of I/R injury. Therefore, only MMP-9 seems to be involved in *early* I/R injury during human liver transplantation and controlling local MMP-9 may thus be a target for reducing this injury during liver transplantation.

In another group of 33 patients the changes in serum MMP-2 and MMP-9, and their composition, were assessed with respect to the *late* phase of I/R injury after OLT (Kuyvenhoven *et al* 2003b). Both MMP-2 and MMP-9 serum levels, and isoform composition, were found to be comparable two days after OLT between patients with more severe I/R injury and those with absent to mild I/R injury. Therefore, serum MMP-2 and MMP-9 do not seem to play a major role in the *late* phase of hepatic I/R injury after OLT.

The time course of serum MMP-2 and MMP-9 during one year after OLT, with emphasis on acute allograft rejection was subsequently assessed (Kuyvenhoven *et al* 2004b). The extracellular matrix may be an important target in the process of acute rejection after OLT and we demonstrated significantly higher total and active/inhibitor-complexed MMP-9 in patients with rejection compared to those without rejection. Moreover, we found a significant correlation between the rejection activity index scored on the liver biopsies and the serum MMP-9 level (Figure 4). Immunohistochemical staining of liver biopsies at one week after OLT showed increased numbers of MMP-9 positive inflammatory cells, notably neutrophils and lymphocytes, in the portal triads of patients with rejection. Serum MMP-2 levels in patients before OLT were significantly higher compared to controls. Also, the MMP-2 content of cirrhotic liver specimens was significantly higher compared to normal liver, indicating an important role of MMP-2 in the development of fibrosis.

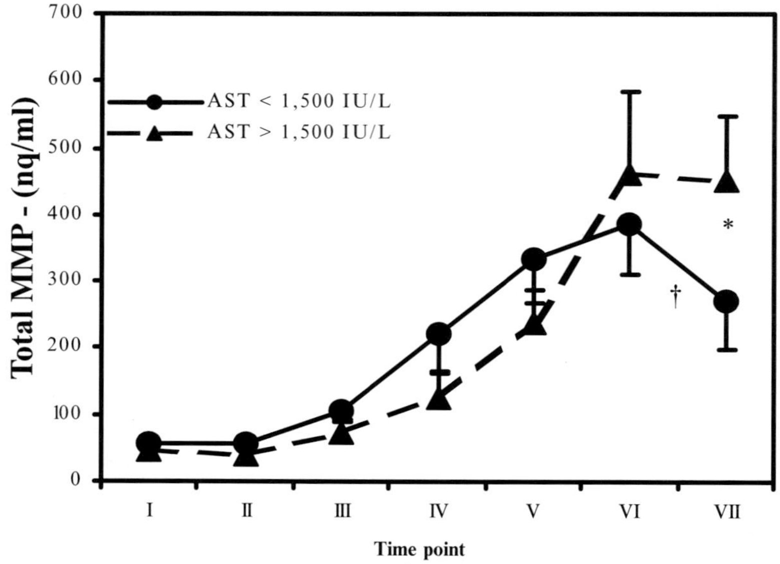

Figure 2: MMP-9 plasma concentrations during orthotopic liver transplantation (OLT). Blood samples were collected at 7 standardized time points: before transplantation (I), after induction of anesthesia (II), 10 minutes before the end of the pre-anhepatic period (III) and anhepatic period (IV), and 5 (V), 30 (VI) and 120 (VII) minutes post-reperfusion. Data are expressed as mean ± S.E.M. AST = serum aspartate aminotransferase •: Patients with a peak AST < 1,500 IU/L; ▲: Patients with a peak AST > 1,500 IU/L. *, P ≤ 0.05 comparing the two groups. †, P ≤ 0.05 comparing MMP-9 concentrations at 30 minutes (VI) and 120 minutes (VII) after reperfusion in the group of patients with a peak AST < 1,500 IU/L.

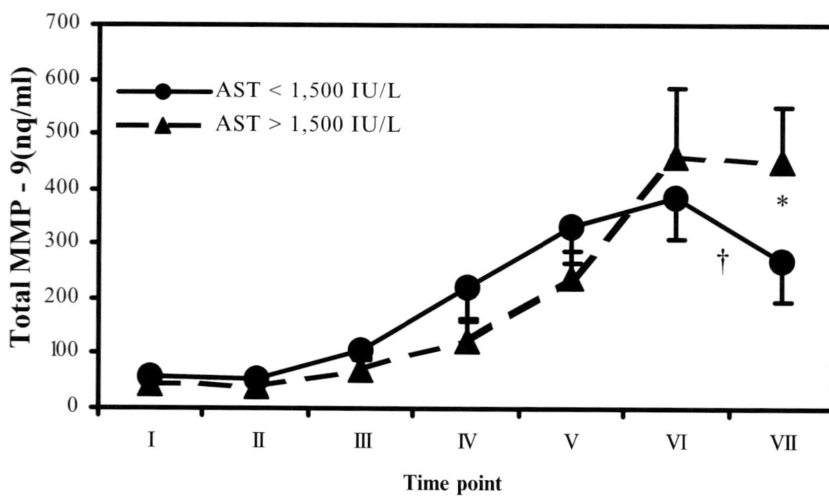

Figure 3: MMP-2 plasma concentrations during orthotopic liver transplantation (OLT). Blood samples were collected at 7 standardized time points: before transplantation (I), after induction of anesthesia (II), 10 minutes before the end of the pre-anhepatic period (III) and anhepatic period (IV), and 5 (V), 30 (VI) and 120 (VII) minutes post-reperfusion. Data are expressed as mean ± S.E.M. AST = serum aspartate aminotransferase •: Patients with a peak AST < 1,500 IU/L; ▲: Patients with a peak AST > 1,500 IU/L.

After OLT serum MMP-2 decreased about 50% but did not return to levels comparable with controls. This latter suggest the presence of persistent extracellular matrix remodeling in some of these patients and reflects probably a multifactorial cause, e.g. return of the original disease in the liver (hepatitis C), low-grade chronic allograft rejection or inflammation.

Finally we performed a study on the influence of the –1306 C/T MMP-2 and –1562 C/T MMP-9 gene promoter polymorphisms in chronic liver disease and transplantation (Kuyvenhoven *et al* 2005). The MMP-2 and MMP-9 protein expression in serum appeared to be independent of the MMP genotype in our total study population. However, in the patients with cirrhosis there was a clear relationship between the higher MMP-2 serum levels with advanced Child-Pugh stage and a more frequent wild-type –1306 CC genotype of MMP-2. In association, a more frequent –1562 CT MMP-9 genotype with an increased serum level was found in the chronic liver disease patients without cirrhosis. The development of *late* phase I/R-injury or rejection after OLT, however, was found to occur unrelated to the MMP-2 and MMP-9 genotype of the donor, the recipient or their MMP-genetic mismatch. Yet, the increased MMP-9 level 1 week after OLT in patients with rejection coincided with a higher donor CT MMP-9 genotype frequency.

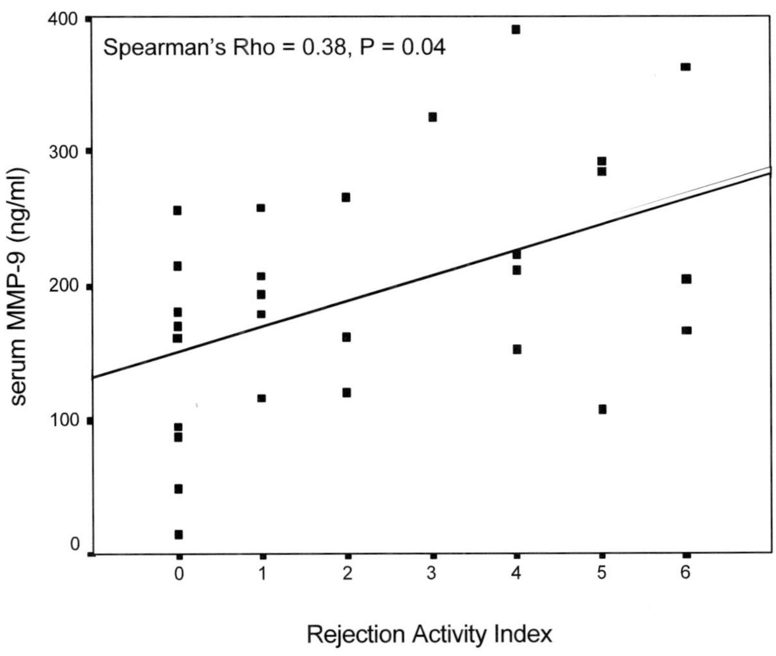

Figure 4: Scatter plot comparing total serum MMP-9 concentration at 1 week after orthotopic liver transplantation with the histopathologic rejection activity index.

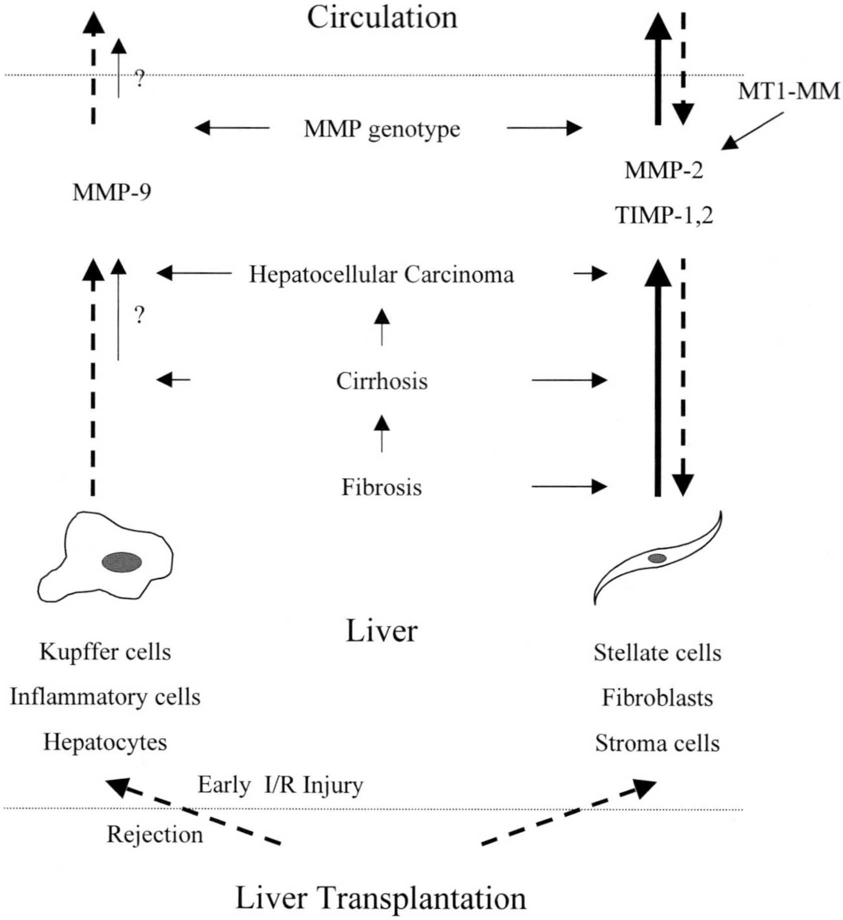

Figure 5: Effect of liver transplantation on the expression of MMP-2 and MMP-9 in chronic liver diseases, as indicated in Figure 1. The broken MMP-directed arrows indicate the strength of the changes observed.

5. CONCLUSIONS

Our studies describe the clinical impact of MMP-2 and MMP-9 in chronic liver disease and the effect of orthotopic liver transplantation, the latter schematically presented in Figure 5. Stellate cells are most likely the key source of MMP-2 and are known to be actively involved in the alteration of extracellular matrix (Benyon and Arthur 2001). The MMP-2 content of cirrhotic liver was higher compared to controls, and serum MMP-2 correlates positively with markers of liver dysfunction. These findings indicate, in concert with other recent publications (Zhou *et al* 2004; Huang *et al* 2005), an important role of MMP-2 in the development and persistence of liver fibrosis. However, in an individual patient, the serum MMP-2 level cannot be used as a single marker for liver function or fibrosis/cirrhosis. Recent studies suggest that the combination of several serum markers related to factors involved in extracellular matrix remodeling and fibrosis, including MMP-2, MMP-9 and TIMP-1, may distinguish between patients without fibrosis and with advanced liver disease (Leroy *et al* 2004; Patel *et al* 2004; Rosenberg *et al* 2004).

End-stage chronic liver disease is often complicated by HCC. In contrast to the earlier study by Hayasaka *et al* (1996) suggesting that serum MMP-9 could be used as a diagnostic marker for HCC, our study clearly demonstrated that serum MMP-9 levels were the same in chronic liver disease patients with or without HCC and thus not discriminative for this end-stage complication. The search for serum markers of HCC, e.g. by serum proteomic profiling through mass spectrometry, has become an important research issue. This is illustrated by a very recent study which revealed that an MMP-cleaved fragment of vitronectin, a glycoprotein involved in cell adhesion and matrix remodeling, identifies HCC in patients with chronic liver disease (Paradis *et al* 2005).

Elevated serum levels of MMP-9, probably derived from neutrophils and Kupffer cells, were found in patients with acute allograft rejection after OLT. MMPs have also been implicated in cold preservation injury to sinusoidal endothelial cells and we have demonstrated high plasma MMP-9 levels in the post-reperfusion period, especially in patients with more severe I/R injury. Therefore, MMP-9 seems to be a key mediator of *early* I/R-injury after OLT. The impact of MMP-9 was recently confirmed in a study on cold preservation injury using genetically deleted MMP-9/KO mice. This genetic deletion of MMP-9 resulted in the disappearance of MMP-9 from the cold preserved liver effluents and this was associated with less sinusoidal endothelial cell rounding, less actin disassembly and a reduction of platelet adhesion resulting in delayed injury to the sinusoidal endothelial cells compared to the wild-type mice (Topp *et al* 2004). Although liver preservation solutions already contain cryptic MMP inhibitors (Upadhya and Strasberg 2000), it remains speculative whether further pharmacological MMP inhibition may prohibit these complications of liver transplantation, due to unfavorable side effects upon chronic application and given the fact that MMPs are not only involved in the injury but also in the regeneration of the liver (Selzner *et al* 2003; Cursio *et al* 2002).

REFERENCES

Arii S, Mise M, Harada T, Fubvrutani M, Ishigami S, Niwano M, Mizumoto M, Fukumoto M, Imamura M, 1996, Overexpression of matrix metalloproteinase 9 gene in hepatocellular carcinoma with invasive potential. *Hepatology.* **24:** 316-322.

Arthur MJ, Stanley A, Iredale JP, Rafferty JA, Hembry RM, Friedman SL, 1992, Secretion of 72 kDa type IV collagenase/gelatinase by cultured human lipocytes. Analysis of gene expression, protein synthesis and proteinase activity. *Biochem J.* **287:** 701-707.

Arthur MJ, 1995, Collagenases and liver fibrosis. *J Hepatol.* **22**(2 Suppl)**:** 43-48.

Arthur MJ, 2000, Fibrogenesis II. Metalloproteinases and their inhibitors in liver fibrosis. *Am J Physiol Gastrointest Liver Physiol.* **279:** G245-G249.

Asfar S, Metrakos P, Fryer J, Verran D, Ghent C, Grant D, Bloch M, Burns P, Wall W, 1996, An analysis of late deaths after liver transplantation. Transplantation. **61:** 1377-1381.

Baramova E, Bajou K, Remacle A, L'Hoir C, Krell H, Weidle U, Noel A, Foidart JM, 1997, Involvement of PA/plasmin system in the processing of pro-MMP-9 and in the second step of pro-MMP-2 activation. *FEBS Lett.* **405:** 157-162.

Batts KP, 1999, Acute and chronic hepatic allograft rejection: pathology and classification. *Liver Transpl Surg.* **5**(4 Suppl 1)**:** S21-S29.

Benyon RC, Iredale JP, Goddard S, Winwood PJ, Arthur MJ, 1996, Expression of tissue inhibitor of metalloproteinases 1 and 2 is increased in fibrotic human liver. *Gastroenterology.* **110:** 821-831.

Benyon RC and Arthur MJ, 1998, Mechanisms of hepatic fibrosis. *J Pediatr Gastroenterol Nutr.* **27:** 75-85.

Benyon RC, Hovell C, Gaca MDA, Jones EH, Iredale JP, Arthur MJ, 1999, Progelatinase A is produced and activated by rat hepatic stellate cells and promotes their proliferation. *Hepatology.* **30:** 977-986.

Benyon RC and Arthur MJ, 2001, Extracellular matrix degradation and the role of hepatic stellate cells. *Semin Liver Dis.* **21:** 373-384.

Bissell DM, Roulot D, George J, 2001, Transforming growth factor beta and the liver. *Hepatology.* **34:** 859-867.

Boeker KH, Haberkorn CI, Michels D, Flemming P, Manns MP, Lichtinghagen R, 2002, Diagnostic potential of circulating TIMP-1 and MMP-2 as markers of liver fibrosis in patients with chronic hepatitis C. *Clin Chim Acta.* **316:** 71-81.

Brown PD, 1998, Matrix metalloproteinases in gastrointestinal cancer. *Gut.* **43:** 161-163.

Bruix J, Sherman M, Llovet J, Beaugrand M, Lencioni R, Burroughs AK, Christensen E, Pagliaro L, Colombo M, Rodes J; EASL Panel of Experts on HCC, 2001, Clinical Management of Hepatocellular Carcinoma. Conclusios of the Barcelona-2000 EASL Conference. *J Hepatol.* **35:** 421-430.

Bumgardner GL and Orosz CG, 1999, Transplantation and cytokines. *Semin Liver Dis.* **19:** 189-204.

Capper SJ, Verheijen J, Smith L, Sully M, Visser H, Hanemaaijer R, 1999, Determination of gelatinase-A (MMP-2) activity using a novel immunocapture assay. *Ann N Y Acad Sci.* **878:** 487-490.

Chambers AF and Matrisian LM, 1997, Changing views of the role of matrix metalloproteinases in metastasis. *J Natl Cancer Inst.* **89:** 1260-1270.

Cheung PY, Sawicki G, Wozniak M, Wang W, Radomski MW, Schulz R, 2000, Matrix metalloproteinase-2 contributes to ischemia-reperfusion injury in the heart. *Circulation.* **101:** 1833-1839.

Clavien PA, 1998, Sinusoidal endothelial cell injury during hepatic preservation and reperfusion. *Hepatology.* **28:** 281-285.

Corcoran ML, Hewitt RE, Kleiner Jr DE, Stetler-Stevenson WG, 1996, MMP-2: expression, activation and inhibition. *Enzyme Protein.* **49:** 7-19.

Cursio R, Mari B, Louis K, Rostagno P, Saint-Paul MC, Giudicelli J, Bottero V, Anglard P, Yiotakis A, Dive V, Gugenheim J, Auberger P, 2002, Rat liver injury after normothermic ischemia is prevented by a phosphinic matrix metalloproteinase inhibitor. *FASEB J.* **16:** 93-95.

Danielsen CC, Wiggers H, Andersen HR, 1998, Increased amounts of collagenase and gelatinase in porcine myocardium following ischemia and reperfusion. *J Mol Cell Cardiol.* **30:** 1431-1442.

Demirci G, Hoshino K, Nashan B, 1999, Expression patterns of integrin receptors and extracellular matrix proteins in chronic rejection of human liver allografts. *Transpl Immunol.* **7:** 229-237.

Duffy MJ and McCarthy K, 1998, Matrix metalloproteinases in cancer: prognostic markers and targets for therapy (review). *Int J Oncol.* **12:** 1343-1348.

Ebata M, Fukuda Y, Nakano I, Katano Y, Fujimoto N, Hayakawa T, 1997, Serum levels of tissue inhibitor of metalloproteinases-2 and of precursor form of matrix metalloproteinase-2 in patients with liver disease. *Liver.* **17:** 293-299.

Falk V, Soccal PM, Grunenfelder J, Hoyt G, Walther T, Robbins RC, 2002, Regulation of matrix metalloproteinases and effect of MMP-inhibition in heart transplant related reperfusion injury. *Eur J Cardiothorac Surg.* **22:** 53-58.

Fan C, Zwacka RM, Engelhardt JF, 1999, Therapeutic approaches for ischemia/reperfusion injury in the liver. *J Mol Med.* **77:** 577-592.

Farmer DG, Amersi F, Kupiec-Weglinski J, Busuttil RW, 2000, Current status of ischemia and reperfusion injury in the liver. *Transplantation Rev.* **14:** 106-126.

Friedman SL, 2000, Molecular regulation of hepatic fibrosis, an integrated cellular response to tissue injury. *J Biol Chem.* **275:** 2247-2250.

Geisler S, Lichtinghagen R, Boker KH, Veh RW, 1997, Differential distribution of five members of the matrix metalloproteinase family and one inhibitor (TIMP-1) in human liver and skin. *Cell Tissue Res.* **289:** 173-183.

Giannelli G, Bergamini C, Marinosci F, Fransvea E, Quaranta M, Lupo L, Schiraldi O, Antonaci S, 2002, Clinical role of MMP-2/TIMP-2 imbalance in hepatocellular carcinoma. *Int J Cancer.* **97:** 425-431.

Goetzl EJ, Banda MJ, Leppert D, 1996, Matrix metalloproteinases in immunity. *J Immunol.* **156:** 1-4.

Gveric D, Hanemaaijer R, Newcombe J, van Lent NA, Sier CF, Cuzner ML, 2001, Plasminogen activators in multiple sclerosis lesions: implications for the inflammatory response and axonal damage. *Brain.* **124:** 1978-1988.

Hall BM, 1991, Cells mediating allograft rejection. *Transplantation.* **51:** 1141-1151.

Hanemaaijer R, Visser H, Konttinen YT, Koolwijk P, Verheijen JH, 1998, A novel and simple immunocapture assay for determination of gelatinase-B (MMP-9) activities in biological fluids: saliva from patients with Sjogren's syndrome contain increased latent and active gelatinase-B levels. *Matrix Biol.* **17:** 657-665.

Harada T, Arii S, Mise M, Imamura T, Higashitsuji H, Furutani M, Niwano M, Ishigami S, Fukumoto M, Seiki M, Sato H, Imamura M, 1998, Membrane-type matrix metalloproteinase-1 (MT1-MTP) gene is overexpressed in highly invasive hepatocellular carcinomas. *J Hepatol.* **28:** 231-239.

Hayasaka A, Suzuki N, Fujimoto N, Iwama S, Fukuyama E, Kanda Y, Saisho H, 1996, Elevated plasma levels of matrix metalloproteinase-9 (92-kd type IV collagenase/ gelatinase B) in hepatocellular carcinoma. *Hepatology.* **24:** 1058-1062.

Hoekstra R, Eskens FA, Verweij J, 2001, Matrix metalloproteinase inhibitors: current developments and future perspectives. *Oncologist.* **6:** 415-427.

Huang CC, Chuang JH, Chou MH, Wu CL, Chen CM, Wang CC, Chen YS, Chen CL, Tai MH, 2005, Matrilysin (MMP-7) is a major matrix metalloproteinase upregulated in biliary atresia-associated liver fibrosis. *Mod Pathol.* **18:** 941-950.

Iredale JP, Benyon RC, Pickering J, McCullen M, Northrop M, Pawley S, Hovell C, Arthur MJ, 1998, Mechanisms of spontaneous resolution of rat liver fibrosis. Hepatic stellate cell apoptosis and reduced hepatic expression of metalloproteinase inhibitors. *J Clin Invest.* **102:** 538-549.

Johnatty RN, Taub DD, Reeder SP, Turcovski-Corrales SM, Cottam DW, Stephenson TJ, Rees RC, 1997, Cytokine and chemokine regulation of proMMP-9 and TIMP-1 production by human peripheral blood lymphocytes. *J Immunol.* **158:** 2327-2333.

Kasahara A, Hayashi N, Mochizuki K, Oshita M, Katayama K, Kato M, Masuzawa M, Yoshihara H, Naito M, Miyamoto T, Inoue A, Asai A, Hijioka T, Fusamoto H, Kamada T, 1997, Circulating matrix metalloproteinase-2 and tissue inhibitor of metalloproteinase-1 as serum markers of fibrosis in patients with chronic hepatitis C. Relationship to interferon response. *J Hepatol.* **26:** 574-583.

Kimizuka K, Fujisaki S, Park Y, Inoue M, Sugitou K, Tomita R, Fukuzawa M, Matsumoto K, 2002, Immunohistochemical changes in matrix metalloproteinase-2 and 9 during small bowel allograft rejection in rats. *Transplant Proc.* **34:** 1047-1048.

Kukan M and Haddad PS, 2001, Role of hepatocytes and bile duct cells in preservation-reperfusion injury of liver grafts. *Liver Transpl.* **7:** 381-400.

Kuo WH, Chou FP, Lu SC, Chu SC, Hsieh YS, 2000, Significant differences in serum activities of matrix metalloproteinase- 2 and -9 between HCV- and HBV-infected patients and carriers. *Clin Chim Acta.* **294:** 157-168.

Kuyvenhoven JP, Lamers CBHW, Hoek B van, 2001, Practical Management of Hepatocellular Carcinoma. *Scan J Gastroenterol.* **36**(Suppl 234)**:** 82-87.

Kuyvenhoven JP, Hoek B van, Blom E, Duijn W van, Hanemaaijer R, Verheijen JH, Lamers CBHW, Verspaget HW, 2003a, Assessment of the clinical significance of serum matrix metalloproteinases MMP-2 and MMP-9 in patients with various chronic liver diseases and hepatocellular carcinoma. *Thromb Haemost.* **89:** 718-725.

Kuyvenhoven JP, Ringers J, Verspaget HW, Lamers CBHW, Hoek B van, 2003b, Serum matrix metalloproteinase MMP-2 and MMP-9 in the late phase of ischemia and reperfusion injury in human orthotopic liver transplantation. *Transplant Proc.* **35:** 2967-2969.

Kuyvenhoven JP, Molenaar IQ, Verspaget HW, Veldman MG, Palareti G, Legnani C, Moolenburgh SE, Terpstra OT, Lamers CBHW, Hoek B van, Porte RJ, 2004a, Plasma MMP-2 and MMP-9 and their inhibitors TIMP-1 and TIMP-2 during human orthotopic liver transplantation. The effect of aprotinin and the relation to ischemia/reperfusion injury. *Thromb Haemost.* **91:** 506-513.

Kuyvenhoven JP, Verspaget HW, Gao Q, Ringers J, Smit VTHBM, Lamers CBHW, Hoek B van, 2004b, Assessment of serum matrix metalloproteinases MMP-2 and MMP-9 after human liver transplantation: increased serum MMP-9 level in acute rejection. *Transplantation.* **77:** 1646-1652.

Kuyvenhoven JP, Hove WR ten, Hoek B van, Meijer MJW, Berg M van den, Reijden JJ van der, Verduyn W, Lamers CBHW, Verspaget HW, 2005, Matrix metalloproteinase (MMP)-2 and MMP-9 gene promoter polymorphisms in chronic liver disease – relation to ischemia/reperfusion injury and rejection after orthotopic liver transplantation. Chapter 7 in Thesis Kuyvenhoven JP: Gelatinases in Chronic Liver Disease. The Clinical Relevance of MMP-2 and MMP-9 in Orthotopic Liver Transplantation: 67-77.

Lentsch AB, Kato A, Yoshidome H, McMasters KM, Edwards MJ, 2000, Inflammatory mechanisms and therapeutic strategies for warm hepatic ischemia/reperfusion injury. *Hepatology.* **32:** 169-173.

Leroy V, Monier F, Bottari S, Trocme C, Sturm N, Hilleret MN, Morel F, Zarski JP, 2004, Circulating matrix metalloproteinases 1, 2, 9 and their inhibitors TIMP-1 and TIMP-2 as serum markers of liver fibrosis in patients with chronic hepatitis C: comparison with PIIINP and hyaluronic acid. *Am J Gastroenterol.* **99:** 271-279.

Lichtinghagen R, Breitenstein K, Arndt B, Kuhbacher T, Boker KH, 1998, Comparison of matrix metalloproteinase expression in normal and cirrhotic human liver. *Virchows Arch.* **432:** 153-158.

Lichtinghagen R, Huegel O, Seifert T, Haberkorn CI, Michels D, Flemming P, Bahr M, Boeker KH, 2000, Expression of matrix metalloproteinase-2 and -9 and their inhibitors in peripheral blood cells of patients with chronic hepatitis C. *Clin Chem.* **46:** 183-192.

Lichtinghagen R, Michels D, Haberkorn CI, Arndt B, Bahr M, Flemming P, Manns MP, Boeker KH, 2001, Matrix metalloproteinase (MMP)-2, MMP-7, and tissue inhibitor of metalloproteinase-1 are closely related to the fibroproliferative process in the liver during chronic hepatitis C. *J Hepatol.* **34:** 239-247.

Lichtman SN and Lemasters JJ, 1999, Role of cytokines and cytokine-producing cells in reperfusion injury to the liver. *Semin Liver Dis.* **19:** 171-187.

Lijnen HR, Silence J, Lemmens G, Collen D, 1998, Regulation of gelatinase activity in mice with targeted inactivation of components of the plasminogen/plasmin system. *Thromb Haemost.* **79:** 1171-1176.

Määttä M, Soini Y, Liakka A, Autio-Harmainen H, 2000, Differential expression of matrix metalloproteinase (MMP)-2, MMP-9, and membrane type 1-MMP in hepatocellular and pancreatic adenocarcinoma: implications for tumor progression and clinical prognosis. *Clin Cancer Res.* **6:** 2726-2734.

Maring JK, Klompmaker IJ, Zwaveling JH, Kranenburg K, Ten Vergert EM, Slooff MJ, 1997, Poor initial graft function after orthotopic liver transplantation: can it be predicted and does it affect outcome? An analysis of 125 adult primary transplantations. *Clin Transplant.* **11:** 373-379.

Milani S, Herbst H, Schuppan D, Grappone C, Pellegrini G, Pinzani M, Casini A, Calabro A, Ciancio G, Stefanini F, 1994, Differential expression of matrix-metalloproteinase-1 and -2 genes in normal and fibrotic human liver. *Am J Pathol.* **144:** 528-537.

Millis JM, 1999, Treatment of liver allograft rejection. *Liver Transpl Surg.* **5**(4 Suppl 1)**:** S98-S106.

Mueller AR, Platz KP, Gebauer B, Schmidt C, Keck H, Lobeck H, Neuhaus P, 1998, Changes at the extracellular matrix during acute and chronic rejection in human liver transplantation. *Transpl Int.* **11**(Suppl 1)**:** S377-S382.

Murawaki Y, Ikuta Y, Idobe Y, Kitamura Y, Kawasaki H, 1997, Tissue inhibitor of metalloproteinase-1 in the liver of patients with chronic liver disease. *J Hepatol.* **26:** 1213-1219.

Murawaki Y, Yamada S, Ikuta Y, Kawasaki H, 1999, Clinical usefulness of serum matrix metalloproteinase-2 concentration in patients with chronic viral liver disease. *J Hepatol.* **30:** 1090-1098.

Murphy G and Docherty AJ, 1992, The matrix metalloproteinases and their inhibitors. *Am J Respir Cell Mol Biol.* **7:** 120-125.

Musso O, Theret N, Campion JP, Turlin B, Milani S, Grappone C, Clement B, 1997, In situ detection of matrix metalloproteinase-2 (MMP2) and the metalloproteinase inhibitor TIMP2 transcripts in human primary hepatocellular carcinoma and in liver metastasis. *J Hepatol.* **26:** 593-605.

Nagase H, Woessner Jr JF, 1999, Matrix metalloproteinases. *J Biol Chem.* **274:** 21491-21494.

Neuberger J, 1999, Incidence, timing, and risk factors for acute and chronic rejection. *Liver Transpl Surg.* **5**(4 Suppl 1)**:** S30-S36.

Nguyen M, Arkell J, Jackson CJ, 2001, Human endothelial gelatinases and angiogenesis. *Int J Biochem Cell Biol.* **33:** 960-970.

Ogata R, Torimura T, Kin M, Ueno T, Tateishi Y, Kuromatsu R, Shimauchi Y, Sakamoto M, Tamaki S, Sata M, Tanikawa K, 1999, Increased expression of membrane type 1 matrix metalloproteinase and matrix metalloproteinase-2 with tumor dedifferentiation in hepatocellular carcinomas. *Hum Pathol.* **30:** 443-450.

Okazaki I, Watanabe T, Hozawa S, Arai M, Maruyama K, 2000, Molecular mechanism of the reversibility of hepatic fibrosis: with special reference to the role of matrix metalloproteinases. *J Gastroenterol Hepatol.* **15**(Suppl)**:** D26-D32.

Opdenakker G, Van den Steen PE, Dubois B, Nelissen I, Van Coillie E, Masure S, Proost P, Van Damme J, 2001, Gelatinase B functions as regulator and effector in leukocyte biology. *J Leukoc Biol.* **69:** 851-859.

Paradis V, Degos F, Dargere D, Pham N, Belghiti J, Degott C, Janeau JL, Bezeaud A, Delforge D, Cubizolles M, Laurendeau I, Bedossa P, 2005, Identification of a new marker of hepatocellular carcinoma by serum protein profiling of patients with chronic liver diseases. *Hepatology.* **41:** 40-47.

Parsons SL, Watson SA, Brown PD, Collins HM, Steele RJ, 1997, Matrix metalloproteinases. *Br J Surg.* **84:** 160-166.

Patel K, Gordon SC, Jacobson I, Hezode C, Oh E, Smith KM, Pawlotsky JM, McHutchison JG, 2004, Evaluation of a panel of non-invasive serum markers to differentiate mild from moderate-to-advanced liver fibrosis in chronic hepatitis C patients. *J Hepatol.* **41:** 935-942.

Preaux AM, Mallat A, Nhieu JT, D'Ortho MP, Hembry RM, Mavier P, 1999, Matrix metalloproteinase-2 activation in human hepatic fibrosis regulation by cell-matrix interactions. *Hepatology.* **30:** 944-950.

Price SJ, Greaves DR, Watkins H, 2001, Identification of novel, functional genetic variants in the human matrix metalloproteinase-2 gene. *J Biol Chem.* **276:** 7549-7558.

Rosenberg WMC, Voelker M, Thiel R, Becka M, Burt A, Schuppan D, Hubscher S, Roskams T, Pinzani M, Arthur MJ; European Liver Fibrosis Group, 2004, Serum markers detect the presence of liver fibrosis: a cohort study. *Gastroenterology.* **127:** 1704-1713.

Sakamoto Y, Mafune K, Mori M, Shiraishi T, Imamura H, Mori M, Takayama T, Makuuchi M, 2000, Overexpression of MMP-9 correlates with growth of small hepatocellular carcinoma. *Int J Oncol.* **17:** 237-243.

Schuppan D, 1990, Structure of the extracellular matrix in normal and fibrotic liver: collagens and glycoproteins. *Semin Liver Dis.* **10:** 1-10.

Schuppan D, Ruehl M, Somasundaram R, Hahn EG, 2001, Matrix as a modulator of hepatic fibrogenesis. *Semin Liver Dis.* **21:** 351-372.

Selzner M, Rudiger HA, Graf R, Clavien PA, 2003, Protective strategies against ischemic injury of the liver. *Gastroenterology.* **125:** 917-936.

Serracino-Inglott F, Habib NA, Mathie RT, 2001, Hepatic ischemia-reperfusion injury. *Am J Surg.* **181:** 160-166.

Sier CF, Casetta G, Verheijen JH, Tizzani A, Agape V, Kos J, Blasi F, Hanemaaijer R, 2000, Enhanced urinary gelatinase activities (matrix metalloproteinases 2 and 9) are associated with early-stage bladder carcinoma: a comparison with clinically used tumor markers. *Clin Cancer Res.* **6:** 2333-2340.

Sternlicht MD and Werb Z, 2001, How matrix metalloproteinases regulate cell behavior. *Annu Rev Cell Dev Biol.* **17:** 463-516.

Strasberg SM, Howard TK, Molmenti EP, Hertl M, 1994, Selecting the donor liver: risk factors for poor function after orthotopic liver transplantation. *Hepatology.* **20:** 829-838.

Takahara T, Furui K, Yata Y, Jin B, Zhang LP, Nambu S, Sato H, Seiki M, Watanabe A, 1997, Dual expression of matrix metalloproteinase-2 and membrane-type 1- matrix metalloproteinase in fibrotic human livers. *Hepatology.* **26:** 1521-1529.

Theret N, Musso O, L'Helgoualc'h A, Campion JP, Clement B, 1998, Differential expression and origin of membrane-type 1 and 2 matrix metalloproteinases (MT-MMPs) in association with MMP2 activation in injured human livers. *Am J Pathol.* **153:** 945-954.

Theret N, Musso O, Turlin B, Lotrian D, Bioulac-Sage P, Campion JP, Boudjema K, Clement B, 2001, Increased extracellular matrix remodeling is associated with tumor progression in human hepatocellular carcinomas. *Hepatology.* **34:** 82-88.

Topp SA, Upadhya GA, Strasberg SM, 2004, Cold preservation of isolated sinusoidal endothelial cells in MMP 9 knockout mice: effect on morphology and platelet adhesion. *Liver Transpl.* **10:** 1041-1048.

Tran T, Poordad F, Nissen N, Martin P, 2002, Hepatocellular Carcinoma: An Update. *Clin Persp Gastroenterology.* **5:** 302-306.

Ueno T, Tamaki S, Sugawara H, Inuzuka S, Torimura T, Sata M, Tanikawa K, 1996, Significance of serum tissue inhibitor of metalloproteinases-1 in various liver diseases. *J Hepatol.* **24:** 177-184.

Upadhya AG, Harvey RP, Howard TK, Lowell JA, Shenoy S, Strasberg SM, 1997, Evidence of a role for matrix metalloproteinases in cold preservation injury of the liver in humans and in the rat. *Hepatology.* **26:** 922-928.

Upadhya GA and Strasberg SM, 1999, Evidence that actin disassembly is a requirement for matrix metalloproteinase secretion by sinusoidal endothelial cells during cold preservation in the rat. *Hepatology.* **30:** 169-176.

Upadhya GA and Strasberg SM, 2000, Glutathione, lactobionate, and histidine: cryptic inhibitors of matrix metalloproteinases contained in University of Wisconsin and histidine/tryptophan/ketoglutarate liver preservation solutions. *Hepatology.* **31:** 1115-1122.

Vierling JM, 1999, Immunology of acute and chronic hepatic allograft rejection. *Liver Transpl Surg.* **5**(4 Suppl 1)**:** S1-S20.

Walsh KM, Timms P, Campbell S, MacSween RN, Morris AJ, 1999, Plasma levels of matrix metalloproteinase-2 (MMP-2) and tissue inhibitors of metalloproteinases -1 and -2 (TIMP-1 and TIMP-2) as noninvasive markers of liver disease in chronic hepatitis C: comparison using ROC analysis. *Dig Dis Sci.* **44:** 624-630.

Wiesner RH, Demetris AJ, Belle SH, Seaberg EC, Lake JR, Zetterman RK, Everhart J, Detre KM, 1998,_Acute hepatic allograft rejection: incidence, risk factors, and impact on outcome. *Hepatology.* **28:** 638-645.

Winwood PJ, Schuppan D, Iredale JP, Kawser CA, Docherty AJ, Arthur MJ, 1995, Kupffer cell-derived 95-kd type IV collagenase/gelatinase B: characterization and expression in cultured cells. *Hepatology.* **22:** 304-315.

Woessner Jr JF, 1991, Matrix metalloproteinases and their inhibitors in connective tissue remodeling. *FASEB J.* **5:** 2145-2154.

Yano M, Omoto Y, Yamakawa Y, Nakashima Y, Kiriyama M, Saito Y, Fuyii Y, 2001, Increased matrix metalloproteinase 9 activity and mRNA expression in lung ischemia-reperfusion injury. *J Heart Lung Transplant.* **20:** 679-686.

Yu Q and Stamenkovic I, 2000, Cell surface localized matrix metalloproteinase-9 proteolytically activates TGF-beta and promotes tumor invasion and angiogenesis. *Genes Dev.* **14:** 163-176.

Zhang B, Ye S, Herrmann S-M, Eriksson P, de Maat M, Evans A, Arveiler D, Luc G, Cambien F, Hamsten A, Watkins H, Henney AM, 1999, Functional polymorphism in the regulatory region of gelatinase B gene in relation to severity of coronary atherosclerosis. *Circulation.* **99:** 1788-1794.

Zhou X, Hovell CJ, Pawley S, Hutchings MI, Arthur MJ, Iredale JP, Benyon RC, 2004, Expression of matrix metaloproteinasse-2 and –14 persists during early resolution of experimental liver fibrosis and might contribute to fibrolysis. *Liver International.* **24:** 492-501.

Ziswiler R, Daniel C, Franz E, Marti HP, 2001, Renal matrix metalloproteinase activity is unaffected by experimental ischemia-reperfusion injury and matrix metalloproteinase inhibition does not alter outcome of renal function. *Exp Nephrol.* **9:** 118-124.

Zucker S, Hymowitz M, Conner C, Zarrabi HM, Hurewitz AN, Matrisian L, Boyd D, Nicolson G, Montana S, 1999,_Measurement of matrix metalloproteinases and tissue inhibitors of metalloproteinases in blood and tissues. Clinical and experimental applications. *Ann N Y Acad Sci.* **878:** 212-227.

Chapter 10

MMPs and ADAMs in Inflammatory Bowel Disease

Alicja Wiercinska-Drapalo, Jerzy Jaroszewicz, Anna Parfieniuk, Anna Moniuszko

Department of Infectious Diseases, Medical University of Bialystok, Zurawia 14 Str., 15-540 Bialystok, Poland.

1. INTRODUCTION

Idiopathic inflammatory bowel disease (IBD) is classified into two distinct disorders: ulcerative colitis (UC) and Crohn's diseases (CD). IBD are chronic inflammatory bowel diseases characterized by repeated episodes of intestinal inflammation and damage following by relapses and intestine wound healing. Although classified together, UC and CD show a different localization and to some extent different pathogenesis. Ulcerative colitis affects colon and the intestine lesions are superficial while Crohn's disease may involve any part of gastrointestinal tract and is characterized by transmural granulomatous infiltrations. The exact pathogenesis of UC and CD is still mysterious. A number of studies suggested that CD is T-cell mediated disorder with excessive Th-1 cell activity associated with pro-inflammatory cytokine overproduction. Less information on pathogenesis of UC is available. Many authors believe that in contrast to CD the predominant immune response type is Th2, however this hypothesis is not fully documented, for example IL-4, classical Th2-type cytokine seems not to increase in UC. The common feature of CD and UC is extracellular matrix (ECM) remodeling associated with ongoing inflammatory responses and intestinal lesions healing.

The regulation of ECM turnover is a dynamic process essential for embryonic development, morphogenesis, reproduction, and tissue resorption and remodeling. The major regulators of collagen synthesis and degradation

U. Lendeckel and Nigel M. Hooper (eds.), Proteases in Gastrointestinal Tissue, 235-254.

are zinc-dependant enodpeptidases - matrix metalloproteinases (MMPs) and their inhibitors (tissue inhibitors of metalloproteinases - TIMPs).

2. MATRIX METALLOPROTEINASES

2.1 Expression, regulation and functions in the gut

The variety of cells in the intestine are able to produce MMPs, among them fibroblasts (MMP-1, 2, 3, 14), macrophages (MMP-1, 3, 9, 12), epithelial cells (MMP-7, 8, 10), neutrophils (MMP-8) and eosinophils (MMP-9). It is believed that the major source of MMP-1 and MMP-3 are macrophages and T-cells-induced MMP production by those cells links mucosal inflammation and tissue destruction in chronic gut diseases (Goetzl *et al* 1996). However in-situ hybridization studies indicate that α-actin positive cells such as myofibroblasts are a main source of MMP mRNAs in the inflamed gut, which is not confirmed in immunochemistry (Pender *et al* 1998). According to hypothesis presented by von Lampe *et al* (2000) MMP produced by α-actin positive cells are not stored within these cells and are secreted and bound to ECM. In contrast with majority of other cells macrophages are able to store pro-MMP.

In physiological condition MMPs are present at low levels and their expression and activation is regulated at the level of gene expression, their precursors activation, interaction with ECM components as well as inhibition by TIPMs (Pender *et al* 2004). The MMP expression "inductors" include (Nagase *et al* 1999) growth factors, cytokines (including TNF-alpha, IL-1β), chemical agents (among them phorbol esters) and oncogenes. On the contrary increased MMPs gene expression may be downregulated by suppressive factors including TGF-beta1, retinoids and glucocrticoids. Recently cell-to-cell and cell-to-ECM interactions were underlined as a important regulators of MMPs gene expression. For example expression of MT1-MMP by fibroblasts in cell-culture is mediated by $\alpha_2\beta_1$ integrin (Seltzer *et al* 1994).

Most of MMPs are secreted from the cell in inactive forms and anchored to the cell surface thus their activity is restrained to cell membrane or extracellular matrix. Secreted MMPs are activated in-vivo by tissue or plasma proteinases or bacterial proteinases, mainly on the cell surface. In 1994 Sato *et al.* (1994) cloned the first membrane-type MMP (MT1-MMP named MMP-14) and they demonstrated it to be an activator of pro-MMP2 (Sato *et al* 1994). The subsequent studies suggested that this process requires both active MT1-MMP and TIMP-2 bound MT1-MMP.

Tissue activity of MMPs is controlled by their endogenous inhibitors (TIMPs) by forming 1:1 complexes with zinc in MMPs. In some disorders the production of MMP exceeds the inhibitory potential of TIMP which results in imbalance between ECM synthesis and breakdown. This process was proposed as a potential etiology of fistulae formation in Crhon's disease (Kirkegaard *et al* 2004).

The most extensively studied function of metalloproteinases, since the first MMP discovery in 1962 (Gross and Lapiere 1962) is degradation of all classes of ECM including collagens, non-collagenous glycoproteins and proteoglycans. In-vitro studies showed considerable overlap in MMP substrates (especially fibronectin, laminins, elastin, type IV collagen), (Sternlicht *et al* 2001). Substrates selectivity in-vivo is regulated by enzyme affinity and compartmentalization. Since MMPs are anchored on the cell membrane, bound to integrins, CD44 or surface proteoglycans they maintain high concentration locally and are able to target specific substrates in the pericellular space.

In spite of the most widely discussed role of MMPs/TIMPs in ECM turnover, recent findings suggested their function in the inflammation and immunity, as a pro-inflammatory cytokines, chemokines and other immune and inflammation regulators (Parks *et al* 2004; McQuibban *et al* 2000 and 2001). Increased or misregulated levels of MMPs as well as TIMPs are observed in the majority immune-related or chronic inflammatory disorders including IBD. However the exact role of MMP family members, which comprises of more then 24 related but distinct proteins, in inflammatory conditions was not yet entirely revealed.

Targeting of immune system by MMPs could be a result of chemokine as well as cytokine activity modulation and gradient formation (McQuibban *et al* 2002). It was shown that selected MMPs are able to convert initial forms of chemotactic factors into antagonistic molecules. For example CC-chemokine ligand 7 (CCL7) is a substrate for MMP-2, which after cleavage looses its chemotactic abilities and functions as chemokine antagonist. Similarly MMP-1, 3 and 14 are capable of cleaving CCL2 which is also mechanism of angiogenesis regulation. (Galvez *et al* 2005). This MMP functions illustrates a possible anti-inflammatory activity of MMPs. Moreover several authors shown MMPs are able to directly or indirectly activate various cytokines engaged in inflammatory and wound healing processes. In in-vitro models it was suggested that MMP-3, 9 as well as 14 are able to activate TGF-β1. Since TGF-β1 is a cytokine of a known anti-inflammatory and immunoupressive activity this could be another mechanism of MMP-mediated immune restrain. On the other hand several MMPs are engaged in pro-inflammatory cytokine activation. Despite the major activator of TNF-α is ADAM17, a number of MMPs (MMP-1, 2, 3, 9 and 17) are capable of processing pro-TNF into active form in-vitro (Mohan *et al* 2002, English *et al* 2000).

Additionally MMP-7 and MMP-12 activate pro-TNF on macrophages. Schonbeck *et al* (1997) showed that at least three of MMP family members, namely MMP-2, 3, 9 can cleave and activated IL-β precursor. Interestingly after IL-1β activation MMP3 is able to degrade this cytokine into inactive form. In conclusions the regulation of immune and inflammation by MMPs is complex, probably bimodal and unrevealed even to the extent whether they act as a pro-inflammatory or anti-inflammatory factors.

2.2 Matrix metalloproteinases in IBD

The hallmark of an IBD is tissue degradation and lesion development resulting from uncontrolled and chronic inflammatory responses. Among the modulators of an IBD activity the role cytokines, growth factors, chemokines, free radicals and recently metalloproteinases and their endogenous inhibitors – TIMPs is underlined. A number of up to date studies pointed to MMPs as the most important proteolytic enzymes engaged in extracellular matrix degradation in inflammatory bowel diseases. Although many authors showed overexpression of majority MMPs in IBD the MMP-1 (collagenase-1) and MMP-3 (stromelysin-1) are believed to be predominant in the IBD pathogenesis.

von Lampe *et al* (2000) studied the expression of various MMPs (MMP-1, MMP-2, MMP-3, MMP-14) as well as TIMPs (TIMP-1 and TIMP-2) in IBD (UC and CD) patients as well as healthy controls at the protein and mRNA levels. They found the low expression of MMP-1 and MMP-3 in normal colonic mucosa. However in inflamed colon samples from IBD patients authors observed that mRNA expression of all studied MMPs was significantly increased in inflamed compared with non-inflamed colonic mucosa. Median expression of MMP-1 increased 20-fold in CD and 42-fold in UC subjects with analogous 15-fold and 43-fold (respectively) increase of MMP-3 expression. The increase in the expression of MMP-2 and MMP-14 mRNA was less pronounced. Analogous data indicating the increase in MMP-1 and MMP-2 expression were obtained by Stallmach *et al*. (2000).

Another major finding arising from the study of von Lampe *et al* (2000) was a strong, positive correlation between the histological degree of acute inflammation and MMP-1, MMP-2 and MMP-3 mRNA expression. The strongest correlation was noted between procollagen type III and MMP-2 mRNA expression. The most prominent expression of MMPs was noted in severely inflamed tissues characterized by ulcerations. In another study Heuschkel *et al* (2000) found the similar relationship between MMP-1 expression and loss of mucosal integrity in children with IBD, with MMP-1 normalization after introduction of eneteral nutrition. Therefore the elevated MMP-1 and MMP-3 expression may reflect acute tissue damage rather than wound healing. The common and quite intriguing feature of reports by von Lampe (2000) and by Heuschkel (2000) was that expression of MMPs and MMPs/TIMPs ratio was comparable between an IBD individuals of different etiology: UC and CD and depended mainly on degree of histological inflammation. It is quite unexpected since different pathogenesis of both of those disorders with presumably Th1 type immunological response predominance in CD and Th2 in UC as well as intestinal fibrosis as a key event occurring in CD but not in ulcerative colitis. However current knowledge of molecular mechanism of fibrosis in IBD is limited and cannot be understood as a simple wound-healing response.

The relationship between MMP-3 expression in intestine tissues and the extent of macroscopic and microscopic inflammation was further evaluated by Louis *et al* (2000). Authors found the strong, significant positive correlations between MMP-3 concentrations in tissue cultures obtained from UC and CD and local concentrations of pro-inflammatory cytokines: IL-1β, IL-6, TNF-α as well as IL-10 (Louis *et al* 2000). Since there are many evidences that TNF-α, IL-1β and to lesser extent IL-6 are able to stimulate several metalloproteases production (Saarialho-Kere *et al* 1996), this finding provides the link between MMPs and local inflammatory processes. Interestingly in this study the correlation between MMP-3 and TNF-α was stronger in UC than in CD, which might indicate the difference in the regulation of MMP-3 production in both of IBD conditions. Moreover increase in IL-10 concentration and its positive correlation with MMP-3 suggests that IL-10 overproduction is not sufficient to suppress MMP-3 significantly. Another suggestion that intestine injury caused by TNF-α in IBD is mediated by MMP overproduction comes from study of Pender *et al* (1998). Authors showed inhibition in MMPs expression (particularly MMP-3) after delivery of TNF-α neutralizing antibody p55 TNF receptor-human IgG fusion protein.

In the recently published study Kirkegaard *et al* (2004) observed that acute fistulising inflammation in CD is characterized by high expression of MMP-3 and MMP-9 coupled with high activity of MMP-2 and MMP-9 in inflammatory, while in chronic fistulae MMP-9 expression diminished with continuous production of MMP-3 with shift to myofibroblastic cells. MMP-3 acts as a proactivator to many substrates including MMP-1, MMP-2, MMP-9 and thus has been identified as a predominant aggressive protease in intestinal inflammation which favors invasiveness. In the fistula samples expression of TIMPs remained low which can in some measure explain high fibrinolytic activity of MMPs and low fibrinogenesis in fistulising intestinal inflammation.

Other report indicated to MMP-8 (collagenase-2), expressed in large intestinal surface epithelial cells, as important metalloproteinase participating in remodeling and homesotatsis of epithelial layer as well as ulcer formation associated with the extensive type I collagen degradation (Pirilla *et al* 2003).

Apart of many evidences suggesting significant role of MMP-1, MMP-3 and MMP-9 in acute inflammation and damage some authors underline its function in intestine lesions healing. In the recent study Salmela *et al* (2004) found that MMP-1, MMP-7 and MMP-10 were expressed by migrating enetrocytes bordering intestinal ulcers. Their production was stimulated by cytokines involved in wound healing i.e. TGF-β, EGF and TNF-α. Authors concluded that above mentioned MMPs are involved in epithelial cell migration during intestinal wound healing and potential therapeutic use of MMP inhibitors should be considered cautiously.

MMP-7 (matrylisin), an MMP contributing to initiation and continuation of tumor growth (Chambers and Matrisian 1997; Adachi *et al* 1999), was also found in epithelil cells in UC. Newell *et al* (2002) showed a switch from focal expression of MMP-7 in UC-related low-grade dysplasia to widespread expression in high-grade dysplasia and invasive cancer. Thus MMP-7 may be implicated in tumorgenesis in the course of UC. In another tissue expression of MMP-7 showed a significant correlation with degree of inflammation in UC (Matsuno *et al* 2003) and could be used as an important marker of activity and subsequent transformation in UC patients.

von Lampe (2000) reported increased mRNA expression of MMP-14, the membrane bound activator of MMP-2, predominantly in ulcerated colonic mucosa in IBD patients. Inflammation without ulceration causes only a minor increase (2-2,5 fold) in both mRNA steady state levels. In ulcerated tissue samples however, both mRNA levels (MMP-2, MMP-14) were increased 9-12 fold compared with non-inflamed mucosa. Expression MMP-14 is also required for neoangiogenesis (Hiraoka *et al* 1998) witch is important factor in ulcer healing.

In the recent years several new MMPs were described of which at least two were implicated in IBD pathogenesis. MMP-19 was cloned in 1997 from liver (Pendas *et al* 1997) and its expression was found in fibroblasts and smooth muscle cells. This metalloproteinase is engaged in degradation of many ECM substrates however was not implicated in activating any of pro-MMPs (Stracke *et al* 2000). Moreover unlike others MMPs the expression of MMP-19 is downregulated during tumorgenesis (Djonov *et al* 2001). In the recent work Bister *et al* (2004) found expression of MMP-19 in non-migrating enterocytes and shedding epithelium in IBD and suggested its role in restoring normal composition of gut ephitelium and mucosa after injury. Another newly described metalloproteinase: MMP-26 (matrylisin-2) is able to cleave fibronectin, vitronectin, fibrinogen and type IV collagen, moreover in-vitro studies shown its capacity of activating MMP-9. In-vivo it was implicated in carcinogenesis (Zhao *et al* 2004). In IBD individuals expression of MMP-26 was detected in migrating enterocytes bordering the sites of intestinal injury and it is probably implicated in regulating enterocyte migration (Bister *et al* 2004).

2.3 Tissue matrix metalloproteinases inhibitors in IBD

Tissue inhibitors of metalloproteinases (TIMPs) are endogenous MMPs inhibitors acting via noncovalent binding of the active forms of MMPs at molar equivalence. TIMP-1 is inducible and TIMP-2 is expressed mainly constitutively. The function of TIMPs in IBD is less known and to some extent ambiguous.

von Lampe (2000) observed significantly increased expression of TIMP-1 mRNA in inflamed, particularly ulcerated colon colon mucosa from IBD patients. mRNA TIMP-2 levels remained unchanged. However the mRNA expression of MMP-1 and MMP-3 overly exceeded the moderate increased expression of their TIMP-1 in inflamed mucosa of IBD patients. Some of other studies did not report the increase in TIMP-1 expression in tissue samples of IBD patients while observing significant increase in MMP-3 expression (Heuschkel *et al* 2000, Louis *et al* 2000, Matsuno *et al* 2003). Thus the elevated MMP-3 with inadequate increase in expression of its endogenous inhibitor – TIMP-1 (i.e. MMP/TIMP ratio imbalance) would favor matrix degradation in IBD.

On the contrary, recently McKaig *et al* (2003) showed higher constitutive expression of TIMP-1, but no TIMP-2 in myofibroblasts cultures established from CD fibrotic intestinal lesions compared to similar cells isolated from UC or normal intestinal tissue. This overexpression may result in the increase in inhibition of MMPs activity and therefore may lead to excessive matrix deposition and stricture formation in Crohn's disease. Moreover authors showed that TIMP-1 expression in myofibroblasts may be regulated in different manner by various isoforms of TGF-β with TGF-β1 and TGF-β2 with stimulatory effect and TGF-β3 with no influence on TIMP-1. We reported the increase in TGF-β1 plasma concentration in UC patients with a significant positive correlation with clinical disease activity and the extent of inflammatory lesions. (Wiercinska-Drapalo *et al* 2001). Furthermore in the next study we showed the decrease in TGF-β1 concentrations after successful UC treatment (Wiercinska-Drapalo *et al* 2003). Taken together it may indicate the role of TGF-β1-regulated TIMP-1 expression in IBD pathogenesis.

The majority of reports on metalloproteinases and their inhibitors in IBD were focused on their role in disease pathogenesis. In several of previous reports the relationship between MMP/TIMP and degree of local inflammation was observed. Going further we investigated the MMP-1 and TIMP-1 plasma concentrations in ulcerative colitis as a possible markers of disease activity. The plasma levels of MMP-1 as well as TIMP-1 in UC were increased in comparison to healthy individuals (Fig. 1). Moreover TIMP-1 concentration was positively associated with endoscopic degree of mucosal injury, clinical activity as well as C-reactive protein concentration. Therefore we concluded that plasma TIMP-1 concentration measurement could be a useful biomarker reflecting UC severity (Wiercinska-Drapalo *et al* 2003).

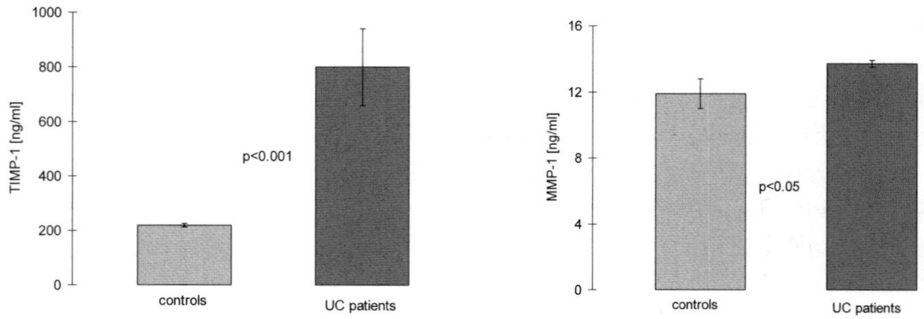

Figure 1: Comparison of mean (±SEM) MMP-1 as well as TIMP-1 plasma concentrations in group of patients with ulcerative colitis and controls.

2.4 Conclusions

Since vast MMP engagement in IBD pathogenesis the therapeutic approaches to control MMP activity and pathways were undertaken. Synthetic MMP inhibitors (i.e. Batimastat, ONO-4847) as well as MMPs signal transduction modulators (i.e. NF-kappa B) were used in IBD animal models with encouraging results (Di Sebastiano *et al* 2001, Naito *et al* 2004, Lawrance *et al* 2003). However the difficulty in drug administration to intestine tissue as well as limited selectivity of synthetic MMPs inhibitors and complexity of their actions resulted in several adverse reacting including bone and joints disorders. Further studies overcoming those obstacles as well as getting deeper insight into MMPs involvement in IBD pathogenesis are required.

In summary, up to date reports demonstrate that several MMPs are upregulated in association with T-cell immune responses and are engaged in different IBD pathogenesis pathways including ongoing mucosal inflammation and injury, but also wound healing, immunomodulation, angiogenesis and tumorgenesis. Overproduction of MMPs and the failure to control their activity by endogenous inhibitors activity (TIMPs) is probably the foremost mechanism of ulcers formation in UC and strictures and fistulae in CD. Thus interfering MMP signal transduction cascade may be an attractive therapeutic option. However since the knowledge on exact role of MMPs and TIMPs in IBD pathogenesis as well as the fact of influence on to some extent divergent pathways is still limited their therapeutic approaches should be undertaken cautiously.

3. ADAM FAMILY MEMBERS

3.1 Introduction and definition

ADAMs are membrane anchored multidomain proteins containing A Disintegrin and A Metalloproteinase domain. Due to the content of the cysteine rich region they are also named MDCs – Metalloproteinase Disintegrin Cysteine rich proteins (Black 1998; Wolfsberg and White 1995, 1996, 1998; http://www.people.virginia.edu/~jw7g/Table_of_the_ADAMs.html). This subfamily of the zinc – dependent metalloproteinases perform several functions in a variety of cells and have now been implicated in an array of developmental and disease processes.

ADAM family are the proteins of the highly phylogenetically conserved basic structure that have been found in various species, including yeast *Schizosaccharomyces pombe*, nematodes *Caenorhabditis elegans* and *Caenorhabditis briggsae*, *Drosophila melanogaster* and vertebrates. It was noted that these proteins contain structures of the metalloproteinase and disintegrin similar to those of the PIII class of the snake venom metalloproteinases (SVMPs) (Blobel 2005, 1992; Niewiarowski *et al* 1994; Yamamoto *et al* 1999). A number of ADAMs occur as different isoforms, including soluble isoforms. Moreover, there is a separate ADAM-TS family of the proteases, similar to the ADAMs, with additional thrombospondin type 1 motif, the expression of which is associated with inflammatory processes http://www.gene.ucl.ac.uk/nomenclature/genefamily/adamts.html; Yamamoto *et al* 1999).

3.2 Molecular structure – model

A typical ADAM's molecule consist of a pro–domain following an N – terminal signal sequence, a metalloproteinase domain, a disintegrin domain, a cysteine – rich domain in which an EGF-like structure is contained. Membrane-bound ADAMs possesses additional transmembrane and cytoplasmic domains (Blobel 2005; Seals *et al* 2003; Wolfsberg *et al* 1995).

The pro – domain is considered to function as intramolecular chaperone (Seals 2003). It keeps the properly folded enzyme in an inactive state until it is removed by pro – proteine convertase or through an autocatalytic removal activating the metalloproteinase domain.

All ADAMs have a metalloproteinase domain, but only half of them contain a zinc – dependent catalytic – site consensus amino acid sequence: HEXGHXXGXXHD and display a protease activity (Yamamoto *et al* 1999; Wolfsberg and White 2003). This motif is present in ADAMs 1, 8-10, 12, 13,

15, 16, 17, 19-21, 24-26, 28, 30 and 33-40 (http://www.people.viginia.edu/~jw7g/Table_of_the_ADAMs.html). The other members that do not contain this motif presumably do not possess protease activity. The catalytic domains mediate the important regulatory process of ectodomain shedding and can cleave and remodel extracellular matrix proteins.

A disintegrin and a cysteine – rich domains (D/C) are responsible for adhesive activities. The name of a disintegrin domain is derived from the resemblance to the snake – venom disintegrins which are short soluble proteins binding to the platelet glycoprotein IIIb/IIa and thus functioning as inhibitors of platelet aggregation. It have been shown, that both, disintegrins and ADAMs disintegrin domains, are sharing the Arg-Gly-Asp (RGD) consensus sequence or RGD – like motif appearing as a key elements of their (integrin – like) receptor recognition site (Blobel 2005, 1992; Niewiarowski *et al* 1994; Yamamoto *et al* 1999). The adhesive domains play a significant role in binding important molecules involved in cell-matrix adhesion (e.g. integrins and syndecans). Moreover D/C can facilitate the removal of the pro – domain from the catalytic domain and are implicated in substrate targeting and determination of a protease-dependent response *in vivo* (Blobel 2005).

The cytoplasmic tails of ADAMs have multiple potential binding partners. Several of them contain signalling motifs, such as phosphorylation sites or proline – rich regions that are capable of binding Src – homology – 3 (SH3) ligands. Therefore they could be involved in signal transduction (Blobel 2005, Seals *et al* 2003).

3.3 Family & function

Until now, 37 ADAM proteins are known. 33 of them have been described as mammalian and 22 of them have been identified in human. An updated list of ADAMs is available online on the White Lab. website (http://www.people.virginia.edu/~jw7g/Table_of_the_ADAMs.html).

The first identified ADAMs appeared to be the subunits of the sperm protein fertilin (ADAM 1 and ADAM 2) (Blobel & White 1990). Now, it is known that ADAM proteins are expressed in the wide variety of cells as it is shown in the table 1. The primarily testis-specific are ADAMs: 2-6, 18, 20, 21, 24-26, 29, 30, 32, 34, 36-40. The testases (ADAMs 24-26, 34, and 36-40) seem to be present in the mouse, but not in the human, genome.

ADAMs are known as a major regulatory proteins of the cell surface. Due to the ability of shedding ligands and receptors involved in cell-cell contact and signalling they can influence on cell to cell interactions. They are also engaged in cleaving and remodelling ECM proteins and adhesion molecules.

ADAM proteases are involved in the processing of broad diversity of substrates, including growth factors, cytokines, cell adhesion molecules and receptors. They are implicated in the activation of precursor forms of proteins by ectodomain shedding, for instance, TNF-α (tumor necrosis factor-α), TGF-β (transforming growth factor-β, HB-EGF (heparin-binding epidermal growth factor), amphiregulin, APP (amyloid precursor protein), Notch, IL6R (interleukin 6 receptor), IL1-RII (interleukin 1 receptor type II), CD 163, GHBP (growth hormone binding protein), L-selectin, the neural recognition molecule L1, close homolog of L1 - CHL1, TNFRI (tumor necrosis factor receptor I), TNFRII (tumor necrosis factor receptor II), the M-CSF receptor (macrophage colony stimulating factor receptor), the low affinity receptor for IgE - CD23, the erbB4 receptor, and type 1 neuregulin (Moss and Bartsch 2004). Hence, it seems they play a key role in regulating diverse extracellular signalling events.

Different ADAM proteins take part in many interactions with various types of cells (Table 1). The studies on ADAM 11, 15, 23 demonstrated that disintergrin domain support integrin mediated cell adhesion (White *et al* 2001). In tissue culture ADAM disintegrin domains are able to interact with group of β1-integrins, as well as β3 and β5-integrin, on the surface of adjoining cells. There are evidences suggesting that selected ADAMs - integrin interactions might require previous integrin activation.

ADAM adhesive domains can also interact with extracellular matrix components. The cysteine-rich domains interact with the Hep-II binding domain of fibronectin. This process requires residues in the Hep-II domain of fibronectin that interact with syndecans. Syndecans and integrins cooperate to foster cell binding to ECM proteins (Ropreager 2001). Therefore the ability of ADAMs to interact with integrins, syndecans and ECM proteins suggests that ADAMs seem to play key role in modulating cell-matrix interactions.

ADAMs are also able to cleave and remodel extracellular matrix proteins. ADAMs 9,10,12,13 have been shown to cleave ECM proteins *in vitro*. ADAM10 and ADAM13 generate specific ECM cleavage products (Table 1) (Alfandari *et al* 2001). ADAM-mediated cleavage of ECM proteins can foster cell migration and release growth factors, previously bound to ECM, for downstream signalling.

To sum it up, we can say that association between ADAMs, integrins, proteoglycans and substrates may regulate shedding. The same way integrins and syndecans can work in *cis* with ADAMs to cleave ECM proteins. ADAM proteins play key roles in both the ectodomain shedding of many cell surface proteins and the cleavage and remodelling of the extracellular matrix making them important components of cell-cell and cell-matrix interactions.

3.4 Regulation

To date, the regulation of ADAM 17 function appears to be the best studied. It was shown that the shedding of ADAM 17 substrates can be stimulated by phorbol esters or phosphatase inhibitor pervanadate *in vitro* (Massague & Pandiella 1993, 1991; Arribas *et al* 1995, 1996). Phorbol esters can irreversibly activate protein kinase C (PKC) due to their ability to mimic diacylglycerol. Hence, *in vivo*, PKC signalling seems to be an important way that affects the activation of ADAM 17 ligands (Sahin *et al* 2004; Peschon *et al* 1998, Jackson *et al* 2003). The other signalling pathways that influence the shedding of ADAM 17 substrates are the receptor-tyrosine-kinase-activated extracellular signal-regulated kinase (ERK) / mitogen-activated protein kinase (MAPK) pathway (Fan & Derynck 1999) and also stimulation of G-protein-coupled receptors (GPCRs) (Lemjabbar *et al* 2003; Gschwind *et al* 2003). Besides, several cytoplasmatic proteins interacting with ADAM 17 have been identified, but the mechanism and effect of this interaction remain obscure (Peiretti *et al* 2003; Nelson *et al* 1999; Zheng *et al* 2002).

Currently little is known about the regulation of other ADAMs. The majority of ADAM proteins have specific signalling motifs, such as phosphorylation sites and proline - rich regions which bind SH3 domains. The ADAMs' general ability of activating many substrates could be modulated by phosphorylation of or binding of accessory proteins to, ADAM cytoplasmatic tails. Modifications of tails may affect their expression at the cell surface, interactions with other surface proteins, stability or ability to cleave specific substrates in respond to particular factors. Many other interactions between ADAMs and cytoplasmatic proteins have been studied. Several of these proteins seem to influence the functions of ADAMs through a mechanism, which so far remains unclear.

It was proved *in vitro* that at least two members of ADAMs family, ADAM 10 and ADAM 19, have constitutive shedding activity (Chesneau *et al* 2003, Sahin *et al* 2004), which could be regulated by the expression levels of these proteins. Furthermore, ADAM 10 has been reported to be activated through a GPCRs pathway (Lemjabbar *et al* 2002, 2003; Yan *et al* 2002). Another interesting interaction occur between the levels of cholesterol and activation of specific shedases, such as ADAM 10 and ADAM 17, which are up-regulated under the conditions of cholesterol removal (Lammich *et al* 1999; Kojro *et al* 2001; Matthews 2003). Moreover, there are reports that several of ADAM proteases have been shown to lose their catalytic activity in the presence of tissue inhibitors of matrix metalloproteinases (TIMPs) (Murphy *et al* 2003).

Table 1: Distribution, functions and substrates of selected ADAMs in human.

ADAM	Species	Distribution	Function	Shed substrates	ECM substrates
ADAM 1 (PH-30 α; Fertilin α)	H. sapiens & other spp.	Sperm and others	Sperm-egg fusion	?	?
ADAM 2 (PH-30 β; Fertilin β)	H. sapiens & other spp.	Sperm	Sperm-egg fusion		
ADAM 3 (Cyritestin; tMDC I)	H. sapiens & other spp.	Sperm	Spermato-genesis		
ADAM 6 (tMDC IV)	H. sapiens & other spp.	Sperm	Spermato-genesis		
ADAM 7 (EAP I)	H. sapiens & other spp.	Epididymis	Spermato-genesis		
ADAM 8 (MS2)	H. sapiens & other spp.	PMN, Macrophage	PMN infiltration		
ADAM 9 (MDC9, meltrin γ)	H. sapiens & other spp.	Lung and others	Signalling	Pro-HB-EGF	Fibronectin, gelatin
ADAM 10 (MADM; kuzbanian)	H. sapiens & other spp.	Brain, spleen and others	Myelin degradat., TNF-α -release	Pro-HB-EGF, Pro- TNF-alpha, Notch, ephrin-A2, delta L1, APP, cellular prion precursor	Type-IV collagen, gelatin
ADAM 11 (MDC)	H. sapiens & other spp.	Breast, ovary and others	Tumor suppressor		
ADAM 12 (meltrin α)	H. sapiens & other spp.	Bone, fetal muscle	Myogenesis	Pro-HB-EGF, ILGF-BP-3, -5	?
ADAM 15 Metargidin; MDC 15)	H. sapiens & other spp.	Macrophage, endothelial cells	Platelet aggregation, atheroscler.	?	Type-IV collagen, gelatin
ADAM 17 (TACE)	H. sapiens & other spp.	Macrophage and others	TNF-α, β-amyloid release	Pro-TNF-α, pro-TGF-α, pro-HB-EGF, pro-amphiregulin, TRANCE, pro-neuregulin-β- 2C, Notch, Fas ligand, fractalkine, L-selectin, type-XVII collagen, TNF-RI, TNF-RII, IL-1RII, IL-6R, Erb-B4/HER4, MCSF-RI, NGF-R (TrkA), GH-R MUC1, APP, cellular prion precursor	?
ADAM 18 (tMDCIII)	H. sapiens & other spp.				
ADAM 19 (meltrin β)	H. sapiens & other spp.	Bone, fetal muscle	Myogenesis, metallo-protease	Pro-neuregulin	?

The expression of mRNA for ADAM proteins in various cells is up – regulated by stimulation with pro–inflammatory factors, such as lipopolysaccharide (LPS), interferon-γ (INF-γ), interleukins 4 (IL-4) and 13 (IL-13) for the gene of ADAM 8 (Yamamoto *et al* 1999, King *et al* 2004), or IL-1 and LPS with reference to ADAM-TS family member – ADAM-TS 1. Hence, the involvement of ADAM proteins in the immune reactions is likely to occur.

3.5 ADAMs in IBD

There is little and ambiguous evidence on the activity of the ADAMs family members in the inflammatory bowel disease (IBD). Up-to-date the function of ADAM 17 (TACE – TNF-α converting enzyme) appears to be the best studied in the pathogenesis of IBD. Current data suggest that inhibition of TACE may provide a potential therapeutic approach in IBD, through subsequent reduction in release of soluble form of TNF-α (Kirkegaard *et al* 2004, Brynskov *et al* 2002, Colón *et al* 2001). However, there are reports providing data on the role of TACE in intestinal epithelial resustitution that promotes the healing of intestinal tract ulcers (Gennett *et al* 2004).

Foegh *et al* (1999) showed the presence of TACE activity in the human colonic mucosa and suggested the increased TACE mRNA expression in colonic biopsy specimens in the course of IBD. The further research (Brynskov *et al* 2002) disclosed significant increase in TACE activity in patients with ulcerative colitis (UC) versus healthy controls. On the contrary, the activity level of TACE observed in colonic mucosa in patients with Crohn's disease (CD) was comparable to that observed in controls. Moreover, this observation was irrespective of disease activity. Furthermore, it was proved that the TACE activity in samples obtained from endoscopically normal areas and endoscopically inflamed areas in IBD were similar. However, in the separate analysis of paired biopsies from patients with IBD was reported, that TACE activity was higher in areas with macroscopically active IBD compared with endoscopically normal areas. The expression of TACE protein in human colonic mucosa was limited to lamina propria mononuclear cells (LPMNC) and epithelial cells in crypts. This findings remained in contrast to the further studies of above mentioned group (Kirkegaard *et al* 2004) concerning TACE activity in the human colonic epithelial cells lines. Latest research showed that the expression of TACE mRNA and protein in the colonic epithelial cells is constitutive. Moreover, TACE activity levels remained similar in involved and non-involved IBD mucosa and healthy controls. The previously noted differences between Crohn's disease and ulcerative colitis were not observed in this study. This may suggest the engagement of LPMNC in the upregulation and increased levels of TACE noted in preceding research in the course of IBD. However, authors hint that constitutive TACE activity levels are sufficient to fulfil the requirements for TNF-α processing in the intestinal epithelial cells during inflammatory response *in vivo*.

Apart from reports on unfavourable role of TACE in the pathogenesis of IBD, there are studies providing with conclusions about beneficial role of this protein to the healing of intestinal tract ulcers (Gennett *et al* 2004, Egan *et al* 2003, Polk 1998). It was suggested that the presumable mechanism of reepithelialization of ulcers occurs through the EGFR activation by TACE.

These divergent reports indicate that possible therapeutic targeting of ADAMs in the course of IBD seems to be limited by wide spectrum of processed substrates. Thus TACE could not be considered as the therapeutic aim until more precise selectivity can be achieved. Hence, the further studies are required to elucidate the role of ADAM proteins in the pathogenesis of IBD and establish their position in the therapeutic targeting.

REFERENCES

Adachi Y, Yamamoto H, Itoh F, Hinoda Y, Okada Y, Imai K, 1999, Contribution of matrilysin (MMP-7) to the metastatic pathway of human colorectal cancers. *Gut.* **45:** 252-258.

Alfandari D, Cousin H, 2001, Xenopus ADAM 13 is a metalloproteinase required for cranial neural crest-cell migration. *Curr Biol.* **11:** 918-930.

Arribas J, Coodly L, Vollmer P, Kishimoto TK, Rose-John S, Massague J, 1996, Diverse cell surface protein ectodomains are shed by a system sensitive to metalloprotease inhibitors. *J Biol Chem.* **271:** 11376-11382.

Arribas J, Massague J, 1995, Transforming growth factor-α and β-amyloid precursor share a secretory mechanism. *J Cell Biol.* **128:** 433-441.

Bister VO, Salmela MT, Karjalainen-Lindsberg ML, Uria J, Lohi J, Puolakkainen P, Lopez-Otin C, Saarialho-Kere U, 2004, Differential expression of three matrix metalloproteinases, MMP-19, MMP-26, and MMP-28, in normal and inflamed intestine and colon cancer. *Dig Dis Sci.* **49:** 653-661.

Black RA, 1998, in *Handbook of Proteolytic Enzymes* (Barrett, A.J., Rawlings, N.D. and Woessner, J.F., eds), pp1315-1317, Academic Press.

Black RA, White JM, 1998, ADAMs: focus on the protease domain. *Curr Opin Cell Biol.* **10:** 654-659.

Blobel CP, 2005, ADAMs: Key Components in EGFR Signalling and Development, Nature. **6:** 32-43.

Blobel CP, Myles DG, Primakoff P, White JM, 1990, Proteolytic processing of a protein involved in sperm-egg fusion correlates with acquisition of fertilization competence. J Cell *Biol.* **111:** 69-78.

Blobel CP, White JM, 1992, Structure, function and evolutionary relationship of proteins containing a disintegrin domain. *Curr Opin Cell Biol.* **4:** 760-765.

Brynskov J, Foegh P, Pedersen G, Ellervik C, Kirkegaard T, Bingham A, Saermark T, 2002, Tumor necrosis factor-□ converting enzyme (TACE) activity in the colonic mucosa of patients with inflammatory bowel disease. *Gut.* **51:** 37-43.

Chambers AF, Matrisian LM, 1997, Changing views of the role of matrix metalloproteinases in metastasis. *J Natl Cancer Inst.* **89:** 1260-70.

Chesneau V, Becherer JD, Zheng Y, Erdjument-Bromage H, Tempst P, Blobel CP, 2003, Catalytic properties of ADAM19. *J. Biol. Chem.* **278:** 22331-22340.

Colón AL, Menchén LA, Hurtado O, De Cristóbal J, Lizasoain I, Leza JC, Lorenzo P, Moro MA, 2001, Implication of TNF-α convertase (TACE/ADAM17) in inducible nitric oxide synthase expression and inflammation in an experimental model of colitis. *Cytokine.* **16:** 220-226.

Di Sebastiano P, di Mola FF, Artese L, Rossi C, Mascetta G, Pernthaler H, Innocenti P, 2001, Beneficial effects of Batimastat (BB-94), a matrix metalloproteinase inhibitor, in rat experimental colitis. *Digestion.* **63:** 234-239.

Djonov V, Hogger K, Sedlacek R, Laissue J, Draeger A, 2001, MMP-19: cellular localization of a novel metalloproteinase within normal breast tissue and mammary gland tumours. *J Pathol.* **195:** 147-155.

Egan LJ, de Lecea A, Lehrman ED, Myhre GM, Eckmann L, Kagnoff MF, 2003, Nuclear factor-κB activation promotes resustitution of wounded intestinal epithelial monolayers. *Am J Physiol Cell Physiol.* **285:** C1028-C1035.

English WR, Puente XS, Freije JM, Knauper V, Amour A, Merryweather A, Lopez-Otin C, Murphy G, 2000, Membrane type 4 matrix metalloproteinase (MMP17) has tumor necrosis factor-alpha convertase activity but does not activate pro-MMP2. *J Biol Chem.* **275:** 14046-14055.

Fan H, Derynck R, 1999, Ectodomain shedding of TGF-α and other transmembrane proteins is induced by receptor tyrosine kinase activation and MAP kinase signaling cascades. *EMBO J.* **18:** 6962-6972.

Galvez BG, Genis L, Matias-Roman S, Oblander SA, Tryggvason K, Apte SS, Arroyo AG, 2005, Membrane type 1-matrix metalloproteinase is regulated by chemokines monocyte-chemoattractant protein-1/ccl2 and interleukin-8/CXCL8 in endothelial cells during angiogenesis. *J Biol Chem.* **280:** 1292-1298.

Goetzl EJ, Banda MJ, Leppert D, 1996, Matrix metalloproteinases in immunity. *J Immunol.* **156:** 1-4.

Gross J, Lapiere CM, 1962, Collagenolytic activity in amphibian tissues: a tissue culture assay. *Proc Natl Acad Sci USA.* **48:** 1014-1022.

Gschwind A, Hart S, Fisher OM, Ullrich A, 2003, TACE cleavage of amphiregulin regulates GPCR-induced proliferation and motility of cancer cells. *EMBO J.* **22:** 2411-2421.

Heuschkel RB, MacDonald TT, Monteleone G, Bajaj-Elliott M, Smith JA, Pender SL, 2000, Imbalance of stromelysin-1 and TIMP-1 in the mucosal lesions of children with inflammatory bowel disease. *Gut.* **47:** 57-62.

Hiraoka N, Allen E, Apel IJ, Gyetko MR, Weiss SJ, 1998, Matrix metalloproteinases regulate neovascularization by acting as pericellular fibrinolysins. *Cell.* **95:** 365-377.

Jackson LF, Qiu TH, Sunnarborg SW, Chang A, Zhang C, Patterson C, Lee DC, 2003, Defective valvulogenesis in HB-EGF and TACE-null mice associated with aberrant BMP signaling. *EMBO J.* **22:** 2704-2716.

King NE, Zimmermann N, Pope SM, Fulkerson PC, Nikolaidis NM, Mishra A, Witte DP, Rothenberg ME, 2004, Expression and regulation of a disintegrin and metalloproteinase (ADAM) 8 in experimental asthma. *Am J Respir Cell Mol Biol.* **31:** 257-65.

Kirkegaard T, Hansen A, Bruun E, Brynskov J, 2004, Expression and localisation of matrix metalloproteinases and their natural inhibitors in fistulae of patients with Crohn's disease. *Gut.* **53:** 701-9.

Kirkegaard T, Pedersen G, Saermark T, Brynskov J, 2004, Tumor necrosis factor-α converting enzyme (TACE) activity in human colonic epithelial cells. *Clin Exp Immunol.* **135:** 146-153.

Kojro E, Gimpl G, Lammich S, Marz W, Fahrenholz F, 2001, Low cholesterol stimulates the nonamyloidogenic pathway by its effect on the (-secretase ADAM 10). *Proc Natl Acad Sci USA.* **98:** 5815-5820.

Lammich S, Kojro E, Postina R, Gilbert S, Pfeiffer R, Jasionowski M, Haass C, Fahrenholz F, 1999, Constitutive and regulated (-secretase cleavage of Alzheimer's amyloid precursor protein by a disintegrin metalloprotease). *Proc Natl Acad Sci* USA **96:** 3922-3927.

Lawrance IC, Wu F, Leite AZ, Willis J, West GA, Fiocchi C, Chakravarti S, 2003, A murine model of chronic inflammation-induced intestinal fibrosis down-regulated by antisense NF-kappa B. *Gastroenterology*. **125:** 1750-1761

Lemjabbar H, Basbaum C, 2002, Platelet activating factor receptor and ADAM10 mediated responses to Staphylococcus aureus in epithelial cells. *Nature Med.* **8:** 41-46.

Lemjabbar H, Li D, Gallup M, Sidhu S, Drori E, Basbaum C, 2003, Tobacco smoke-induced lung cell proliferation mediated by tumor necrosis factor (-converting enzyme and amphiregulin. *J Biol Chem.* **278:** 26202-26207.

Louis E, Ribbens C, Godon A, Franchimont D, De Groote D, Hardy N, Boniver J, Belaiche J, Malaise M, 2000, Increased production of matrix metalloproteinase-3 and tissue inhibitor of metalloproteinase-1 by inflamed mucosa in inflammatory bowel disease. *Clin Exp Immunol.* **120:** 241-246.

Massague J, Pandiella A, 1993, A membrane-anchored growth factors. *Annu Rev Biochem.* **62:** 515-541.

Matsuno K, Adachi Y, Yamamoto H, Goto A, Arimura Y, Endo T, Itoh F, Imai K, 2003, The expression of matrix metalloproteinase matrilysin indicates the degree of inflammation in ulcerative colitis. *J Gastroenterol.* **38:** 348-54.

Matthews V, Schuster B, Schutze S, Bussmeyer I, Ludwig A, Hundhausen C, Sadowski T, Saftig P, Hartmann D, Kallen KJ, Rose-John S, 2003, Cellular cholesterol depletion triggers shedding of the human interleukin-6 receptor by ADAM10 and ADAM17 (TACE). *J Biol Chem.* **278:** 38829-38839.

McKaig BC, McWilliams D, Watson SA, Mahida YR, 2003, Expression and regulation of tissue inhibitor of metalloproteinase-1 and matrix metalloproteinases by intestinal myofibroblasts in inflammatory bowel disease. *Am J Pathol.* **162:** 1355-1360.

McQuibban GA, Butler GS, Gong JH, Bendall L, Power C, Clark-Lewis I, Overall CM, 2001, Matrix metalloproteinase activity inactivates the CXC chemokine stromal cell-derived factor-1. *J Biol Chem.* **276:** 43503-43508.

McQuibban GA, Gong JH, Tam EM, McCulloch CA, Clark-Lewis I, Overall CM, 2000, Inflammation dampened by gelatinase A cleavage of monocyte chemoattractant protein-3. *Science.* **289:** 1202-1206.

McQuibban GA, Gong JH, Wong JP, Wallace JL, Clark-Lewis I, Overall CM, 2002, Matrix metalloproteinase processing of monocyte chemoattractant proteins generates CC chemokine receptor antagonists with anti-inflammatory properties in vivo. *Blood.* **100:** 1160-1167.

Mohan MJ, Seaton T, Mitchell J, Howe A, Blackburn K, Burkhart W, Moyer M, Patel I, Waitt GM, Becherer JD, Moss ML, Milla ME, 2002, The tumor necrosis factor-alpha converting enzyme (TACE): a unique metalloproteinase with highly defined substrate selectivity. *Biochemistry*. **41:** 9462-9469.

Moss ML, Bartsch JW, 2004, Therapeutic Benefits from Targeting of ADAM Family Members. *Biochemistry*. **43:** 7227-7235.

Murphy G, Knauper V, Lee MH, Amour A, Worley JR, Hutton M, Atkinson S, Rapti M, Williamson R, 2003, Role of TIMPs (tissue inhibitors of metalloproteinases) in pencellular proteolysis: the specificity is in the detail. *Biochem Soc Symp*. 65-80.

Myhre GM, Toruner M, Abraham S, Egan LJ, Metalloprotease disintegrin-mediated ectodomain shedding of EGFR ligands promotes intestinal epithelial restitution. *AJP-GI* **287:** 1213-1219.

Nagase H, Woessner JF, 1999, Matrix metalloproteinases. *J Biol Chem.* **274:** 21491-21494.

Naito Y, Takagi T, Kuroda M, Katada K, Ichikawa H, Kokura S, Yoshida N, Okanoue T, Yoshikawa T, 2004, An orally active matrix metalloproteinase inhibitor, ONO-4817, reduces dextran sulfate sodium-induced colitis in mice. *Inflamm Res.* **53:** 462-468.

Nelson KK, Schlondorff J, Blobel CP, 1999, Evidence for an interaction of the metalloprotease-disintegrin tumor necrosis factor α convertase (TACE) with mitotic arrest deficient 2 (MAD2), and of the metalloprotease-disintegrin MDC9 with a novel MAD2-related protein, MAD2β. *Biochem J.* **343:** 673-680.

Newell KJ, Matrisian LM, Driman DK, 2002, Matrilysin (matrix metalloproteinase-7) expression in ulcerative colitis-related tumorigenesis. *Mol Carcinog* **34:** 59-63.

Niewiarowski S, McLane MA, Kloczewiak M, Stewart GJ, 1994, Disintegrins and other naturally occurring antagonists of platelet fibrinogen receptors. *Semin Hematol.* **31:** 289-300.

Pandiella A, Massague J, 1991, Cleavage of the membrane precursor for transforming growth factor alpha is a regulated process. *Proc Natl Acad Sci U S A.* **88:** 1726-1730.

Parks WC, Wilson CL, Lopez-Boado YS, 2004, Matrix metalloproteinases as modulators of inflammation and innate immunity. *Nat Rev Immunol.* **4:** 617-629.

Peiretti F, Deprez-Beauclair P, Bonardo B, Aubert H, Juhan-Vague I, Nalbone G, 2003, Identification of SAP97 as an intracellular binding partner of TACE. *J Cell Sci.* **116:** 1949-1957.

Pendas AM, Knauper V, Puente XS, Llano E, Mattei MG, Apte S, Murphy G, Lopez-Otin C, 1997, Identification and characterization of a novel human matrix metalloproteinase with unique structural characteristics, chromosomal location, and tissue distribution. *J Biol Chem.* **272:** 4281-4286.

Pender SL, Breese EJ, Gunther U, Howie D, Wathen NC, Schuppan D, MacDonald TT, 1998, Suppression of T cell-mediated injury in human gut by interleukin 10: role of matrix metalloproteinases. *Gastroenterology.* **115:** 573-583.

Pender SL, Fell JM, Chamow SM, Ashkenazi A, MacDonald TT, 1998, A p55 TNF receptor immunoadhesin prevents T cell-mediated intestinal injury by inhibiting matrix metalloproteinase production. *J Immunol.* **160:** 4098-4103.

Pender SL, MacDonald TT, 2004, Matrix metalloproteinases and the gut - new roles for old enzymes. *Curr Opin Pharmacol.* **4:** 546-50.

Peschon JJ, Slack JL, Reddy P, Stocking KL, Sunnarborg SW, Lee DC, Russell WE, Castner BJ, Johnson RS, Fitzner JN, Boyce RW, Nelson N, Kozlosky CJ, Wolfson MF, Rauch CT, Cerretti DP, Paxton RJ, March CJ, Black RA, 1998, An essential role for ectodomain shedding in mammalian development. *Science* **282:** 1281-1284.

Polk DB, 1998, Epidermal growth factor receptor-stimulated intestinal epithelial cell migration requires phospholipase C activity. *Gastroenterology.* **114:** 493-502.

Prilla E, Ramamurthy NS, Sorsa T, Salo T, Hietanen J, Masi P, 2003, Gelatinase A (MMP-2), Collagenase 2 (MMP-8) and Laminin-5 y2-Chain Expression in Murine Inflammatory Bowel Disease (Ulcerative Colitis). *Dig Dis Sci.* **48:** 93-8.

Ropreager AC, 2001, Molecular interactions of syndecans during development. *Semin Cell Dev Biol.* **12:** 107-116.

Saarialho-Kere UK, Vaalamo M, Puolakkainen P, Airola K, Parks WC, Karjalainen-Lindsberg ML, 1996, Enhanced expression of matrilysin, collagenase and stromelysin-1 in gastrointestinal ulcers. *Am J Pathol.* **148:** 519-26.

Sahin U, Weskamp G, Kelly K, Zhou HM, Higashiyama S, Peschon J, Hartmann D, Saftig P, Blobel CP, 2004, Distinct roles for ADAM10 and ADAM17 in ectodomain shedding of six EGFR-ligands. *J Cell Biol.* **164:** 769-779.

Salmela MT, Pender SL, Karjalainen-Lindsberg ML, Puolakkainen P, Macdonald TT, Saarialho-Kere U, 2004. Collagenase-1 (MMP-1), matrilysin-1 (MMP-7), and stromelysin-2 (MMP-10) are expressed by migrating enterocytes during intestinal wound healing. *Scand J Gastroenterol.* **39:** 1095-1104.

Sato H, Takino T, Okada Y, Cao J, Shinagawa A, Yamamoto E, Seiki M, 1994, A matrix metalloproteinase expressed on the surface of invasive tumour cells. *Nature.* **370:**61-65.

Schonbeck U, Mach F, Bonnefoy JY, Loppnow H, Flad HD, Libby P, 1997, Ligation of CD40 activates interleukin 1beta-converting enzyme (caspase-1) activity in vascular smooth muscle and endothelial cells and promotes elaboration of active interleukin 1beta. *J Biol Chem.* **272:** 19569-19574.

Seals DF, Courtneidge SA, 2003, The ADAMs family of metalloproteases: multidomain proteins with multiply functions. *Genes Dev.* **17:** 7-30.

Seltzer JL, Lee AY, Akers KT, Sudbeck B, Southon EA, Wayner EA, Eisen AZ, 1994, Activation of 72-kDa type IV collagenase/gelatinase by normal fibroblasts in collagen lattices is mediated by integrin receptors but is not related to lattice contraction. *Exp Cell Res.* **213:** 365-374.

Stallmach A, Chan CC, Ecker KW, Feifel G, Herbst H, Schuppan D, Zeitz M, 2000, Comparable expression of matrix metalloproteinases 1 and 2 in pouchitis and ulcerative colitis. *Gut.* **47:** 415-422.

Sternlicht MD, Werb Z, 2001, How matrix metalloproteinases regulate cell behavior? *Annu Rev Cell Dev Biol.* **17:** 463-516.

Stracke JO, Fosang AJ, Last K, Mercuri FA, Pendas AM, Llano E, Perris R, Di Cesare PE, Murphy G, Knauper V, 2000, Matrix metalloproteinases 19 and 20 cleave aggrecan and cartilage oligomeric matrix protein (COMP). *FEBS Lett.* **478:** 52-56.

van Deventer SJH, 2002, A place for TACE, *Gut.* **51:** 5-6.

von Lampe B, Barthel B, Coupland SE, Riecken EO, Rosewicz S, 2000, Differential expression of matrix metalloproteinases and their tissue inhibitors in colon mucosa of patients with inflammatory bowel disease. *Gut.* **47:** 63-73.

White JM, 2003, ADAMs: modulators of cell - cell and cell - matrix interactions. *Curr Opin Cell Biol.* 15, 598-606.

Wiercinska-Drapalo A, Flisiak R, Prokopowicz D, 2001, Effect of ulcerative colitis activity on plasma concentration of transforming growth factor beta1. *Cytokine.* **14:** 343-346.

Wiercinska-Drapalo A, Flisiak R, Prokopowicz D, 2003, Effect of ulcerative colitis treatment on transforming growth factor beta(1) in plasma and rectal mucosa. *Regul Pept.* **113:** 57-61.

Wiercinska-Drapalo A, Jaroszewicz J, Flisiak R, Prokopowicz D, 2003, Plasma matrix metalloproteinase-1 and tissue inhibitor of metalloproteinase-1 as biomarkers of ulcerative colitis activity. *World J Gastroenterol.* **9:** 2843-2845.

Wolfsberg TG, Primakoff P, Myles DG, White JM,1995, ADAM, a novel family of membrane proteins containing A Disintegrin And Metalloprotease domain: multipotential functions in cell-cell and cell- matrix interactions. *J Cell Biol.* **131:** 275-278.

Wolfsberg TG, Straight PD, Gerena RL, Huovila AP, Primakoff P, Myles DG, White JM, 1995, ADAM, a widely distributed and developmentally regulated gene family encoding membrane proteins with a disintegrin and metalloprotease domain. *Dev Biol.* **169:** 378-383.

Wolfsberg TG, White JM, 1996, ADAMs in fertilization and development. *Dev Biol.* **180:** 389-401.

Wolfsberg TG, White JM, 1998, in *Handbook of Proteolytic Enzymes* (Barrett, A.J., Rawlings, N.D. and Woessner, J.F., eds), pp1310-1313, Academic Press.

Yamamoto S, Higuchi Y, Yoshiyama K, Shimizu E, Kataoka M, Hijiya N, Matsuura K, 1999, ADAM family proteins in the immune system. *Immunol Today.* **20:** 278-284.

Zhao H, Bernardo MM, Osenkowski P, Sohail A, Pei D, Nagase H, Kashiwagi M, Soloway PD, DeClerck YA, Fridman R, 2004, Differential inhibition of membrane type 3 (MT3)-matrix metalloproteinase (MMP) and MT1-MMP by tissue inhibitor of metalloproteinase (TIMP)-2 and TIMP-3 rgulates pro-MMP-2 activation. *J Biol Chem.* **279:** 8592-85601.

Zheng Y, Schlondorff J, Blobel CP, 2002, Evidence for regulation of the tumor necrosis factor α-convertase (TACE) by protein-tyrosine phosphatase PTPH1. *J Biol Chem.* **277:** 42463-42470.

Chapter 11

Chemokines and Matrix Metalloproteinases in Colorectal Cancer

Gayle G. Vaday and Stanley Zucker
Northport Veterans Affairs Medical Center, Department of Research, Northport, NY; Stony Brook University, Department of Medicine, Stony Brook, NY

1. INTRODUCTION

Scientific exploration of cancer in the past century has primarily focused on the concept of uncontrolled growth of cancer cells with little attention to the non-neoplastic component of tumors. More recent studies brought to light the important positive and negative effects of the local host response to cancer.

The tumor microenvironment is a specialized niche that provides the survival signals necessary for cancer cells to undergo proliferation, neovascularization, invasion, and metastasis. The tumor microenvironment thus provides the fertile soil for tumor growth and the selective survival advantages necessary for dissemination to other organs (Seed and Soil Hypothesis) (Fidler 2002; Paget 1889).

Beginning in the early stages and continuing throughout tumor development, cancer cells secrete multiple cytokines, growth factors, and proteases to re-shape their surrounding connective tissue. This leads to the formation of a 'reactive' stroma that supports tumor progression by inducing reactions such as angiogenesis and inflammation. Stromal cells, such as fibroblasts, leukocytes, and endothelial cells, become activated and release additional growth factors and proteases to foster tumor growth. The extracellular matrix (ECM), another component of tumor stroma, acts as a scaffold for structural support, as well as a specialized reservoir of macromolecules, proteases and their inhibitors, growth factors, and cytokines. By inducing compositional changes in the ECM, cancer cells regulate and modify the contextual information needed for cell proliferation, migration, and invasion, thereby controlling their own fate. The reciprocal (paracrine)

U. Lendeckel and Nigel M. Hooper (eds.), Proteases in Gastrointestinal Tissue, 255-300.

dialogue between cancer cells and tumor stroma is a shared feature among solid tumors. Cancer cell-derived factors may also function in an autocrine manner through feedback loops involving secreted molecules and cell-surface receptors. Thus, cancer progression relies on the cell-cell and cell-matrix crosstalk regulated by pro-malignant factors, stemming from the early stages of tumor development, all the way to metastatic tumor growth.

Metastasis, the spread of cancer cells from a primary tumor to distant organs and their subsequent persistent growth, is the major cause of death from most types of solid tumors, including colorectal cancer (McLeod *et al* 2000). An estimated 145,000 new cases of colorectal cancer will be diagnosed in the United States in 2005, accounting for 10% of all cancer deaths (Jemal *et al* 2005). Approximately 50% of all colorectal cancer diagnoses are made when the cancer has already disseminated to lymph nodes (Dukes' stage C) or distant organs (Dukes' stage D), the most common site being the liver, while the remainder of cases consist of localized disease (Duke's stages A & B). The survival rates of colorectal cancer cases drop precipitously when comparing localized disease to node-positive and metastatic disease (McLeod *et al* 2000). Despite significant improvements in surgical techniques and systemic therapies with new categories of drugs, the foremost clinical challenge in treating colorectal cancer remains the prevention and treatment of metastatic disease. In order to develop more targeted therapies that may be used in conjunction with current therapeutic modalities, it is imperative to characterize the molecular signature of both primary and metastatic colorectal tumors and identify new prognostic markers that may be used in conjunction with the standard pathological Duke's staging. These goals may be achieved through the recent advances of cDNA microarray, comparative genomic hybridization, and proteomic technologies, all of which can identify potential tumor markers at different stages of disease.

In this chapter, we will discuss two important families of pro-malignant factors involved in tumor progression: chemokines and matrix metalloproteinases (MMPs). Numerous research and review articles have been published in the last few years on the significance of chemokines and MMPs in cancer progression. Chemokines, as potent chemoattractants and inducers of cell proliferation, and MMPs, as efficient ECM-degrading enzymes, have both been implicated in colorectal cancer biology. Both types of molecules are prominent regulatory molecules in the tumor microenvironment and are considered key factors in cancer dissemination and metastasis. In addition, chemokines found in tumors can induce the expression of MMPs, while MMPs have been shown to proteolytically cleave chemokines and alter their activities, suggesting that chemokines and MMPs can cooperatively regulate one another in a tumor setting. Herein, we will present recent contributions in the chemokine and MMP fields, their potential use as prognostic markers, and new perspectives on how chemokine antagonists and MMP inhibitors may be applied clinically in the treatment of colorectal cancer.

2. CHEMOKINE BIOLOGY

Chemokines are a superfamily of small (~8-14 kDa) proteins that act as chemotactic factors in the migration of leukocytes, hematopoietic stem cells, and a variety of other cell types, including cancer cells. Induced by inflammatory cytokines and growth factors, chemokines are best known for their ability to recruit leukocytes into specific sites where tissue is inflamed or injured, creating a navigational trail of signals for efficient movement within a target tissue (Luster 1998; Rollins 1997). Over 50 chemokines have been discovered thus far. Chemokines are grouped into four highly conserved groups—CXC, CC, C, and CX3C—based on the positioning of the first two cysteine residues at the amino terminus. Chemotaxis toward chemokines is regulated by the expression of chemokine receptors, which are seven-transmembrane, G protein-coupled receptors expressed on the surface of many cell types (Zlotnik and Yoshie, 2000). The CC and CXC chemokines and their receptors are listed in Table I. The flexible N-terminal region of a chemokine sequence is believed to be important in receptor activation because modifications (e.g. truncation; elongation) to this region have been shown to decrease agonist activity (Loetcher and Clark-Lewis, 2001). In general, the chemokine system is promiscuous in the sense that most receptors bind to more than one ligand, and most ligands bind to more than one receptor. There are some exceptions to this trend, as some receptors bind to a single ligand. However, since many chemokines are redundant in their effects on cellular responses, the chemokine system is considered a robust mechanism of modulating cellular behavior (Mantovani 1999).

The rapid pace of chemokine discovery in the last two decades led to the problematic issue of several groups giving different names to the same newly-described molecule. Since most chemokines possess more than one function, this problem in nomenclature created a great deal of confusion for those working in the chemokine field. In 2000, Zlotnik and Yoshie proposed a new chemokine classification system that grouped chemokines and their receptors into families based on their highly conserved N-terminal cysteine moieties (Zlotnik and Yoshie, 2000). In this review, we will refer to each chemokine based on the new classification system. A broader categorization of chemokine receptors provides a general indication of their principal functions, based on whether or not they are constitutively produced or are inducible. Constitutively expressed chemokine receptors are generally involved in basal cell trafficking and homing, while inducible receptors tend to function primarily in inflammatory reactions (Proudfoot 2002).

3. CHEMOKINES IN COLORECTAL CANCER

The chemokine network encompasses a myriad of functions in cancer, which may be narrowed down to at least five areas of tumor biology: 1) regulation of the leukocyte infiltrate and manipulation of the immune response; 2) inflammation-induced carcinogenesis; 3) regulation of angiogenesis; 4) effects on cell survival and tumor growth; 5) control of cancer metastasis. We will discuss each of these areas in the broader picture of cancer biology, and relate how these chemokine functions relate specifically to colorectal cancer.

3.1 Leukocyte infiltration

Leukocytes are a major constituent of the tumor stroma. Leukocyte recruitment into tumors is largely influenced by the chemokines produced by cancer cells, primarily those from the CC chemokine family (Balkwill and Mantovani, 2001; Bottazzi *et al* 1983). While macrophages and lymphocytes are the predominant leukocyte subtypes found in tumor stroma, eosinophils, granulocytes, natural killer cells, and B cells also infiltrate into some tumor types (Brigati *et al* 2002; Coussens and Werb, 2002).

Leukocyte infiltration into tumors can lead to two very divergent outcomes: either an anti-tumor immune response, or an immunosuppressive environment that promotes tumor growth. While chemokines may certainly contribute to anti-tumor immunity, the progression of some cancers to advanced stages likely results, in part, from an inefficient anti-tumor response and skewing toward immunosuppression or the evasion of tumor-specific immunity. Overproduction of TH2 cytokines (e.g. IL-4, IL-10), together with TH2 chemokines (e.g. CCL22, CCL18, CCL24), contributes to a TH2 polarization in tumors. It is important to note that CCL2, the chemokine with perhaps the highest levels of expression among all solid tumors, has been shown to specifically cause TH2 polarization (Gu *et al* 2000). Since polarized TH2 responses are not as effective as TH1 responses in combating tumors and viral infections, chronic exposure of chemokine-recruited T lymphocytes to TH2 mediators can lead to cancer cell escape of an immune response (Balkwill and Mantovani, 2001; Mantovani *et al* 2004a).

Table 1: Human CC and CXC Chemokines.

Systemic Name	Common Name	Receptors
CCL1	I-309	CCR8
CCL2	MCP-1/MCAF	CCR2
CCL3	MIP-1α/LD78α	CCR1,CCR5
CCL3L1	MIP-1α/DL78β	CCR1, CCR3, CCR5
CCL4	MIP-1β	CCR1, CCR2, CCR5
CCL5	RANTES	CCR1, CCR3, CCR5
CCL7	MCP-3	CCR1, CCR2, CCR3, CCR5
CCL8	MCP-2	CCR1, CCR2, CCR3, CCR5
CCL11	Eotaxin	CCR2, CCR3
CCL13	MCP-4	CCR1, CCR2, CCR3
CCL14	HCC-1	CCR1, CCR3, CCR5
CCL15	HCC-2/Lkn-1/MIP-1δ	CCR1, CCR3
CCL16	HCC-4/LEC	CCR1
CCL17	TARC	CCR4
CCL18	DC-CK1/PARC/AMAC-1	Unknown
CCL19	MIP-3β/ELC/exodus-3	CCR7
CCL20	MIP-1α/LARC/exodus-1	CCR6
CCL21	6Ckine/SLC/exodus-2	CCR7
CCL22	MDC/STCP-1	CCR4
CCL23	MPIF-1/MIP-3	CCR1
CCL24	MPIF-2/eotaxin-2	CCR3
CCL25	TECK	CCR9
CCL26	Eotaxin-3	CCR3, CCR10
CCL27	CTACK/Eskine	CCR10
CCL28	MEC	CCR10
CXCL1	GROα/MGSA-α	CXCR2
CXCL2	GROβ/MGSA-β	CXCR2
CXCL3	GROγ/MGSA-γ	CXCR2
CXCL4	PF4	CXCR3B
CXCL5	ENA-78	CXCR2
CXCL6	GCP-2	CXCR1, CXCR2
CXCL7	NAP-2	CXCR2
CXCL8	IL-8	CXCR1, CXCR2
CXCL9	Mig	CXCR3
CXCL10	IP-10	CXCR3
CXCL11	I-TAC	CXCR3
CXCL12	SDF-1α/β	CXCR4
CXCL13	BLC/BCA-1	CXCR5
CXCL14	BRAK/bolekine	Unknown

In addition to skewing the T cell-mediated immune response in the TH2 direction, TH2 cytokines and chemokines are also attributed to the skewing of tumor-associated macrophages (TAM) toward the type II (M2) phenotype (Mills *et al* 2000). TAMs are considered integral components of the intratumoral, inflammatory-like environment that promotes tumor progression. In contrast to activated type I macrophages, which are potent effector cells in the eradication of tumor cells and secretion of pro-inflammatory cytokines, type II macrophages downregulate inflammatory and TH1 immune responses through the production of IL-10 (Mantovani *et al* 2002).

There are conflicting studies concerning the role of leukocyte infiltrates in tumor progression, contesting the relationship between high TAM content and patient prognosis. In a recent study by Bingle *et al.*, the majority of cancer cases studied that demonstrated high levels of TAM were correlated with a poor prognosis. However, there were some cases in which a greater TAM infiltrate correlated with a better prognosis (Bingle *et al* 2002). The seminal work by Mantovani and colleagues (Mantovani *et al* 2004b) led to the conclusion that while a high TAM content is indicative of a worse diagnosis in some cancers, such as breast cancer, an important balance likely exists between macrophages that either promote or inhibit cancer. A similar balance between pro- and anti-tumor lymphocyte activities is also likely (Balkwill 2004). Thus, through their ability to chemoattract leukocytes, chemokines present in tumors play a central role in determining the outcome of tumor immunity, depending on the tumor type.

In colon carcinoma, higher numbers of tumor-associated mononuclear cells have been shown to be associated with good prognosis. High tumor-associated mononuclear cell number was also found to correlate with tumor differentiation, as well-differentiated tumors demonstrate a significantly higher density of mononuclear leukocytes than poorly- or moderately-differentiated colon cancers (Norazmi *et al* 1990). Further investigation of the leukocyte infiltrates and IL-10 levels in colorectal tumors compared to breast tumors showed that colorectal tumors exhibited the presence of activated T lymphocytes, low numbers of suppressor (type II) macrophages, and low IL-10 production. In contrast, breast tumors had higher levels of suppressor (type II) macrophages and IL-10 production, as well as poorer activation of T cells (Toomey *et al* 1999). Thus, chemokine-mediated recruitment of mononuclear cells into established colon tumors could lead to inhibition of tumor progression, implicating the use of chemokines in cancer immunotherapy.

Indeed, transfecting the gene encoding CCL2 (monocyte chemoattractant protein-1; MCP-1) into the highly metastatic murine colon carcinoma cell line CT-26 results in significantly fewer lung metastases and an augmented susceptibility to lysis by activated macrophages (Huang *et al* 1994). CCL2 and CCL22 (liver and activation-regulated chemokine; LARC) gene expression is enhanced in the draining lymph nodes of mice bearing mouse colon 26 (C26) adenocarcinoma tumors, resulting in augmented dendritic cell migration and accumulation (Wang *et al* 2003). Anti-CCL2 antibodies decrease the rate of tumor regression, confirming the direct role of CCL2 in regulating tumor rejection (Huang *et al* 1994).

Another example of the applicability of chemokines in cancer immunotherapy is CCL21, a potent chemoattractant for naïve T cells and mature dendritic cells that is produced in lymphoid organs. C26 cells expressing both CCL21 and a costimulatory molecule, the TNF-like molecule LIGHT, were shown to induce a synergistic anti-tumor response that completely eradicated tumors in mice (Hisada *et al* 2004; Nakahara and Sakata, 2003). When expressed locally within a tumor, a fusion protein constructed with CCL21 and IL-2 was demonstrated to lower tumorigenicity of the mouse colon carcinoma cell line CT-26 (Nakahara and Sakata, 2003). Local delivery of recombinant CCL21 expressed in vaccinia virus was also shown to induce T cell infiltration into tumors derived from CT-26 cells, correlating with a reduction in tumor size (Flanagan *et al* 2004). Similar gene therapy studies that involved local expression of the gene encoding the chemokine CXCL9 (monokine induced by IFN-γ; MIG), together with immunotherapy using an antibody-IL-2 fusion protein, led to reduction in tumor burden, suppression of experimental lung metastases, and a prolonged life span of mice bearing CT26 tumors (Ruehlmann *et al* 2001). A number of other chemokines have been examined as potential candidate molecules in experimental immunotherapy in colon carcinoma, with many reporting regression or reduced tumorigenicity in murine models (Homey *et al* 2002).

Considering the effectiveness of chemokines in recruiting effector T lymphocytes into tumors in experimental colon cancer models for an efficient anti-tumor response, it appears that chemokines are a rational choice for the development for new clinical therapies, in combination with other conventional cancer therapies (Homey *et al* 2002). Aggressive, advanced colon carcinomas, such as the CT-26 mouse model, likely maintain low levels of chemokine expression, much like in the normal state. It is known that chemokine production in the colon is increased in response to inflammation (Banks *et al* 2003; Yang *et al* 2002). Thus, chemokines, other cytokines or costimulatory molecules, and the recruitment of effector leukocytes might be exploited as a modality for promoting an immune response in colon cancer.

3.2 Inflammation-induced carcinogenesis

A causal relationship between inflammation and cancer has long been recognized. Historically, cancer development within a tuberculous scar in the lung was an established clinical observation. The infiltration of leukocytes, the production of proinflammatory cytokines and chemokines (e.g. TNF-α; IL-1; CXCL8), matrix degrading enzymes, and growth factors, and the release of reactive oxygen species collectively promote carcinogenesis. Cell proliferation, cell survival, angiogenesis, cell migration, and DNA damage are all affected in some way by a chronic inflammatory environment, resulting in a tendency to develop cancer (Balkwill *et al* 2005; Balkwill and Mantovani, 2001; Coussens and Werb, 2002). Although exploiting chemokines as immunotherapeutic agents may be useful in treating existing colorectal carcinoma, the role of chemokines in attracting leukocytes is detrimental in inflammatory bowel diseases (IBD) associated with carcinogenesis, including ulcerative colitis and Crohn's disease.

The causal link between inflammation and cancer has led to an evolution of anti-inflammatory agents for chemoprevention. Epidemiological studies have shown that the chronic use of nonsteroidal anti-inflammatory drugs (NSAIDs), namely aspirin, correlates with a reduced risk of developing colorectal cancer by up to 50% (Koehne and Dubois, 2004). Protection against cancer in several other organ sites has also been linked to the use of aspirin (Chang *et al* 2004; Garber 2004; Wang *et al* 2004b). However, NSAID use was associated with life-threatening cardiovascular events in a colorectal adenoma chemoprevention trial (Bresalier *et al* 2005; Howard and Dellafontaine, 2004). Thus, the identification and characterization of novel therapeutic agents that specifically target other major inflammatory molecules is highly pertinent in inflammation-associated colorectal cancer.

The predisposition of individuals with IBD to colorectal cancer may be attributed to local chronic inflammation characterized by the presence of leukocyte infiltrates, mainly composed of neutrophils, lymphocytes, monocytes/macrophages, and plasma cells. Oxidative stress, brought about by inflammatory cell release of reactive oxygen and nitrogen species, directly causes DNA damage leading to mutations or methylation of important regulatory or tumor suppressor genes (e.g. *p53*). Free radicals also target other metabolic processes by acting on RNA, proteins, and lipids. Neutrophils and macrophages recruited into the tissue generate free radicals that promote a pro-oxidant environment (Itzkowitz and Yio, 2004). Indeed, colorectal tissue specimens of patients with ulcerative or Crohn's colitis demonstrate increased expression of nitric oxide synthase (NOS) and reactive oxygen and nitrogen species (Rachmilewitz *et al* 1993). The direct action of reactive oxygen and nitrogen species has been shown in animal models of chemical-induced colonic injury, in which oxygen radical scavengers and cyclooxygenase-2 inhibitors attenuate colonic inflammation. In addition to free radicals, inflammatory cells also release a number of other pro-inflammatory molecules, including TNF-α, growth factors, angiogenic factors, and proteases (Itzkowitz and Yio, 2004).

A central player in the progression of colitis to cancer that has recently been identified is the transcription factor NF-κB, which consists of multiple closely related protein dimers that bind a common DNA sequence motif. In resting cells, NF-κB dimers are retained in the cytoplasm by specific inhibitors, called the IκB proteins. The IκB kinase (IKK) complex becomes activated in response to proinflammatory cytokines, leading to phosphorylation of NF-kB-bound IκBs, followed by ubiquitin-dependent degradation of IkBs, and the opportunity for free NF-κB dimers to enter the nucleus and activate the expression of several genes that are important in cell survival and growth. In an elegant study using a mouse model of colitis-associated cancer, Greten *et al* showed that deletion of the gene IKKβ in intestinal epithelial cells resulted in a decrease in tumor incidence and an increase in epithelial apoptosis, while IKKβ gene deletion in myeloid cells resulted in reduced expression of proinflammatory cytokines and chemokines (Greten *et al* 2004).

Considering the major role of inflammatory cells in promoting the transformation of inflamed colonic tissue in IBD to cancer, the importance of chemokines in driving the recruitment process is evident. In ulcerative colitis, several CXC and CC chemokines are expressed at significantly higher mRNA and protein levels than in normal colonic mucosa, with CXC chemokines (e.g. CXCL1; CXCL8) increased up to 50-fold and CC chemokines (e.g. CCL2; CCL5) increased up to 5-fold. Dexamethasone was shown to inhibit secretion of chemokines by in vitro culture of colonoscopic mucosal biopsy specimens taken from patients with ulcerative colitis (Yang *et al* 2002). In addition, chemokine expression is higher in patients with active gut inflammation than in patients with quiescent disease. Interestingly, patients with Crohn's disease demonstrate more marked levels of chemokine expression than patients with ulcerative colitis, even when the levels of disease activity are nearly identical (Banks *et al* 2003). It appears that novel anti-chemokine therapies designed to suppress the infiltration of inflammatory cells in IBD will prove to be a valuable strategy not only in treating colitis, but also in preventing carcinogenesis.

3.3 Regulation of angiogenesis

Angiogenesis, or the outgrowth of new blood vessels, is a critical process in the growth of a tumor. Tumors produce a chaotic vascular organization of capillaries and lymphatics. Although the vascular network is not as severely disrupted as it is in a wound, many interactions that occur in wound healing also occur between tumor and stromal cells. Neoplastic cells produce an array of cytokines and chemokines that are mitogenic and/or are chemoattractants for inflammatory leukocytes, fibroblasts, and endothelial cells. Activated fibroblasts and inflammatory cells secrete proteolytic enzymes, cytokines, and chemokines. These factors potentiate tumor growth and stimulate angiogenesis, enabling the metastatic spread of tumor cells through either venous or lymphatic vessels (Balkwill 2004; Coussens and Werb, 2002). Tumors have thus been described as "wounds that do not heal" (Dvorak 1986).

The disorganized network of the tumor vasculature results in areas of hypoxia, or poor oxygenation. Interestingly, tumor-associated macrophages tend to localize to areas of hypoxia. By downregulating expression of the chemokine receptors (CCR1; CCR2; CCR5) and the cognate chemokines (CXCL8; CCL5) that initially recruited them into a tumor, monocytes/macrophages become less apt to migrate out and thus are retained in the tumor. Expression of tumor cell-derived chemokines, like CCL2, may also be downregulated, leading to a retention and specific distribution of macrophages in a tumor, thus underscoring the capability of chemokines to specifically direct cell migration. In addition to chemokine-mediated recruitment, the proangiogenic factor vascular endothelial growth factor (VEGF), which is produced by tumor cells, endothelial cells, and macrophages, also functions as a chemoattractant, directing tumor-associated macrophages toward areas of hypoxia (Mantovani *et al* 2004a; Murdoch *et al* 1999).

Tumor cells metabolically adapt to hypoxia, as evidenced by a correlation between large areas of hypoxia and poor prognosis (Hockel and Vaupel, 2001). Under hypoxic conditions, gene expression of the transcriptional activator molecule hypoxia-inducible factor (HIF)-1 is upregulated. HIF-1 is a heterodimeric protein composed of a constitutively expressed HIF-1β subunit and an O_2-regulated HIF-1α subunit. Studies have shown that HIF-1α is overexpressed in human colon cancer tissue (Zhong *et al* 1999), and nude mice bearing xenografts of human colon cancer cells overexpressing HIF-1 demonstrate increased tumor growth and angiogenesis (Ravi *et al* 2000). HIF-1α controls the gene expression of angiogenic factors, most notably VEGF, as well as the chemokine receptor CXCR4 (Semenza 2003; Staller *et al* 2003). CXCR4 is implicated as a crucial factor in endothelial cell morphogenesis and angiogenesis, and its overexpression has been shown to promote tumor vascularization (Darash-Yahana *et al* 2004). Thus, the recruitment of macrophages to hypoxic areas in a tumor is part of a perpetual cycle in which the expression of proangiogenic factors, like VEGF and CXCR4, affects both tumor and stromal cells to promote cancer progression.

While CC chemokines play a major role in leukocyte chemoattraction into tumors, the CXC chemokine family is important in either promoting or inhibiting angiogenesis. The key characteristic that determines whether a CXC chemokine is angiogenic or angiostatic is the presence of a specific amino acid sequence, Glu-Leu-Arg (ELR), positioned immediately before the first cysteine residue. Angiogenic chemokines are ELR^+, while angiostatic chemokines are ELR^-. The exception to the ELR rule is the CXCR4 ligand CXCL12, which is ELR^-, yet demonstrates angiogenic activity. Work by Robert Strieter and colleagues have delineated the breakdown of chemokines into the angiogenic and angiostatic groups (Streiter *et al* 2004). A recent article demonstrating the ability of CXCL9 gene therapy to induce angiostatic effects in murine CT26 tumors further supports the potential for ELR- chemokines to be used as a novel therapeutic intervention, through inhibition of angiogenesis (Ruehlmann *et al* 2001).

3.4 Effects on tumor cell survival and growth

Chemokine production by tumors may directly affect cell survival and growth by functioning as growth and survival factors, mainly through autocrine mechanisms. Autocrine growth factors bind to receptors on the same cells that produced them, causing the cells to proliferate. Several different chemokine receptors and their matching chemokines have been characterized for their proliferative effects on tumor cells. Melanoma tumors are perhaps the best example of a cancer that supports its own growth and survival. By secreting elevated levels of CXCL1 and CXCL8 and overexpressing the receptor CXCR2 (compared to normal, non-malignant tissue), melanoma tumors control an autocrine stimulation program that enhances survival and proliferation (Dhawan and Richmond, 2002; Schadendorf *et al* 1993). Autocrine loops involving growth stimulation by CXCL1 and CXCL8, as well as the chemokine/receptor pair CCL20/CCR6, have also been reported in pancreatic cancer (Kleeff *et al* 1999; Takamori *et al* 2000).

The chemokine receptor that is most commonly detected on human and murine cancer cells is CXCR4. In the last five years, an extensive string of articles on the role of CXCR4 and its ligand CXCL12 in tumor biology have been published. Many cancers, including prostate (Taichman *et al* 2002), glioblastoma (Barbero *et al* 2003), bladder (Eisenhardt *et al* 2005), and pancreatic (Marchesi *et al* 2004), have been shown to proliferate in response to CXCL12, in some cases through an autocrine manner. CXCR4 may also mediate paracrine responses that promote tumor progression, as revealed in ovarian cancer cells, which release TNF-α in response to CXCL12 (Scotton *et al* 2002). The resultant TNF-α can subsequently promote tumor growth by inducing the production of other cytokines and proteases in the tumor microenvironment.

CXCL12 regulates cell survival in a number of cell types, including hematopoietic stem cells and T lymphocytes. The survival of cancer cells from hematopoietic (Tavor *et al* 2004) and solid (Marchesi *et al* 2004;

Scotton *et al* 2002) tumors is also affected by CXCL12, as the chemokine has been shown to support cell proliferation and inhibit apoptosis in serum-starved, sub-optimal growth conditions. This survival advantage provided by CXCL12 and CXCR4 may aid in the spread and growth of cancer cells to other sites where conditions may not be optimal (Kulbe *et al* 2004). The essential role of CXCR4 in tumor growth has been clearly proven using a CXCR4 antagonist, AMD3100, which inhibited the growth of brain tumors in mice when administered systemically (Rubin *et al* 2003).

CXCL8 is known to play a prominent role in colon cancer cell growth and survival. CXCL8, which is produced constitutively by colon epithelial cells and upregulated in IBD, functions as an autocrine growth factor for several human colon carcinoma cell lines. Incubation of colon carcinoma cells with a CXCL8 antagonist peptide or anti-CXCL8 antibodies results in attenuated cell proliferation (Brew *et al* 2000). Moreover, the degree of CXCL8 and CXCR2 expression also correlates with the metastatic potential of different colon carcinoma cells, suggesting that this chemokine/receptor pair is a key determinant in the aggressiveness of disease (Li *et al* 2001).

The identification of CXCR4 expression in normal and inflamed human colonic mucosa and in human colon cancer tissue and cell lines was reported several years ago. Ottaiano *et al* demonstrated that CXCR4 expression was significantly higher in cancerous colonic lesions and adenomatous polyps compared to non-cancerous lesions and hyperplastic polyps (Ottaiano *et al* 2004). Since CXCL12 is expressed constitutively in most normal tissues, including colon, it is thought that CXCL12/CXCR4 maintains a physiological role in normal gut homeostasis, likely through an autocrine-mediated loop. Ironically, CXCL12 expression is reduced in primary colon carcinoma, compared to adjacent non-malignant tissue, suggesting that CXCL12 might act as a "tumor-suppressor-like" protein (Shibuta *et al* 1997). However, a recent manuscript by Zeelenberg *et al* found that CXCR4 is required for the growth of colon carcinoma micrometastases. The authors used an intrakine method, in which a CXCL12 DNA construct that encodes an additional KDEL amino acid sequence is transduced into CT-26 cells, causing the retention of CXCR4 protein in the endoplasmic reticulum. Using an experimental metastasis model, their findings showed that CXCR4-deficient CT-26 cells are able to colonize lung and liver, but their growth is impaired, resulting in reduced metastasis. The authors concluded that CXCL12 is required for metastatic colon carcinoma outgrowth in distal organs (Zeelenberg *et al* 2003). Indeed, the proliferation of colon carcinoma cell lines is augmented by CXCL12, suggesting that the presence of CXCL12 in target organs of metastasis may foster the growth and survival of disseminated colon carcinoma cells (Ottaiano *et al* 2004).

3.5 Control of cancer metastasis

As discussed in Section 2, chemokines are best known for their ability to provide directional cues for the leukocytes to migrate into inflamed tissues and for the homing of hematopoietic stem cells into bone marrow. Chemokines are secreted by resident tissue cells, resident and recruited leukocytes, and cytokine-activated endothelial cells in response to inflammation. Chemokines are retained on heparan sulfate proteoglycans on the surface of endothelium and are deposited into the extracellular matrix. A chemokine concentration gradient is thereby formed around the inflammatory focus. Leukocytes rolling on the apical surface of vascular endothelium are brought into contact with bound chemokines, which then activate leukocyte integrins, leading to firm adherence and extravasation across the endothelial barrier and basement membrane. The recruited leukocytes may become desensitized to further encounters with chemokines because of high local concentrations, resulting in their retention at the specific site where their effector functions are needed. Thus, chemokines provide intrinsic signals to leukocytes for their recruitment to a specific organ site, as well as their navigation within the target tissue (Luster 1998; Rollins 1997; Vaday *et al* 2001).

The century-old Paget "seed and soil" theory of metastasis was based on the observation that metastatic cancer has a strong tendency to occur in specific organs (Paget 1889). Cancer's predilection for select organs is likely explained by the theory that metastatic organs provide the optimal conditions for disseminated tumor cells to colonize, survive, and proliferate, although knowledge about the mechanisms regulating this phenomenon are still limited. A mechanism most recently ascribed to organ-specific cancer metastasis is the paradigm of chemokine-mediated cell migration or homing. Since chemokine signaling results in the directional migration and specific arrival of cells, like leukocytes or hematopoietic cells, at a target destination, chemokines have emerged as crucial molecules in the metastatic process.

Initial studies by Mueller *et al* on the chemokine receptor profile in normal versus malignant breast tissue served as a starting block for a steady stream of papers to follow. The breast cancer study revealed that the mRNA expression of two specific chemokine receptors, CXCR4 and CCR7, was absent or low in normal mammary gland and mammary epithelial cell lines, but was detectable in high amounts in malignant breast tissue and breast cancer cell lines. A further examination of the mRNA levels of CXCL12, the ligand for CXCR4, and CCL19 and CCL21, the ligands for CCR7, demonstrated a pattern corresponding to the organs to which breast cancer most commonly metastasizes. Finally, administering antibodies against CXCR4 led to a decrease in metastasis in nude mice (Muller *et al* 2001). Thus, the organ-specific expression of certain chemokines, whose corresponding chemokine receptors are overexpressed on cancer cells, has developed into a model mechanism of metastasis.

Numerous articles from a growing list of cancer types have been published on the expression and role of CXCR4 or CCR7, describing what has now become a commonality among cancers that metastasize. Higher constitutive expression of CXCL12 in liver, lung, lymph node, and bone marrow and exclusive expression of CCL19 and CCL21 in lymphoid organs prompted investigations into metastatic cancers that "home" to those organs (Muller *et al* 2001). High CCR7 expression is associated with lymphatic metastasis and poor prognosis in gastric cancer (Mashino *et al* 2002), non-small cell lung carcinoma (Takanami 2003), and esophageal (Ding *et al* 2003) and head and neck squamous cell carcinoma (Wang *et al* 2004a). Examples of cancer types that exhibit high CXCR4 expression associated with metastases and poor prognosis include prostate (Sun *et al* 2003), pancreatic (Koshiba *et al* 2000), and osteosarcoma (Laverdiere *et al* 2005). A recent study using DNA microarray techniques to identify a bone metastasis gene expression signature in breast cancer confirmed CXCR4 as one of the decisive genes that predicts a propensity for bone metastasis (Kang *et al* 2003). The recent focus on CXCR4 as a pro-metastatic gene that predicts poor prognosis in cancer has resulted in the suggestion that chemokine receptor antagonists may be applied in clinical therapy.

As discussed in Section 3.4, CT-26 murine colon carcinoma cells were shown to express CXCR4, and the receptor facilitates the outgrowth, but not the colonization and invasion, of micrometastases in an experimental model of metastasis (Zeelenberg *et al* 2003). Another study examining the inhibitory effects of anti-CXCR4 antibodies on colon cancer cells showed an inhibition of CXCL12-induced adhesion, migration, and proliferation (Ottaiano *et al* 2004). Overexpression of another chemokine receptor, CCR6, in small liver metastases of colon carcinoma suggests that its liver-specific ligand, CCL20, may also be involved in the spread of colon cancer to liver (Dellacasagrande *et al* 2003). However, no clinical associations of CCR6 and colon cancer have been published to date. The association of CXCR4 expression with clinical outcome in colorectal cancer patients was addressed in two separate studies. High CXCR4 expression in specimens from patients with stage I/II disease was associated with an increased risk for local recurrence and/or metastasis. High CXCR4 expression in stage IV colorectal cancer patients was associated with a reduced overall median survival (Kim *et al* 2005) or a reduced 3-year survival rate (Schimanski *et al* 2005). Interestingly, CCR7 was not found to be associated with poor prognosis in colorectal cancer, despite its pronounced expression in cancer tissue and the presence of lymph node metastases (Schimanski *et al* 2005). These findings suggest that while CCR7 may play a minor role in the metastasis of colorectal cancer to lymph nodes, CXCR4 mediates the spread and arrival of cancer cells at specific organs, promotes their growth and survival, and thereby affects clinical outcome.

4. THERAPEUTIC APPLICATIONS OF CHEMOKINES IN CANCER

As discussed above, chemokines are clearly involved in many processes of cancer progression, implicating their suitability as cancer therapeutic targets. The versatility and redundancy of chemokines in a number of different diseases, like inflammatory diseases and HIV infection, has led to the generation of several chemokine receptor antagonists or chemokine-inhibiting strategies, and thus laid the groundwork for testing in cancer models (De Clercq and Schols, 2001). Clinical trials have shown the safety and efficacy of chemokine receptor antagonists (Hendrix *et al* 2000). The chemokine network is complex. Although it is unlikely that an individual chemokine or chemokine receptor antagonist would solely overcome the progression of cancer in humans, preclinical testing of such antagonists in animal models of cancer has shown promising applicability in cancer therapies.

Met-CCL5, a CCL5 analogue with the initiating methionine retained at the amino terminus, has demonstrated potent antagonistic effects on the receptors CCR1 and CCR5 (Proudfoot *et al* 1999; Proudfoot *et al* 1996). In a study by Robinson *et al* the daily administration of Met-CCL5 to mice bearing 410.4 murine carcinoma tumors led to a marked inhibition of tumor growth (Robinson *et al* 2003). 410.4 tumor cells express CCL5, and infiltrating leukocytes express the cognate receptors CCR1 and CCR5. The effects of Met-CCL5 were attributed to a decrease in inflammatory cell infiltration, which has been linked to better prognosis in breast cancer. The application of CCL5 receptor antagonists may also prove effective in other cancer types expressing CCL5 and/or its receptors, such as melanoma (Mrowietz *et al* 1999) and prostate cancer (Konig *et al* 2004). We have found that T AK-779, a small-molecule antagonist of CCR5, inhibits CCL5-induced cell proliferation and invasion of human prostate cancer cell lines (Vaday *et al* 2005).

The small-molecule antagonist AMD3100, which specifically inhibits CXCR4 function, has proven to be well-tolerated in clinical trials (Hendrix *et al* 2000). A recent study by Rubin *et al* showed that the administration of AMD3100 in intracranial glioblastoma and medulloblastoma xenografts resulted in increased apoptosis and reduced tumor cell proliferation (Rubin *et al* 2003). AMD3100 has subsequently been tested in a murine breast cancer model, showing substantial inhibition of tumor growth (Smith *et al* 2004). AMD3100 was also shown to inhibit CXCR4-mediated motility and development of acute myelogenous leukemia stem cells in transplanted NOD/SCID mice (Tavor *et al* 2004). To our knowledge, the only AMD3100 clinical trial published to date in cancer patients involved the administration of AMD3100 to patients with multiple myeloma or non-Hodgkin's lymphoma (Devine *et al* 2004). AMD3100 effectively caused the rapid mobilization of $CD34^{+}$ cells in patients who had previously received chemotherapy. Considering that CXCR4 has been shown to be critical in the colonization of metastatic colorectal cancer cells (Zeelenberg *et al* 2003), there is a strong rationale to test CXCR4 antagonists like AMD3100 in colorectal carcinoma animal models.

Antibody-based therapies may be another mode of inhibiting chemokine function in new cancer therapies. Muller *et al* published the first study in which antibodies against CXCR4 inhibited the metastasis of human breast cancer xenografts (Muller *et al* 2001). Anti-CXCR4 antibodies have also proven effective at preventing tumor growth, angiogenesis, and metastasis in prostate cancer xenograft models (Darash-Yahana *et al* 2004; Sun *et al* 2005). Attacking the SDF-1/CXCR4 axis from the other end using anti-SDF-1 antibodies demonstrated inhibition of metastasis of non-small cell lung carcinoma cells (Phillips *et al* 2003). A major hurdle in developing antibodies against chemokines or their receptors for clinical use is the requirement to humanize such antibodies, and still maintain inhibitory function.

Other modes of antagonizing chemokine function that may be applied to cancer therapy include small peptide antagonists and RNA interference (RNAi). Several peptidic compounds, ranging from 9- to 18-mers, have been identified as CXCR4 antagonists (De Clercq and Schols, 2001) and demonstrated inhibition of CXCR4-mediated activities in cancer cell lines (Koshiba *et al* 2000), as well metastasis of breast cancer xenografts (Liang *et al* 2004). RNAi experiments using small interfering RNA (siRNA) to silence CXCR4 gene expression have also shown effectiveness at abrogating breast tumor growth and metastasis *in vivo* (Lapteva *et al* 2005; Liang *et al* 2005). The rapidly advancing field of RNAi is now striving toward application of the RNAi technology in the clinical arena.

On the opposite spectrum, chemokines may be applied as immunotherapeutic agents, to promote the infiltration of host cells that have the capability to combat tumors (Homey *et al* 2002). The potent ability of chemokines to chemoattract effector cells of the immune system has proven effective at increasing the anti-tumor response in colorectal cancer studies, as noted in Table 2. The duality in chemokine function in cancer and the apparent therapeutic benefits of exploiting chemokines thus warrant more extensive understanding of chemokine signaling and specific chemokine functions related to colorectal cancer.

Table 2: Chemokines Implicated in Colorectal Cancer.

Chemo-kine(s)	Cellular Effect	Reference(s)
CCL2	⇓ lung metastases of CT-26 cells and ⇑ susceptibility to lysis	Huang *et al* 1994
CCL2; CCL22	⇑ dendritic cell accumulation in lymph nodes in C26 tumor model	Wang *et al* 2003
CCL3	⇑ dendritic cell accumulation in lymph nodes in C26 tumor model	Nakashima *et al* 1996
CCL21	⇑ anti-tumor response to C26 tumors when combined with LIGHT	Hisada *et al* 2004
CCL21	⇑ anti-tumor response and ⇓ tumorigenesis when fused to IL-2	Nakahara and Sakata, 2003
CCL21	⇑ T cell infiltration and ⇓ tumor size in CT-26 tumor model	Flanagan *et al* 2004
CXCL9	angiostatic, ⇓ lung metastases, and ⇑ life span in CT-26 tumor model	Ruehlmann *et al* 2001
CXCL10	angiostatic, ⇓ lung metastases, and ⇑ life span in CT-26 tumor model	Narvaiza *et al* 2000
CXCL8	⇑ proliferation of HCT116A, HT29, CaCo2 cells	Brew *et al* 2000
CXCL8	⇑ metastatic potential	Li *et al* 2001
CXCL12	required for metastatic CT-26 tumor outgrowth in distal organs	Zeelenberg *et al* 2003
CXCL12	⇑ adhesion, migration, and proliferation	Ottaiano *et al* 2004
CCL20	⇑ metastasis to liver	Dellacasagrande *et al* 2003
CXCL12	High CXCR4 receptor associated with ⇓ survival	Kim *et al* 2005 Schimanski *et al* 2005

5. MMP BIOLOGY AND CHEMISTRY

The first member of the MMP family, interstitial collagenase, was discovered to be the enzyme responsible for the dissolution of the collagen-rich tadpole tail during frog development (Gross and Lapiere, 1962). Collagenases and other enzymes with different substrate specificities were subsequently found to mediate proteolysis in a number of normal and pathological conditions, including arthritis, wound healing, and congestive heart failure. Since collagens constitute the major structural proteins in all tissues and the primary barrier encountered by migrating tumor cells, the secretion of collagenolytic enzymes by cancer cells is considered a pivotal mechanism of cancer dissemination.

Over 20 related enzymes comprise the MMP family, all sharing common functional domains and zinc-dependent catalytic activity. MMPs are grouped either according to their preferred substrate specificity, or according to a numbering system based on their sequential order of discovery (Chambers and Matrisian, 1997). Collectively, MMPs are capable of cleaving all extracellular matrix components (Nagase and Woessner, 1999; Woessner 1991). Some substrate specificities are distinct, but more often, MMPs overlap in their target substrates. The basic structure of MMPs is comprised of the following homologous domains: (1) a signal peptide that targets the MMPs to the secretory pathway; (2) a pro-domain that keeps the enzymes latent by occupying the active site; (3) a zinc-binding catalytic site; (4) a hemopexin domain that mediates interactions with substrates, as well as substrate specificity; and (5) a hinge region linking the catalytic and hemopexin domain.

Additional characteristics separate MMPs into other subgroups. MMP-7, or matrilysin, lacks the hemopexin domain and is the smallest MMP in size. The membrane-type MMPs are expressed on the cell surface via a 20-amino acid transmembrane domain and a small cytoplasmic domain (MT1-, MT2-, MT3-, and MT5-MMP), or via a glycosylphosphatidylinositol anchor (MT4- and MT6-MMP). MMP-2 (gelatinase A) and MMP-9 (gelatinase B) contain fibronectin-like domain repeats that mediate substrate binding.

Two sequence motifs that are highly conserved in the protein structure of MMPs are each important regulating the catalytic activity of the enzymes. The catalytic domain of all MMPs contains the consensus motif VAAHExGHxxGxxH, whose three histidine residues coordinate with the zinc ion in the active center for enzymatic activity (Birkedal-Hansen 1995; Stoker and Bode, 1995). The cysteine residue found in the PRCGxPD motif of the pro-domain also coordinates interactions with the zinc ion in the active site and confers latency to the MMPs (Birkedal-Hansen 1995; Nagase and Woessner, 1999).

MMP activity is tightly controlled through several different mechanisms. In general, MMPs are expressed in very low amounts, and their transcription is regulated either positively or negatively by oncogenes, cytokines, and growth factors (Sternlicht *et al* 1999; Zucker *et al* 2002). Cell-cell and cell-matrix interactions may also affect MMP gene expression (Hidalgo and Eckhardt, 2001). MMPs are synthesized as zymogens and thus require conversion to an enzymatically active form. Activation is accomplished through proteolytic removal of the pro-domain, or through conformational changes leading to disruption of pro-domain interactions with the catalytic site. Certain MMPs that contain furin-like recognition domains in their propeptides (MMP-11, MT-MMPs, MMP-28) can be activated intracellularly by members of the subtilisin family of serine proteases. Extracellular activation of MMPs can be mediated by proteolytic cleavage of the pro-domain by serine proteases, such as plasmin, or by other active MMPs (Sato *et al* 1994; Zucker *et al* 2002). For example, active MMP-3 is capable of activating proMMP-9 and proMMP-1. The activation of MMP-2 on the cell surface by MT1-MMP also exemplifies the diverse ways in which MMP activity is regulated (Cao *et al* 1998).

Active MMPs are inhibited in vivo by endogenous inhibitors, such as α2-macroglobulin and the tissue inhibitors of metalloproteinases (TIMP) family. The TIMP family consists of four members (TIMP-1, -2, -3, and -4), which vary in their affinities and specificities. TIMPs inhibit MMP activity by binding to the active site. A notable exception is the ability for stochastic concentrations of TIMP-2 to enhance MT1-MMP-induced activation of MMP-2 on the cell surface.

6. MMPs IN CANCER

MMPs contribute to all stages of tumor progression, from tumorigenesis to metastasis, through their ability to degrade ECM (Chambers and Matrisian, 1997; Goss *et al* 1998; Sternlicht and Werb, 2001). In tumor invasion, the ECM is viewed as a physical barrier against cell migration. MMPs play a major role in breaking down the ECM barrier, allowing the tumor cells to make their passage through the stroma and facilitating metastasis. Indeed, metastatic tumors demonstrate an increase in type IV collagenolytic activity and MMP expression (Liotta *et al* 1980). In addition to creating a path for migrating tumor cells, MMP degradation of ECM can also lead to liberation of growth factors, such as TGF-β, and other biologically active molecules that affect cell proliferation, invasion, and survival (Imai *et al* 1997).

MMP enzymatic activity extends beyond ECM, as several other soluble and membrane-bound proteins have been shown to be cleavable by MMPs. The cleavage of E-cadherin by MMP-3 and -7 has been shown to generate a soluble fragment that stimulates cell migration (Noe *et al* 2001). As we will discuss later in this chapter, certain MMPs readily cleave chemokines, such as CXCL12, which could have profound effects on chemokine-mediated processes in cancer (McQuibban *et al* 2001a). Other cytokines or growth factors are also subject to MMP cleavage, leading to the generation of mitogenic molecules (Schonbeck *et al* 1998; Yu and Stamenkovic, 2000), or alternatively, leading to inactivation of the growth factor. The ability of MMPs to cleave plasminogen and generate angiostatin, a potent inhibitor of angiogenesis, further demonstrates the multiple levels, and often conflicting ways, in which MMPs can affect cancer progression.

Although cancer cells can certainly contribute to their own fate by producing MMPs in tumors, it is believed that stromal cells produce large amounts of MMPs as well. The first report supporting this concept showed stromal fibroblasts, but not the cancer cells themselves, expressing MMP-11 in human breast cancer (Basset *et al* 1990). MMP-1, -2, -3, -9, and MT1-MMP mRNA has also been demonstrated in fibroblasts in close proximity to invading cancer cells (Nelson *et al* 2000; Polette *et al* 1996). It is believed that MMPs produced by stromal cells bind to docking sites on the surface of cancer cells, thereby equipping the cancer cells with enzymes on the cell membrane to facilitate invasion (Cao *et al* 1998; Yu and Stamenkovic, 2000). The discovery of extracellular matrix metalloproteinase inducer (EMMPRIN) by Biswas *et al* is an excellent example of the cooperative effort and reciprocal communication between cancer cells and stromal cells in tumors (Biswas *et al* 1995). EMMPRIN is a plasma membrane glycoprotein that is expressed by all epithelial cancer cells. Upon binding to fibroblasts through an unidentified receptor, EMMPRIN stimulates fibroblasts to produce MMP-1, -2, and -3. The secreted MMP-1 can then bind to EMMPRIN on the tumor cell, thereby arming the cancer cell with cell-surface MMPs for highly localized proteolysis (Guo *et al* 2000). The observation that overexpression of EMMPRIN in cancer cells markedly enhances tumor growth in vivo further supports the importance of EMMPRIN in cancer (Zucker *et al* 2001).

7. ROLE OF SPECIFIC MMPs IN COLORECTAL CANCER

A comprehensive list of the MMPs and TIMPs implicated in colorectal cancer is shown in Table 3. An important consideration in analyzing MMP data is the variety of techniques employed in MMP analysis, all of which may yield conflicting results. For example, measurements of MMP mRNA in tissue by cDNA microarray, Northern blot, RT-PCR, and *in situ* hybridization may not necessarily reflect the concomitant protein levels. Differences in sensitivity of cDNA or RNA probes may also result in variations of apparent MMP levels. Since cells are capable of binding to or endocytosing MMPs, positive detection by immunohistochemical staining does not exclusively indicate cell production of MMPs. Tissue microarrays are also limited in the small area analyzed per tissue section. Gelatin zymography, a highly sensitive technique for demonstrating MMP-2 and MMP-9 activity, may not be entirely accurate if MMP autoactivation occurs due to prolonged frozen storage of specimens.

Prominent findings from selected publications on the role of specific MMPs in colorectal cancer are discussed below.

MMP-1. It has been reported that the presence of MMP-1 in colorectal cancer tissues is associated with poor prognosis, independent of Dukes' stage (Murray *et al* 1996). Shiozawa *et al.* later confirmed these findings by using a range of techniques, including immunohistochemical staining, fluorescent *in situ* hybridization, and RT-PCR (Shiozawa *et al* 2000). While MMP-1 was not found in benign colon adenomas, high levels of MMP-1 expression were observed in invasive cancer, which correlated with the degree of invasiveness, lymph node involvement, and metastasis to the liver. MMP-1 was localized to both cancer and stromal cells. Positive correlations between high MMP-1 levels and hematogenous metastasis and between low MMP-1 levels and prolonged survival suggest that patients with colorectal cancer might benefit from using MMP inhibitors to prevent metastasis (Bendardaf *et al* 2003; Sunami *et al* 2000). The increase in MMP-1 levels in colon carcinoma may be due in part to the induction of MMP-1 by glycine-extended gastrin, which enhances invasion of colon cancer cells (Baba *et al* 2004). Of interest, colon cancer patients with polymorphism in the promoter region of MMP-1 had significantly worse survival (Zinzindohoue *et al* 2005). In contrast, hereditary nonpolyposis colorectal cancers exhibited lower expression of MMP-1 and MMP-9 in the fibroblastic stroma, which correlated with a less invasive and metastatic phenotype (Behrens *et al* 2003).

MMP-2. Active MMP-2 is not found in most normal tissues, but is significantly increased in some malignancies, including colorectal cancer. Paulsom *et al* first demonstrated enhanced distribution of MMP-2 in colorectal cancer by in situ RNA:RNA hybridization. In this study, MMP-2 mRNA was expressed in the majority (10 of 12 tumors) of tumors examined, localizing primarily in the stromal cells, rather than in the malignant cells (Paulsom *et al* 1992). These findings were confirmed in another study by Parsons *et al* which further showed by gelatin zymography that the ratio of active MMP-2 to proMMP-2 is 20-fold higher in colorectal cancer specimens compared to non-malignant specimens. Increased levels of MMP-2, along with MMP-9, IGF-II, and TGF-α, were found to be accurate predictors of hepatic metastasis (Parsons *et al* 1998). In contrast to other reports (Table 2), Sis *et al.* reported that although MMP-2 expression was found to correlate with the lymphatic invasion and stage, immunohistochemical staining for MMP-2 was not a significant indicator of survival (Sis *et al* 2004). Polymorphisms in the MMP-2 promoter have also been reported to be linked to colorectal cancer development (Xu *et al* 2004). Tutton *et al* conducted a recent study to determine the correlation between plasma MMP-2 and MMP-9 levels and colorectal cancer, as well as any changes following surgical resection. Plasma MMP-2 was significantly elevated in patients with colorectal cancer, and marked reductions of plasma MMP-2 levels were observed in specimens obtained from patients who underwent curative resections at all stages. Thus, plasma MMP-2 levels may be used as a non-invasive indicator of advanced colorectal cancer, or as a surrogate for disease status following curative resection (Langenskiold *et al* 2005; Tutton *et al* 2003).

MMP-3. Increased MMP-3 expression in colorectal tumors has been hypothesized to play a role in an enzymatic cascade that promotes disease progression. The co-expression of urokinase plasminogen activator (uPA) with MMP-9 in colorectal tumors is thought to be responsible for the generation of plasmin from plasminogen. Plasmin, in turn, converts proMMP-3 to MMP-3, which then activates proMMP-9 (Inuzuka *et al* 2000).

Microsatellite instability (MSI) involves proximal (right side) poorly differentiated colon tumors with mucinous or medullary architecture and peritumoral lymphocyte infiltrates. MSI is strongly associated with hereditary non-polyposis colon cancer and 16% of sporadic colorectal cancers. The presence of MSI has been shown to confer a survival advantage independent of other prognostic factors (Bubb *et al* 1996). Interestingly, colorectal adenocarcionomas with high MSI were found to have a significantly lower expression of MMP-3 than those with low or null MSI. More detailed analysis of the MMP-3 gene indicated that mutations, mainly nucleotide insertions and/or deletions, in the promoter region were found, possibly the result of the defective mismatch repair mechanism in sporadic colorectal cancers (Moran *et al* 2002).

MMP-7. Studies have invariably found that MMP-7 is expressed in the majority of colonic adenocarcinomas (Newell *et al* 1994). Increased levels of MMP-7 (as measured by immunohistochmistry and in situ hybridization) correlate with the presence of lymph node or distal metastasis (Adachi *et al* 1999). Experimental models of colorectal cancer using the SW480 human colon cancer cell line, which does not express endogenous MMP-7, further defined the significance of MMP-7. SW480 cells transfected with activated MMP-7 cDNA and implanted into nude mice demonstrated an increase in tumorigenicity and metastasis (Witty *et al* 1994). Further experiments to inhibit MMP-7 gene expression using an antisense oligonucleotide approach resulted in decreased tumor formation and metastasis, signifying that MMP-7 is necessary for colorectal cancer progression (Hasegawa *et al* 1998; Witty *et al* 1994). Interestingly, chronic exposure to MMP-7 was found to select for cancer cells that are resistant to apoptosis, and thereby not susceptible to chemotherapeutic drugs (Vargo-Gogola *et al* 2002). Overexpression of the transcription factor E1A-F early in colorectal neoplasia is believed to be a contributing factor in the upregulation of MMP-7 (Boedefeld *et al* 2005). Epidermal growth factor has also been shown to upregulate MMP-7 expression in colon cancer cells through an increase in PEA3 transcription factor activity (Lynch *et al* 2004).

The multiple intestinal neoplasia (Min) mouse, a model of familial adenomatous polyposis, was generated by ethylnitrosurea mutagenesis (Moser *et al* 1990). The Min phenotype is marked by truncation of the adenomatous polyposis coli (APC) gene, leading to the formation of numerous polyps of the small and large bowel (Su *et al* 1992). MMP-7 mRNA was found to be highly expressed in Min mice, localizing exclusively to the carcinoma cells.

Experiments were performed in the Matrisian lab to generate Min mice that are deficient in MMP-7. MMP-7-deficient Min developed >50% fewer polyps than wild-type Min mice with normal MMP-7 expression, providing strong evidence of the role of MMP-7 early colonic adenomas and transformation to invasive cancer (Wilson *et al* 1997).

MMP-9. High levels of MMP-9 mRNA and protein expression in adenomas, tumors, and plasma have been demonstrated in colon cancer (Mook *et al* 2004; Zucker *et al* 1995). It has also been observed that colon, but not rectal, tumors have higher MMP-9 expression levels than healthy tissue (Roeb *et al* 2001). A high ratio of MMP-9 mRNA in colon tumors versus normal intestinal mucosa was shown to be associated with shorter disease-free survival and with overall survival (Zeng *et al* 1996). The proMMP-9 levels in colonic adenomas were high compared to normal mucosal tissue, possibly representing a functional role for MMP-9 in early pre-malignant stages. Similarly, polyps with severe dysplasia show an increase in MMP-9 compared to polyps with mild to moderate dysplasia (Parsons *et al* 1998). Increased MMP-9 in colorectal cancer has been localized primarily to the inflammatory cells typically seen in and around neoplasms, rather than in the carcinoma cells (Nielsen *et al* 1999).

In a study of patients with Dukes' D colorectal cancer, patients with increased plasma levels of proMMP-9 or MMP-9/TIMP-1 complexes had significantly shorter survival than patients with normal plasma levels of these proteins (Zucker *et al* 1995). Similar studies by Tutton *et al* later confirmed the potential use of plasma MMP-9 levels as an indicator of advanced colon cancer (Tutton *et al* 2003), although any elevation in MMP-9 levels may be transient, depending on the timing of specimen collection.

Table 3: Characterization of MMPs and TIMPs in human colorectal cancer.

MMPs	Methods	Conclusions	References
-1	ZYMO; ELISA; IHC; ISH, RT-PCR	⇑ MMP-1 correlated with invasiveness and Dukes' stage and metastasis	Baker *et al* 2000; Baker and Leaper, 2003; Shiozawa *et al* 2000; Sunami *et al* 2000; van Stappen *et al* 1990
-1	IHC	MMP-1 correlated with poor prognosis	Murray *et al* 1996
-1	ZYMO, ELISA	⇑ active MMP-1 in cancer	Garbett *et al* 1999
-2	ZYMO, Northern, ELISA, IHC, RT-PCR	⇑MMP-2 in colon cancer correlated with Dukes stage, tumor grade, & angiogenesis	Barozzi *et al* 2002; Bodey *et al* 2000; Heslin *et al* 200; Karakiulakis *et al* 1997; Liabakk *et al* 1996; Matsuyama *et al* 2002; Moran *et al* 2002; Papadopoulou *et al* 2001
-2	ZYMO, ELISA, Activity Assays	⇑ active MMP-2 in cancer	Baker *et al* 2000; Garbett *et al* 1999
-2	ISH, IHC	⇑ stromal MMP-2 in cancer	Gallegos *et al* 1995; Poulsom *et al* 1992
-2	IHC	MMP-2 levels did not correlate with liver metastasis	Mukai, 1999 #2653
-2	IHC	⇑ mmp-2 correlated with more invasive cancer	Kikuchi *et al* 2000; Masaki *et al* 2003
-2	IHC, ZYMO	⇑ MMP-2 and loss of basement membrane during progression from adenoma-to-carcinoma	Parsons *et al* 1998; Tomosugi *et al* 1996; Zeng *et al* 1999
-2	RT-PCR	⇑ MMP-2/ TIMP-2 ratio in cancer	Parsons *et al* 1998; Tomita and Iwata, 1996; Zeng *et al* 1999
-2	ZYMO	⇑ pro & active MMP-2 in areas of tumor invasion	Emmert-Buck *et al* 1994

MMPs	Methods	Conclusions	References
-3	IHC	⇑ MMP-3 in cancer	Baker *et al* 2000; Bodey *et al* 2000; Moran *et al* 2002; Roeb *et al* 2004
-3	IHC	⇑MMP-3 in tumor stromal cells	Gallegos *et al* 1995
-7	FISH	⇑ MMP-7 in cancer	McDonnell *et al* 1991
-7	FISH, ZYMO, Northern, IHC, RT-	⇑ MMP-7 correlated with ⇑ stage	Adachi *et al* 1999; Ichikawa *et al* 1998; Ishikawa *et al* 1996; Kumar and Baglioni, 1991; Masaki *et al* 2001; Mori *et al* 1995; Zeng *et al*
-7	RT-PCR	⇑ MMP-7 early event in adenoma to carcinoma pathway	Heslin *et al* 2001
-9	Northern	⇑ MMP-9 RNA correlated with metastasis, dukes' stage and poor survival	Zeng *et al* 1996
-9	Zymo, ISH, IHC, RT-PCR	⇑ MMP-9 in cancer and adenomas	Bodey *et al* 2000; Liabakk *et al* 1996; Moran *et al* 2002; Parsons *et al* 1998
-9	ISH	⇑ MMP-9 correlated with increased angiogenesis	Kim and Kim, 1999
-9	ZYMO, ELISA, Activity Assays	⇑ active MMP -9 in cancer	Baker *et al* 2000; Garbett *et al* 1999; Waas *et al* 2003
-9	Zymo	⇑ MMP-9 corrleated with tumor grade and survival	Karakiulakis *et al* 1997; Matsuyama *et al* 2002; Zeng *et al* 1996
-9	Zymo; Western	⇑ MMP-9 in hepatic metastasis	Roeb *et al* 2001
-9	IHC	⇑ MMP- 9 in colon cancer, not in recal cancer	Jeziorska *et al* 1994
-10	IHC	⇑ MMP-9 especially at invasive tumor marginand inversely correlated with type iv collagen	Bodey *et al* 2000
-11	Noerthern, FISH	⇑ MMP-10 in cancer	Porte *et al* 1995

Table 3: Characterization of MMPs and TIMPs in human colorectal cancer (continued).

MMPs	Methods	Conclusions	References
-12	FISH, Nortrhern	⇑ MMP-12 correlates with improved prognosis	Yang *et al* 2001
-13	IHC	MMP-13 expression correlated with poor survival	Leeman *et al* 2002; Roeb *et al* 2004
-14	IHC, FISH	⇑ MT1-MMP In cancer and localization to cancer cells	Bendardaf *et al* 2003; Ohtani *et al* 1996
-14	IHC	⇑ MMP-14 correlated with more invasive cancer and prognosis	Kikuchi *et al* 2000
TIMP-1	FISH	⇑ TIMP-1 correlated with Dukes' stage and poor survival	Baker *et al* 2000; Garbett *et al* 1999; Joo *et al* 1999
TIMP-1	IHC	⇑ TIMP-1 correlates with progression from adenoma to adenocarcinoma and more invasive	Kikuchi *et al* 2000; Tomita and Iwata, 1996
TIMP-2	ISH, IHC	⇑ stromal TIMP-2 in cancer	Poulsom *et al* 1992
TIMP-2	IHC	⇑ TIMP-2 during progression from adenoma to adenocarcinoma	Tomosugi *et al* 1996
TIMP-2	IHC	TIMP-2 levels did not correlate with liver metastasis	Mukai *et al* 1999
TIMP-2	FISH, Western	⇑ MMP-2:TIMP-2 ratio correlated with advanced stage	Chan *et al* 2001

after colorectal surgery (de Hingh *et al* 2004). The balance between MMP-9 and RECK, a membrane-anchored regulator of MMPs, has also been proposed as an indicator of prognosis (Takeuchi *et al* 2004). The importance of measuring plasma, as opposed to serum, levels of MMPs should be emphasized due to the probability of artifact caused by the release of MMP-9 by neutrophils in clotted blood.

MMP-12. Although the majority of MMPs function as key promoters of cancer growth and progression, MMP-12 has been implicated in the inhibition of tumor growth. Known as macrophage metalloelastase, MMP-12 is expressed by TAM in response to granulocyte-macrophage colony-stimulating factor (GM-CSF) derived from tumor cells (Dong *et al* 1997). MMP-12 cleaves plasminogen, resulting in the generation of angiostatin, an endogenous inhibitor of tumor neovascularization (O'Reilly *et al* 1994). Overexpression of tumor MMP-12 mRNA in colorectal cancer patients has been shown to correlate with increased survival, due to a decrease in tumor vascularization (Yang *et al* 2001).

MMP-13. MMP-13 interacts with several other MMPs or proteases, either in its proenzyme form to generate the activated enzyme, or in it's active form, such as through its activation of proMMP-9 (Knauper *et al* 1996). In a recent study by Leeman *et al* MMP-13 protein expression in colorectal tumor biopsy specimens was localized to the tumor cell cytoplasm in >90% of the cases examined. Gelatin zymography showed that MMP-13 levels were significantly higher in colorectal tumors than in non-malignant tissues. Moreover, increased levels of MMP-13 correlated with poor survival (Leeman *et al* 2002).

MMP-14 (MT1-MMP). MT1-MMP expression is believed to play a critical role in the transformation of colon cancer from adenoma to carcinoma in situ and metastatic cancer. Northern blot and immunohistochemical staining analyses have demonstrated that increasing levels of MT1-MMP mRNA and protein expression correlate with increasing colon cancer stage. Takahashi *et al* showed that MT1-MMP was expressed in the majority (>90%) of colon cancers analyzed in a cDNA microarray study. Furthermore, low MT1-MMP expression is considered a marker of good prognosis in advanced colorectal carcinoma.

The regulation of MT1-MMP expression has been attributed to the oncogenic transcriptional activator β-catenin. Deregulation of the WNT signaling pathway due to mutation in the APC gene leads to the nuclear accumulation of β-catenin, which then interacts with members of the T-cell factor (TCF) family of DNA-binding proteins to function as a composite transcriptional activator. The MT1-MMP gene is a target of the β-catenin/TCF complex, and its upregulation is mediated through a TCF binding site in its promoter. In addition, the gene encoding the laminin-5 γ2 chain is also a β-catenin target. Fragments of laminin-5 γ2 chain resulting from MT1-MMP cleavage are potent inducers of epithelial cell migration. Hlubek *et al* and Murai *et al* demonstrated that the coordinated expression of β-catenin, laminin-5 γ2 chain, and MT1-MMP in the invasive regions of colorectal cancer tissue is indicative of promigratory activity (Hlubek *et al* 2004; Murai *et al* 2004).

MMP-19 and MMP-28. In contrast to many previously characterized MMPs, MMP-19 and MMP-28 appear to be downregulated in tumor epithelium during malignant transformation of the colon and may play a role in tissue homeostasis (Bister *et al* 2004).

TIMPs. Although TIMPs are endogenous inhibitors of MMP activity, increased TIMP expression has been associated with colorectal cancer progression. High levels of plasma TIMP-1 are indicative of short survival and recurrence of disease in colorectal cancer patients (Holten-Anderson *et al* 2000). Similarly, elevated TIMP-1 tumor levels in patients with colon cancer were shown to correlate with poor prognosis (Joo *et al* 1999; Lu *et al* 1991). A recent cDNA microarray study also showed that TIMP-1 mRNA expression is significantly higher in colorectal cancer versus normal tissue, and that higher TIMP-1 mRNA expression is a distinguishing marker of early invasive colorectal carcinoma compared to colorectal adenoma (Nosho *et al* 2005). Interestingly, plasma levels of TIMP-2 have been found to be higher in patients with Dukes stage A compared with patients with advanced Dukes stages (Larsen *et al* 2005). Ring *et al.* also reported a distinct distribution of TIMP-2, with more TIMP-2 found in localized than in disseminated tumors (Ring *et al* 1997). Recently Curran *et al.* examined the major MMPs and TIMPs by immunochemistry in a series of stage III colorectal cancer specimens (Curran *et al* 2004). The MMP/TIMP profile defined by hierarchical cluster analysis of histochemical scores identified a distinct group of colorectal cancers associated with poor prognosis (18 months) versus a good prognosis group (49 months).

Several studies have reported conflicting findings on which cells in the colorectal tumor microenvironment express TIMPs. While it is debatable whether carcinoma cells express TIMP-1 and TIMP-2, it is known that these TIMPs are expressed in the stromal compartment of colorectal carcinomas, predominantly by fibroblast-like cells localized to the invasive front of the tissue (Holten-Anderson *et al* 2005).

The overexpression of TIMPs in colorectal cancer seems paradoxical, considering their ability to inhibit MMP-regulated activities. However, besides inhibiting MMPs, TIMP-1 has also been implicated in cell proliferation and inhibition of apoptosis (Guedez *et al* 1998a; Guedez *et al* 1998b; Li *et al* 1999). As discussed above, TIMP-2 complexes with MT1-MMP and MMP-2 to promote localized proteolysis. Thus, it is likely that TIMPs play dual, contrasting roles in colorectal cancer.

8. MMP INHIBITORS IN CANCER

Enhanced expression of MMPs in cancer, coupled with their ability to degrade connective tissue barriers provided a logical role for these enzymes in cancer metastasis. The pharmaceutical industry developed numerous MMP inhibitors (MMPIs) in the1990s with the anticipation of reaping the harvest of blockbuster anticancer drugs. Chemists achieved considerable success in designing MMPIs that are orally active, achieve effective blood levels, and display high specificity for MMPs, while generally sparing other types of proteases. However, higher MMPI doses inhibited other metalloproteinases know as ADAMs. Although some specificity for subgroups of MMPs was attained, none of the MMPIs in clinical trials were highly specific for individual MMPs. Testing of MMPIs in animal models of colorectal cancer resulted in inhibition of tumor growth and metastases and prolongation of survival (see Figure 3). A preliminary trial of marimastat in patients with colon cancer resulted in a decreased rate of rise in carcinoembryonic antigen (CEA) (Primrose *et al* 1999).

Based on the success of MMPIs in preclinical models and phase I/II human trials, five pharmaceutical companies initiated phase III clinical trials of MMPIs in patients with lung (Leighl *et al* 2005; Shepherd *et al* 2002), breast (Sparano *et al* 2002), gastric (Bramhall *et al* 2002), pancreatic (Bramhall *et al* 2001; Moore *et al* 2003), colorectal (King *et al* 2003) and prostate cancer. Based on the non cytotoxic nature of MMPIs, most of these clinical trials included the combination of standard chemotherapy with or without the addition of an MMPI. In contrast to the excitement generated by data from phase I and II trials of MMPIs, the phase III trials employing marimastat (produced by British Biotech), prinomastat (produced by Agouron/Pfizer) and BMS-275291 (produced by Bristol-Myers Squibb) (Leighl *et al* 2005) failed to demonstrate improvement in overall survival, response rate, progression-free survival or quality of life assessment (Pavlaki and Zucker, 2003). Subgroup analysis in patients with advanced gastric cancer who had been treated with marimastat and chemotherapy demonstrated that those who had received prior chemotherapy had a small (13%), but significant increase in survival at 2 years (Bramhall *et al* 2002) One of the unanticipated problems with MMPIs has been the high incidence of joint pain side effects that resulted in modification of drug dosage in ~30% of patients on marimastat and prinomastat. One double blind placebo control study of the use of adjuvant marimastat in patients with inoperable colorectal metastases to the liver reported a significant survival advantage in a small subgroup of patients with musculoskeletal side effects (King *et al* 2003); this was not the case in breast cancer (Sparano *et al* 2004). BMS-275291was not associated with joint toxicity, but still lacked efficacy in patients with advanced non small cell lung cancer. Clinical trials with BAY-129566 in lung cancer and pancreatic cancer (MMPI versus gemcitabine) were prematurely terminated because of lower survival in MMPI-treated patients (Moore *et al* 2003). These disappointing results are a reminder that the path to curing human cancer is treacherous with unanticipated hazards encountered at every turn.

The crucial question is whether the lack of success with MMPIs to date in cancer patients is due to: 1) the drugs were employed too late in the clinical progression of disease (advanced/metastatic cancer), whereas preclinical studies have suggested optimal response in early stages of cancer (Bergers *et al* 1999), 2) the drugs lacked specificity and inhibited MMPs that might have anti-tumoral activity e.g. MMP-12, 3) the high incidence of rheumatoid side effects compromised achieving effective drug levels, or 4) MMPIs are not effective agents for treatment of cancer. Based on competitive/financial pressures on pharmaceutical companies, it is of concern that the industry may be reluctant to initiate trials of MMPIs in early stage cancer where drug effectiveness is more likely to be manifest, but where outcome results will be delayed.

Several pharmacologic agents have been demonstrated to have both anti-tumor and indirect anti-MMP activity. In these cases, it is difficult to determine whether the inhibition of MMPs is causal in the anti-tumor effect. For example, troglitazone, a selective ligand and agonist of PPAR-γ, which inhibits the proliferation of cancer cells, also has effects on MMPs. Troglitazone treatment of colon cancer cells strongly inhibited the production of MMP-7 and adhesion to ECM proteins; a role for troglitazone in cancer prevention and treatment was proposed (Sunami *et al* 2002). Likewise, the anti-angiogenic and anti-metastatic effects of interferon-α in colon cancer are accompanied by inhibition of MMP-9 expression (Ozawa *et al* 2001). Tetracyclines and non antibiotic derivatives of tetracycline have demonstrated anti-tumor effects in animal models of cancer and in patients with Kaposi's sarcoma (Cianfrocca *et al* 2002). It is unclear whether these effects are due to the inhibitory effects of tetracyclines on MMP activity or on cell proliferation (Lokeshwar *et al* 2002).

Natural agents have also been demonstrated to exert profound inhibitory effects on MMPs. These include: epigallocatechin gallate, a green tea polyphenol with chemopreventive properties (Demeule *et al* 2000; Pezzato *et al* 2004), hyperforin, the major lipophilic constituent of St. John's wort

(Dona *et al* 2004), and caffeic acid phenethyl ester derived from honey bee propolis (Liao *et al* 2003).

9. MMP-CHEMOKINE INTERACTIONS

Since an extensive array of MMPs and chemokines is found in tumors, it is likely that MMPs and chemokines interact, either directly or indirectly. Such interactions could reciprocally affect gene expression, enzymatic or chemotactic activity, and receptor/substrate interactions. For example, cells from different origins have been shown to upregulate MMP production in response to chemokines (Azenshtein *et al* 2002; Janowska-Wieczorek-A. *et al* 2000; Robinson *et al* 2002). Chemokines have also been described as putative substrates of MMPs, resulting in modified chemokines with altered capabilities to bind their receptors (Van Damme *et al* 2004). Although MMPs are best known for their ability to degrade the major ECM components, it is important to consider that chemokines produced by tumor and stromal cells bind to ECM components and are likely to encounter MMPs. Thus, in the context of a tumor microenvironment, MMPs may act on chemokines, cleaving the native protein to modify its pro- or anti-tumor activities. One should also consider the enzymatic actions of other proteases, namely the serine protease CD26/dipeptidyl peptidase IV (DPP IV), which modulates the activity of several different chemokines by enzymatic processing (Van Damme *et al* 2004). Thus, the potential for chemokine modification by proteases has important implications in the growth of a tumor. In this section, we will discuss prominent findings on the enzymatic cleavage of chemokines by MMPs, and the implications of MMP-modified chemokines in cancer progression.

Naturally-occurring variants of chemokines, which are generally truncated by several amino acids residues, have been identified. An excellent example is CXCL8, of which several natural variants have been found. Van den Steen *et al*. demonstrated that MMP-9 may be at least one of the proteases responsible for the truncation of CXCL8. The authors proved that MMP-9 cleaves the first six amino acids from the amino terminus of CXCL8, converting CXCL8 (1-77 aa) to CXCL8 (7-77 aa) (Van den Steen *et al* 2000). Remarkably, the resultant CXCL8 (7-77 aa) demonstrated at least 10-fold higher activity than the native CXCL8. Other chemokines known to exist naturally in truncated or modified forms include CXCL7, CXCL1, and CXCL5. However, in contrast to the augmentation of CXCL8 activity by MMP-9 processing, these chemokines become degraded and hence inactivated by MMP-9 enzymatic action (Van den Steen *et al* 2003). The inability of MMP-9 to cleave CCL5 and CCL8, and the lack of functional alterations to MMP-9-cleaved CXCL6, confirm that MMP proteolysis of chemokines is, in fact, selective and specific (Van den Steen *et al* 2000). Cleavage of CXCL12 by several different MMPs also results in inactivation of chemotactic function and receptor binding capability, implicating the robustness of the MMP family in modulating chemokine function (McQuibban *et al* 2001b).

A recently described method of discovering novel substrates of MMPs was reported by Overall and colleagues. Assuming the importance of MMP substrate binding to exosites outside the catalytic domain of the enzyme, a yeast two-hybrid system was employed, using the MMP hemopexin C domain as bait (Overall *et al* 2002). Remarkably, a number of chemokines have been found to bind the hemopexin domain and subsequently become targets for cleavage by the same MMP. Several MMPs, including MMP-2, MT1-MMP, MMP-1, and MMP-3 were found to cleave CCL7 (McQuibban *et al* 2000), while the closely related chemokines CCL2, CCL8, and CCL13 varied in their susceptibility to the same MMPs (McQuibban *et al* 2002). More advanced technologies for degradomic screening have led to the identification of novel substrates of MT1-MMP, such as CXCL8 (Tam *et al* 2004). A significant discovery resulting from these studies is that some truncated chemokine products can serve as potent antagonists of their cognate chemokine receptors (McQuibban *et al* 2002). This point was clearly proven in different animal models of inflammation, showing that the administration of MMP-processed CC chemokines, like CCL7 and CCL2, dampen the inflammatory response. Thus, while MMPs and chemokines play significant roles in the early stages of inflammation, MMP-chemokine interactions likely also function in a self-attenuating mechanism as inflammation wanes. How such a mechanism of MMP-chemokine checkpoints applies in cancer is as yet unknown. Redundancies in MMP and chemokine activities and receptor/substrate binding, the vast assortment of MMPs and chemokines produced in tumors, and differential responses by malignant and stromal cells to MMP-modified chemokines, are all factors that make it difficult to delineate how MMP-chemokine interactions impact on tumor progression. Either the augmentation or inactivation of chemokine functions by MMPs could affect all aspects of cancer progression, including angiogenesis and metastasis. Thus, it is abundantly clear that delineation of MMP-chemokine interactions and resultant chemokine products would lead to the identification of pertinent molecules to target in new cancer therapeutic modalities (Van Damme *et al* 2004).

10. CONCLUSIONS

Over a decade ago, Opdenakker and Van Damme coined the term "countercurrent principle of invasion" to describe the involvement of chemokines in the directional movement of tumor and host cells. Since invasive tumor cells move away from the primary tumor site, while leukocytes are drawn toward the tumor, the two cell populations move in opposing "currents". The countercurrent concept stresses that tumor-derived chemokines likely play a detrimental role in tumor progression, as opposed to being involved in the host anti-tumor response (Opdenakker and Van Damme, 1992a; Opdenakker and Van Damme, 1992b). Chemokines are fundamentally involved in trafficking migratory cells, as well as facilitating proteolysis through induction of protease gene expression. Chemokines and MMPs also interact through direct proteolysis of chemokines by MMPs to yield either bioactive chemokine variants or deactivated chemokine fragments. Thus, the chemokine and MMP networks converge in multiple crossroads that can dramatically affect the progression of cancer.

Both chemokines and MMPs are implicated in the progression of colorectal carcinoma. For example, colorectal tumor cells are responsible for producing increased amounts of MMP-7, whereas tumor-infiltrating inflammatory cells produce high levels of MMP-9. The chemokine CXCL8/IL-8 is an important growth factor for colon cancer cells, and the CXCL12/CXCR4 axis is considered a critical mechanism of colorectal cancer metastasis.

To date, clinical trials of broad spectrum MMPIs have failed to demonstrate their efficacy in advanced colorectal, lung, gastric, prostate, breast, and pancreatic cancers. We propose that future development of MMPIs as therapeutic agents in cancer should entail the following: 1) development of MMPIs with higher specificity associated with low incidence of musculoskeletal side effects, 2) trials of MMPIs in earlier stage cancer, and 3) development of surrogate markers to monitor the inhibitory effect of MMPIs in tissues. The application of chemokine receptor antagonists or chemokine immunotherapy in cancer treatment has yet to move far beyond the preclinical stages. The myriad effects of MMPs and chemokines on biologic functions complicate our ability to understand the role of individual molecules in physiologic and pathologic states. However, it is becoming more evident from the rapidly advancing field that the inhibition of both chemokines and MMPs is recognized as a promising avenue for novel cancer therapies.

ACKNOWLEDGEMENTS

This work was supported by a Merit Review Grant, Merit Review Entry Program Award, and Research Enhancement Award Program (REAP) grant from the Department of Veterans Affairs, an RO1-CA79866 grant from the National Institutes of Health, and a Targeted Research Opportunity Grant from the Research Foundation of SUNY, Stony Brook University.

REFERENCES

Adachi Y, Yamamoto H, Itoh F, Hinoda Y, Okada Y and Imai K, 1999, Contribution of matrilysin (MMP-7) to the metastatic pathwayof human colorectal cancers. *Gut* **45:** 252-258.

Azenshtein E, Luboshits G, Shina S, Neumark E, Shahbazian D, Weil M, Wigler N, Keydar I and Ben-Baruch A, 2002, The CC chemokine RANTES in breast carcinoma progression: regulation of expression and potential mechanisms of promalignant activity. *Cancer Res.* **62:** 1093-1102.

Baba M, Itoh K and Tatsuta M, 2004, Glycine-extended gastrin induces matrix metallo-proteinase-1- and -3-mediated invasion of human colon cancer cells through type I collagen gel and matrigel. *Int J Cancer.* **111:** 23-31.

Balkwill F, 2004, Cancer and the chemokine network. *Nat Rev Cancer.* **4:** 540-550.

Balkwill F, Charles K, A and Mantovani A, 2005, Smoldering and polarized inflammation in the initiation and promotion of malignant disease. *Cancer Cell.* **7:** 211-217.

Balkwill F and Mantovani A, 2001, Inflammation and cancer: back to Virchow? *Lancet* 357, 539-545.

Banks C, Bateman A, Payne R, Johnson P and Sheron N, 2003, Chemokine expression in IBD. *J Pathol.* **199:** 28-35.

Barbero S, Bonavia R, Bajetto A, Porcile C, Pirani P, Ravetti JL, Zona GL, Spaziante R, Florio T and Schettini G, 2003, Stromal Cell-derived Factor 1alpha stimulates human glioblastoma cell growth through the activation of both extracellular signal-regulated kinases 1/2 and Akt. *Cancer Res.* **63:** 1969-1974.

Basset P, Bellocq JP, Wolf C, Stoll I, Hutin P, Limacher JM, Podhajcer OL, Chenard MP, Rio MC and Chambon P, 1990, A novel metalloproteinase gene specifically expressed in stromal cells of breast carcinomas. *Nature.* **348:** 699-704.

Behrens P, Mathiak M, Mangold E, Kirdorf S, Wellmann A, Fogt F, Rothe M, Florin A and Wernert N, 2003, Stromal expression of invasion-promoting, matrix-degrading proteases MMP-1 and -9 and the Ets 1 transcription factor in HNPCC carcinomas and sporadic colorectal cancers. *Int J Cancer.* **107:** 183-188.

Bendardaf R, Lamlum H, Vihinen P, Ristamaki R, Laine J and Pyrhonen S, 2003, Low collagenase-1 (MMP-1) and MT1-MMP expression levels are favourable survival markers in advanced colorectal carcinoma. *Oncology.* **54:** 337-346.

Bergers G, Javaherian K, Lo KM, Folkman J, Hanahan D,1999, Effect of angiogenesis inhibitors on multistage carcinogenesis in mice. *Science.* **284:** 808-812.

Bingle L, Brown NJ and Lewis CE, 2002, The role of tumour-associated macrophages in tumour progression: implications for new anticancer therapies. *J Pathol.* **196:** 254-265.

Birkedal-Hansen H, 1995, Proteolytic remodeling of extracellular matrix. *Curr Opin Cell Biol.* **7:** 728-735.

Bister VO, Salmela MT, Karjalainen-Lindsberg ML, Uria J, Lohi J, Puolakkainen P, Lopez-Otin C and Saariahlo-Kere U, 2004, Differential expression of the matrix metalloproteinases, MMP-19, MMP-26, and MMP-28, in normal and inflamed intestine and colon cancer. *Dig Dis Sci.* **49:** 653-661.

Biswas C, Zhang Y, DeCastro R, Guo H, Nakamura T, Kataoka H and Nabeshima K , 1995, The human tumor cell-derived collagenase stimulating factor (renamed EMMPRIN) is a member of the immunoglobulin superfamily. *Cancer Res.* **55:** 434-439.

Boedefeld WM, Soong R, Weiss H, Diasio RB, Urist MM, Bland KI and Heslin MJ, 2005, E1A-F is overexpressed earl yin human colorectal neoplasia and associated with cyclooxygenase-2 and matrix metalloproteinase-7. *Mol Carcinog.* **43:** 13-17.

Bottazzi B, Polentarutti N, Acero R, Balsari A, Boraschi D, Ghezzi P, Salmona M and Mantovani A, 1983, Regulation of the macrophage content of neoplasms by chemoattractants. *Science.* **220:** 210-212.

Bramhall SR, Hallissey MT, Whiting J, Scholefield J, Tierney G, Stuart RC, Hawkins RE, McCulloch P, Maughan T, Brown PD, Fielding JW, 2002, Marimastat as maintenance therapy for patietns with advanced gastric cancer: a randomised trial. *Brit J Cancer.* **86:** 1864-1870.

Bramhall SR, Rosemurgy AS, Brown PD and Buckels JAC, 2001, Marimastat as first line therapy for patients with unresected pancreatic cancer: A randomzed trial. *J Clin Oncol.* **19:** 3447-3455.

Bresalier RS, Sandler RS, Quan H, Bolognese JA, Oxenius B, Horgan K, Lines C, Riddell R, Morton D, Lanas A, Konstam MA, Baron JA; Adenomatous Polyp Prevention on Vioxx (APPROVe) Trial Investigators, 2005, Cardiovascular events associated with rofecoxib in a colorectal adenoma chemoprevention trial. *N Engl J Med.* **352:** 1092-1102.

Brew R, Erikson JS, West DC, Kinsella AR, Slavin J and Christmas SE, 2000, Interleukin-8 as an autocrine growth factor for human colon carcinoma cells in vitro. *Cytokine.* **12:** 78-85.

Brigati C, Noonan D, Albini A and Benelli R, 2002, Tumors and inflammatory infiltrates: friends or foes? *Clin Exp Metastasis.* **19:** 247-258.

Bubb VJ, Curtis LJ, Cunningham C, Dunlop MG, Carothers AD, Morris RG, White S, Bird CC and Wyllie AH, 1996, Microsatellite instability and the role of hMSH2 in sporadic colorectal cancer. *Oncogene.* 1996, 2641-2649.

Cao J, Drews M, Lee HM, Conner C, Bahou WF and Zucker S, 1998, The propeptide domain of membrane type I matrix metalloproteinase is required for binding of tissue inhibitor of metalloproteinases and for activation of pro-gelatinase A. *J Biol Chem* **273:** 34745-34752.

Chambers AF and Matrisian LM, 1997, Changing views of the role of matrix metalloproteinases in metastasis. *J Natl Cancer Inst.* **89:** 1260-1270.

Chang ET, Zheng T, Weir EG, Borowitz M, Mann RB, Spiegelman D and Mueller NE, 2004, Aspirin and the risk of Hodgkin's lymphoma in a population-based case-control study. *J Natl Cancer Inst.* **96:** 305-315.

Cianfrocca M, Cooley TP, Lee JL, Rudek MA, Scadden DT, Ratner L, Pluda JM, Figg WD, Krown SE and Dezube BJ, 2002, Matrix metalloprteinase inhibitor Col-3 in the treatment of AIDS-related Kaposi's sarcoma: A phase I AIDS malignancy consortium study. *J Clin Oncol.* **20:** 153-159.

Coussens LM and Werb Z, 2002, Inflammation and cancer. *Nature.* **420:** 860-867.

Curran S, Dundas SR, Buxton J, Leeman MF, Ramsay R and Murray GI, 2004, Matrix metalloproteinase/tissue inhibitors of matrix metalloproteinase phenotype identifies poor prognosis colorectal cancers. *Clin Cancer Res.* **10:** 8229-8234.

Darash-Yahana M, Pikarsky E, Abramovitch R, Zeira E, Pal B, Karplus R, Beider K, Avniel S, Kasem S, Galun E, Peled A, 2004, Role of high expression levels of CXCR4 in tumor growth, vascularization, and metastasis. *FASEB J.* **18:** 1240-1242.

De Clercq E and Schols D, 2001, Inhibition of HIV infection by CXCR4 and CCR5 chemokine receptor antagonists. *Antivir Chem Chemother.* **12 Suppl. 1:** 19-31.

de Hingh I, Waas ET, Lomme R, Wobbes T and Hendriks T, 2004, Circulating matrix metalloproteinase-9 is transiently elevated after colorectal surgery. *Int J Colorect Dis.* **19:** 446-450.

Dellacasagrande J, Schreurs OJ, Hofgaard PO, Ombolt H, Steinsvoll S, Schenck K, Bogen B, and Dembic Z, 2003, Liver metastasis of cancer facilitated by chemokine receptor CCR6. *Scand J Immunol.* **57:** 534-544.

Demeule M, Brossard M, Page M, Gingras D, and Beliveau R, 2000, Matrix metalloproteinase inhibition by green tea catechins. *Biochim Biophys Acta.* **1478:** 51-60.

Devine SM, Flombenberg N, Vesole DH, Liesveld J, Weisdorf D, Badel K, Calandra G, and DiPersio JF, 2004, Rapid mobilization of CD34+ cells following administration of the CXCR4 antagonist AMD3100 to patients with multiple myeloma and non-Hodgkin's lymphoma. *J Clin Oncol.* **22:** 1095-1102.

Dhawan P and Richmond A, 2002, Role of CXCL1 in tumorigenesis of melanoma. *J Leuko Biol.* **72:** 9-18.

Ding Y, Shimada Y, Maeda M, Kawabe A, Kaganoi J, Komoto I, Hashimoto Y, Miyake M, Hashida H, and Imamura M, 2003, Association of CC chemokine receptor 7 with lymph node metastasis of esophageal squamous cell carcinoma. *Clin Cancer Res.* **9:** 3406-3412.

Dona M, Dell'Aica I, Pezzato E, Sartor L, Calabrese F, Della Barbera M, Donella-Deana A, Appendino G, Borsarini A, Caniato R *et al*, 2004, Hyperforin inhibits cancer invasion and metastasis. *Cancer Res.* **64:** 6225-6232.

Dong Z, Kumar R, Yang X and Fidler IJ, 1997, Macrophage-derived metalloelastase is responsible for the generation of angiostatin in Lewis lung carcinoma. *Cell.* **88:** 801-810.

Dvorak HF, 1986, Tumors: wounds that do not heal. Similarities between tumor stroma generation and wound healing. *N Engl J Med.* **315:** 1650-1659.

Eisenhardt A, Frey U, Tack M, Rosskopf D, Lummen G, Rubben H and Siffert W, 2005, Expression analysis and potential functional role of the CXCR4 chemokine receptor in bladder cancer. *Eur Urol.* **47:** 111-117.

Fidler IJ, 2002, The pathogenesis of cancer metastasis: the 'seed and soil' hypothesis revisited. *Nat Rev Cancer* **3:** 1-6.

Flanagan K, Glover RT, Horig H, Yang W and Kaufman HL, 2004, Local delivery of recombinant vaccinia virus expressing secondary lymphoid chemokine (SLC) results in a CD4 T-cell dependent antitumor response. *Vaccine.* **22:** 2894-2903.

Garber K, 2004, Aspirin for cancer chemoprevention: still a headache? *J Natl Cancer Inst.* **96:** 252-253.

Goss KJ, Brown PD and Matrisian LM, 1998, Differing effects of endogenous and synthetic inhibitors of metalloproteinases on intestinal tumorigenesis. *Int J Cancer.* **78:** 629-635.

Greten FR, Eckmann L, Greten TF, Park JM, Li Z-W, Egan LJ, Kagnoff MF and Karin M, 2004, IKKbeta links inflammation and tumorigenesis in a mouse model of colitis-associated cancer. *Cell.* **118:** 285-296.

Gross J and Lapiere CM, 1962, Collagenolytic activity in amphibian tissues; a tissue culture assay. *Proc Natl Acad Sci U S A.* **48:** 1014-1022.

Gu L, Tseng S, Horner RM, Tam C, Loda M and Rollins BJ, 2000, Control of TH2 polarization by the chemokine monocyte chemoattractant protein-1. *Nature.* **404:** 407-411.

Guedez L, Courtemanch L and Stetler-Stevenson W, 1998a, Tissue inhibitor of metalloproteinase (TIMP)-1 induces differentiation and an antiapoptotic phenotype in germinal center B cells. *Blood.* **92:** 1342-1349.

Guedez L, Stetler-Stevenson WG, Wolff L, Wang J, Fukushima P, Mansor A and Stetler-Stevenson M, 1998b, In vitro suppression of programmed cell death of B cells by tissue inhibitor of metalloproteinases-1. *J Clin Invest.* **102:** 2002-2010.

Guo H, Li R, Zucker S and Toole BP, 2000, EMMPRIN (CD147), an inducer of matrix metalloproteinase synthesis, also binds interstitial collagenase to the tumor cell surface. *Cancer Res.* **60:** 888-891.

Hasegawa S, Koshikawa N, Momiyama N, Moriyama K, Ichikawa Y, Ishikawa T, Mitsuhashi M, Shimada H and Miyazaki K, 1998, Matrilysisn-specific antisense oligonucleotide inhibits liver metastasis of human colon cancer cells in a nude mouse model. *Int J Cancer.* **76:** 812-816.

Hendrix CW, Flexner C, MacFarland RT, Giandomenico C, Fuchs EJ, Redpath E, Bridger G and Henson GW, 2000, Pharmacokinetics and safety of AMD2100, a novel antagonist of the CXCR4 chemokine receptor, in human volunteers. *Antimicrob Agents Chemother.* **44:** 1667-1673.

Hidalgo M and Eckhardt SG, 2001, Development of matrix metalloproteinase inhibitors in cancer therapy. *J Natl Cancer Inst.* **93:** 178-193.

Hisada M, Yoshimoto T, Kamiya S, Magami Y, Miyaji H, Yoneto T, Tamada K, Aoki T, Koyanagi Y and Mizuguchi J, 2004, Synergistic antitumor effect by coexpression of chemokine CCL21/SLC and costimulatory molecule LIGHT. *Cancer Gene Ther.* **11:** 280-288.

Hlubek F, Spaderna S, Jung A, Kirchner T and Brabletz T, 2004, Beta-catenin activates a coordinated expression of the proinvasive factors laminin-5 gamma2 chain and MT1-MMP in colorectal carcinomas. *Int J Cancer.* **108:** 321-326.

Hockel M and Vaupel P, 2001, Tumor hypoxia: definitions and current clinical, biologic, and molecular aspects. *J Natl Cancer Inst.* **93:** 266-275.

Holten-Anderson MN, Hansen U, Brunner N, Nielsen HJ, Illemann M and Nielson BS, 2005, Localization of tissue inhibitor of metalloproteinases 1 (TIMP-1) in human colorectal adenoma and adenocarcinoma. *Int J Cancer.* **113:** 198-206.

Holten-Anderson MN, Stephens RW, Nielsen HJ, Murphy G, Christensen IJ, Stetler-Stevenson W and Brunner N, 2000, High preoperative plasma tissue inhibitor of metalloproteinase-1 levels are associated with short survival of patients with colorectal cancer. *Clin Cancer Res.* **6:** 4292-4299.

Homey B, Muller A and Zlotnik A, 2002, Chemokines: agents for the immunotherapy of cancer? *Nat Rev Immunol.* **2:** 175-184.

Howard PA and Dellafontaine P, 2004, Nonsteroidal anti-inflammatory drugs and cardiovascular risk. *J Am Coll Cardiol.* **43:** 519-525.

Huang S, Singh RK, Xie K, Gutman M, Berry KK, Bucana CD, Fidler IJ and Bar-Eli M, 1994, Expression of the JE/MCP-1 gene suppresses metastatic potential in murine colon carcinoma cells. *Cancer Immunol Immunother.* **39:** 231-238.

Imai K, Hiramatsu A, Fukushima D, Pierschbacher MD and Okada Y, 1997, Degradation of decorin by matrix metalloproteinase: identification of the cleavage sites, kinetic analysis and transforming growth factor beta-1 release. *Biochem J.* **322:** 809-814.

Inuzuka K, Ogata Y, Nagase H and Shirouzu K, 2000, Significance of coexpression of urokinase-type plasminogen activator, and matrix metalloproteinase 3 (stromelysin) and 9 (gelatinase B) in colorectal carcinoma. *J Surg Res.* **93:** 211-218.

Itzkowitz SH and Yio X, 2004, Colorectal cancer in inflammatory bowel disease: the role of inflammation. *Am J Physiol Gastrointest Liver Physiol.* **287:** G7-G17.

Janowska-Wieczorek-A, Marquez LA, Dobrowsky A, Ratajczak MZ and Cabuhat ML, 2000, Differential MMP and TIMP production by human marrow and peripheral blood CD34+ cells in response to chemokines. *Exp Hematol.* **28:** 1274-1285.

Jemal A, Murray T, Ward E, Samuels A, Tiwari RC, Ghafoor A, Feuer EJ and Thun MJ, 2005, Cancer statistics, 2005. *CA Cancer J Clin.* **55:** 10-30.

Joo YE, Seo KS, Kim HS, Rew JS, Park CS and Kim SJ, 1999, Role of tissue inhibitors of metalloproteinases (TIMPs) in colorectal carcinoma. *J Korean Med Sci.* **14:** 417-423.

Kang Y, Siegel PM, Shu W, Drobnjak M, Kakonen SM, Cordon-Cardo C, Guise TA and Massague J, 2003, A multigenic program mediating breast cancer metastasis to bone. *Cancer Cell.* **3:** 537-549.

Kim J, Takeuchi H, Lam ST, Turner RR, Wang HJ, Kuo C, Foshag L, Bilchik AJ and Hoon DSB, 2005, Chemokine receptor CXCR4 expression in colorectal cancer patients increases the risk for recurrence and for poor survival. *J Clin Oncol.* **23:** 2744-2753.

King J, Zhao J, Clingan P and Morris D, 2003, Randomised double blind placebo control study of adjuvant treatment with the metalloproteinase inhibitor, Marimastat in patients with inoperable colorectal hepatic metastases: significant survival advantage in patients with musculoskeletal side-effects. *Anticancer Res.* **23:** 639-646.

Kleeff J, Kusama T, Rossi DL, Ishiwata T, Maruyama H, Friess H, Buchler MW, Zlotnik A and Korc M, 1999, Detection and localization of MIP-3a/LARC/Exodus, a macrophage proinflammatory chemokine, and its CCR6 receptor in human pancreatic cancer. *Int J Cancer.* **81:** 650-657.

Knauper V, Will H, Lopez-Otin C, Atkinson SJ, Stanton H, Hembry RM and Murphy G, 1996, Cellular mechanism for human procollagenase-3 (MMP-13) activation. *J Biol Chem.* **271:** 17124-17131.

Koehne C-H and Dubois RN, 2004, COX-2 inhibition and colorectal cancer. *Sem Oncol.* **31:** 12-21.

Konig JE, Senge T, Allhoff EP and Konig W, 2004, Analysis of the inflammatory network in benign prostate hyperplasia and prostate cancer. *Prostate.* **58:** 121-129.

Koshiba T, Hosotani R, Miyamoto Y, Ida J, Tsuji S, Nakajima S, Kawaguchi M, Kobayashi H, Doi R, Hori T, Fujii N, Imamura M, 2000, Expression of stromal cell-derived factor 1 and CXCR4 ligand receptor system in pancreatic cancer: a possible role for tumor progression. *Clin Cancer Res.* **6:** 3530-3535.

Kulbe H, Levinson NR, Balkwill F and Wilson JL, 2004, The chemokine network in cancer--much more than directing cell movement. *Int J Dev Biol.* **48:** 289-296.

Langenskiold M, Holmdahl L, Falk P and Ivarsson ML, 2005, Increased plasma MMP-2 protein expression in lymph node-positive patients with colorectal cancer. *Int J Colorect Dis.* **20:** 245-252.

Lapteva N, Yang AG, Sanders DE, Strube RW and Chen SY, 2005, CXCR4 knockdown by small interfering RNA abrogates breast tumor growth in vivo. *Cancer Gene Ther.* **12:** 84-89.

Larsen MB, Stephens RW, Brunner N, Nielsen HJ, Engelholm LH, Christensen IJ, Stetler-Stevenson W and Hoyer-Hansen G, 2005, Quantification of tissue inhibitor of metalloproteinase 2 in plasma from healthy donors and cancer patients. *Scand J Immunol.* **61:** 449-450.

Laverdiere C, Hoang BH, Yang R, Sowers R, Qin J, Meyers PA, Huvos AG, Healey JH and Gorlick R, 2005, Messenger mRNA expression levels of CXCR4 correlate with metastatic behavior and outcome in patients with osteosarcoma. *Clin Cancer Res.* **11:** 2561-2567.

Leeman MF, McKay JA and Murray GI, 2002, Matrix Metalloproteinase 13 activity is associated with poor prognosis in colorectal cancer. *J Clin Pathol.* **55:** 758-762.

Leighl NB, Paz-Ares L, Douillard JY, Peschel C, Arnold A, Depierre A, Santoro A, Betticher DC, Gatzemeir U, Jassem J, Crawford J, Tu D, Bezjak A, Humphrey JS, Voi M, Galbraith S, Hann K, Seymour L, Shepherd FA, 2005, Randomized Phase III study of matrix metalloproteinase inhibitor BMS-275291 in combination with paclitaxel and carboplatin in advanced non-small-cell lung cancer: National Cancer Institute of Canada-Clinical Trials Group Study BR.18. *J Clin Oncol.* **23:** 2831-2838.

Li A, Varney ML and Singh RK, 2001, Expression of interleukin 8 and its receptors in human colon carcinoma cells with different metastatic potentials. *Clin Cancer Res.* **7:** 3298-3304.

Li G, Fridman R and Kim HR, 1999, Tissue inhibitor of metallproteinase-1 inhibits apoptosis of human breast epithelial cells. *Cancer Res.* **59:** 6267-6275.

Liang Z, Wu T, Lou H, Yu X, Taichman RS, Lau SK, Nie S, Umbreit J and Shim H, 2004, Inhibition of breast cancer metastasis by selective synthetic polypeptide against CXCR4. *Cancer Res.* **64:** 4302-4308.

Liang Z, Yoon Y, Votaw J, Goodman MM, Williams LT and Shim H, 2005 Silencing of CXCR4 blocks breast cancer metastasis. *Cancer Res.* **65:** 967-971.

Liao HF, Chen YY, Liu JJ, Hsu ML, Shieh HJ, Liao HJ, Shieh CJ, Shiao MS and Chen YJ, 2003, Inhibitory effect of caffeic acid phenethyl ester on angiogenesis, tumor invasion, and metastasis. *J Agric Food Chem.* **51:** 7907-7912.

Liotta LA, Tryggavason K, Gabrisa S, Hart I, Foltz CM and Shafie S, 1980, Metastatic potetial correlates with enzymatic degradation of basement membrane collogen. *Nature.* **284:** 67-68.

Loetcher P and Clark-Lewis I, 2001, Agonistic and antagonistic activities of chemokines. *J Leukoc Biol.* **69:** 881-884.

Lokeshwar BL, Selzer MG, Zhu BQ, Block NL and Golub LM, 2002, Inhibition of cell proliferation, invasion, tumor growth, and metastasis by an oral, non-antimicrobial tetracycline analog (COL-3) in a metastatic prostate cancer model. *Int J Cancer.* **98:** 297-309.

Lu X, Levy M, Weinstein IB and Santella RM, 1991, Immunologic quantification of levels of Tissue Inhibitor of Metalloproteinase-1 in human colon cancer. *Cancer Res.* **51:** 6231-6235.

Luster AD, 1998, Chemokines–chemotactic cytokines that mediate inflammation. *N Engl J Med.* **338:** 436-445.

Lynch CC, Crawford HC, Matrisian LM and McDonnell S, 2004, Epidermal growth factor upregulates matrix metalloproteinase-7 expression through activation of PEA3 transcription factors. *Int J Oncol.* **24:** 1565-1572.

Mantovani A, 1999, The chemokine system: redundancy for robust outputs. *Immunol Today* **20:** 254-257.

Mantovani A, Allavena P, Sozzani S, Vecchi A, Locati M and Sica A, 2004a, chemokines in the recruitment and shaping of the leukocyte infiltrate of tumors. *Sem Cancer Biol.* **14:** 155-160.

Mantovani A, Sica A, Sozzani S, Allavena P, Vecchi A and Locati M, 2004b, The chemokine system in diverse forms of macrophage activation and polarization. *Trends Immunol.* **25:** 677-686.

Mantovani A, Sozzani S, Locati M, Allavena P and Sica A, 2002, Macrophage polarization: tumor-associated macrophages as a paradigm for polarized M2 mononuclear phagocytes. *Trends Immunol.* **23:** 549-555.

Marchesi F, Monti P, Leone BE, Zerbi A, Vecchi A, Piemonti L, Mantovani A and Allavena P, 2004, Increased survival, proliferation, and migration in metastatic human pancreatic tumor cells expressing functional CXCR4. *Cancer Res.* **64:** 8420-8427.

Mashino K, Sadanaga N, Yamaguchi H, Tanaka F, Ohta M, Shibuta K, Inoue H and Mori M, 2002, Expression of chemokine receptor CCR7 is associated with lymph node metastasis of gastric carcinoma. *Cancer Res.* **62:** 2937-2941.

McLeod HL, McKay JA, Collie-Duguid ESR and Cassidy J, 2000, Therapeutic opportunities from tumour biology in metastatic colon cancer. *Eur J Cancer.* **36:** 1706-1712.

McQuibban GA, Butler G, Gong J-H, Bendall L, Powers C, Clark-Lewis I and Overall CM, 2001a, Matrix metalloproteinase activity inactivates the CXC chemokine stromal cell-derived factor-1. *J Biol Chem.* **276:** 43503-43508.

McQuibban GA, Butler GS, Gong JH, Bendall L, Power C, Clark-Lewis I and Overall CM, 2001b, Matrix metalloproteinase activity inactivates the CXC chemokine stromal cell-derived factor-1. *J Biol Chem.* **276:** 43505-43508.

McQuibban GA, Gong JH, Tam EM, McCulloch CAG, Clark-Lewis I and Overall CM, 2000, Inflammation dampened by gelatinase A cleavage of monocyte chemoattractant protein-3. *Science.* **289:** 1202-1206.

McQuibban GA, Gong JH, Wong JP, Wallace JL, Clark-Lewis I and Overall CM, 2002, Matrix metalloproteinase processing of monocyte chemoattractant proteins generates CC chemokine receptor antagonists with anti-inflammatory properties in vivo. *Blood.* **100:** 1160-1167.

Mills CD, Kincaid K, Alt J, Heilman MJ and Hill AM, 2000, M-1/M-2 macrophages and the Th2/Th2 paradigm. *J Immunol.* **164:** 6166-6173.

Mook ORF, Frederiks WM and Van Noorden CJF, 2004, The role of gelatinases in colorectal cancer progression and metastasis. *Biochim Biophys Acta.* **1705:** 69-89.

Moore MJ, Hamm J, Dancey J, Eisenberg PD, Dagenais M, Fields A, Hagan K, Greenberg B, Colwell B, Zee B, Tu D, Ottaway J, Humphrey R, Seymour L; National Cancer Institute of Canada Clinical Trials Group, 2003, Comparison of Gemcitabine versus matrix metalloproteinase inhibitor BAY 12-9566 in patients with advanced or metastatic adenocarcinoma of the pancreas: a phase III trial of the National Cancer Institute of Canada Clinical Trials Group. *J Clin Oncol.* **21:** 3296-3302.

Moran A, Iniesta P, de Juan C, Gonzalez-Quevedo R, Sanchez-Pernaute A, Diaz-Rubio E, Ramon y Cajal S, Torres A, Balibrea JL and Benito M, 2002, Stomelysin-1 promoter mutations impair gelatinase B activation in high microsatellite instability sporadic colorectal tumors. *Cancer Res.* **62:** 3855-3860.

Moser AR, Pitot HC and Dove WF, 1990, A dominant mutation that predisposes to multiple intestinal neoplasia in the mouse. *Science.* **247:** 322-324.

Mrowietz U, Schwenck U, Maune S, Bartels J, Kupper M, Fichtner I, Schroder J-M and Schadendorf D, 1999, The chemokine RANTES is secreted by human melanoma cells and is associated with enhanced tumour formation in nude mice. *Br J Cancer.* **79:** 1025-1031.

Muller A, Homey B, Soto H, Ge N, Catron D, Buchanan ME, McClanahan T, Murphy E, Yuan W, Wagner SN, Wagner SN, Barrera JL, Mohar A, Verastegui E, Zlotnik A, 2001, Involvement of chemokine receptors in breast cancer metastasis. *Nature.* **410:** 50-56.

Murai S, Umemiya T, Seiki M and Harigaya K, 2004, Expression and localization of membrane-type-1 matrix metalloproteinase, CD 44, and laminin-5gamma2 chain during colorectal carcinoma tumor progression. *Virchows Arch.* **445:** 271-278.

Murdoch C, Monk PN and Finn A, 1999, Functional expression of chemokine receptor CXCR4 on human epithelial cells. *Immunology.* **98:** 36-41.

Murray G, Duncan M, O'Neil P, Melvin WT and Fothergill JE, 1996, Matrix metalloproteinase-1 is associated with poor prognosis in colorectal cancer. *Nat Med.* **2:** 461-462.

Nagase H and Woessner F, 1999, Matrix metalloproteinases. *J Biol Chem.* **274:** 21491-21494.

Nakahara K and Sakata T, 2003, Augmented antitumor activity of a secondary lymphoid-tissue chemokine (SLC)-interleukin (IL) 2 fusion protein in mouse. *J Gene Med.* **5:** 463-471.

Nelson AR, Fingleton B, Rothenberg ML and Matrisian LM, 2000, Matrix metalloproteinases: Biologic activity and clinical implications. *J Clin Oncol.* **18:** 1135-1139.

Newell KJ, Witty JP, Rodgers WH and Matrisian LM, 1994, Expression and localization of matrix-degrading metalloproteinases during colorectal tumorigenesis. *Molec Carcinogenesis.* **10:** 199-206.

Nielsen BS, Timshel S, Kjeldsen L, Sehested M, Pyke C, Rorregaard N and Dano K, 1999, 92 kDa type IV collagenase (MMP-9) is expressed in neutrophils and macrophages but not in malignant epithelilal cells in human colon cancer. *Int J Cancer.* **365:** 57-62.

Noe V, Fingleton B, Jacobs K, Crawford HC, Vermeulen S, Steelant W, Bruyneel E, Matrisian LM and Mareel M, 2001, Release of an invasion promoter E-cadherin fragment by matrilysin and stromelysin-1. *J Cell Sci.* **114:** 111-118.

Norazmi MN, Hohmann AW, Skinner JM, Jarvis LR and Bradley J, 1990, Density and phenotype of tumour-associated mononuclear cells in colonic carcinomas determined by computer-assisted video image analysis. *Immunology.* **69:** 282-286.

Nosho K, Yoshida M, Yamamoto H, Taniguchi H, Adachi Y, Mikami M, Hinoda Y and Imai K, 2005, Association of Ets-related transcriptional factor E1AF expression with over-expression of matrix metalloproteinases, COX-2 and iNOS in the early stage of colorectal carcinogenesis. *Carcinogenesis.* **26:** 892-899

Opdenakker G and Van Damme J, 1992a, Chemotactic factors, passive invasion and metastasis of cancer cells. *Immunol Today.* **13:** 463-464.

Opdenakker G and Van Damme J, 1992b, Cytokines and proteases in invasive processes: molecular similarities between inflammation and cancer. *Cytokine.* **4:** 251-258.

O'Reilly MS, Holmgren L, Shing Y, Chen C, Rosenthal RA, Moses M, Lane WS, Cao Y, Sage EH and Folkman J, 1994, Angiostatin: A novel angiogenesis inhibitor that mediates the suppression of metastasis by a Lewis lung carcinoma. *Cell.* **79:** 315-328.

Ottaiano A, di Palma A, Napolitano M, Pisano C, Pignata S, Tatangelo F, Botti G, Acquaviva AM, Castello G, Ascierto PA Iaffaioli RV, Scala S, 2004, Inhibitory effects of anti-CXCR4 antibodies on human colon cancer cells. *Cancer Immunol Immunother.* **54:** 781-791.

Overall CM, McQuibban GA and Clark-Lewis I, 2002, Discovery of chemokine substrates for matrix metalloproteinases by exosite scanning: a new tool for degradomics. *Biol Chem.* **383:** 1059-1066.

Ozawa S, Shinohara H, Kanayama HO, Bruns CJ, Bucana CD, Ellis LM, Davis DW and Fidler IJ, 2001, Suppression of angiogenesis and therapy of human colon cancer liver metastasis by systemic administration of interferon-alpha. *Neoplasia.* **3:** 154-64.

Paget S, 1889, The distribution of secondary growths in cancer of the breast. *Lancet.* **1:** 571-573.

Parsons SL, Watson SA, Collins HM, Grifffin NR, Clarke PA and Steele RJC, 1998, Gelatinase (MMP-2 and -9) expression in gastrointestinal malignancy. *Brit J Cancer.* **78:** 1495-1502.

Paulsom R, Pignatelli M, Stetler-Stevenson WG, Liotta LA, Wright PA, Jeffery RE, Longcroft JM, Rogers L and Stamp GW, 1992, Stromal expression of 72 Kda type IV collagenase (MMP-2) and TIMP-2 mRNAs in colorectal neoplasia. *Am J Pathol.* **141:** 389-96.

Pavlaki M and Zucker S, 2003, Matrix metalloproteinase inhibitors (MMPIs): The beginning of phase I or the termination of phase III clinical trials. *Cancer Metast Rev.* **22:** 177-203.

Pezzato E, Sartor L, Dell'Aica I, Dittadi R, Gion M, Belluco C, Lise M and Garbisa S, 2004, Prostate carcinoma and green tea: PSA-triggered basement membrane degradation and MMP-2 activation are inhibited by (-)epigallocatechin-3-gallate. *Int J Cancer.* **112:** 787-792.

Phillips RJ, Burdick MD, Lutz M, Belperio JA, Keane MP and Streiter RM, 2003, The stromal derived factor-1/CXCL12-CXC chemokine receptor 4 biological axis in non-small cell lung cancer metastases. *Am J Respir Crit Care Med.* **167:** 1676-1686.

Polette M, Nawrocki B, Gilles C, Sato H, Seiki M, Tournier JM and Birembaut P, 1996, MT-MMP expression and localization in human lung and breast cancer. *Virchows Arch.* **428:** 29-35.

Primrose J, Bleiberg H, Daniel F, Van Belle S, Mansi JL, Seymour M, Johnson PW, Neoptelemos JP, Baillet M, Barker K, Berrington A, Brown PD, Millar AW, Lynch KP, 1999, Marimastat in recurrent colorectal cancer: exploratory evaluation of biological activity by measurement of carcinoembryonic antigen. *Br J Cancer.* **79:** 509-514.

Proudfoot, AEI, 2002, Chemokine receptors: multifaceted therapeutic targets. *Nat. Rev. Immunol.* **2:** 106-115.

Proudfoot AEI, Buser R, Borlat F, Alouani S, Soler D, Offord RE, Schroder J-M, Power CA and Wells TN, 1999, Amino-terminally modified RANTES analogues demonstrate differential effects on RANTES receptors. *J Biol Chem.* **274:** 32478-32485.

Proudfoot AEI, Power CA, Hoogewerf AJ, Montjovent MO, Borlat F, Offord RE and Wells TN, 1996, Extension of recombinant human RANTES by the retention of the initiating methionine produces a potent antagonist. *J Biol Chem.* **271:** 2599-2603.

Rachmilewitz D, Stamler JS, Bachwich D, Karmeli F, Ackerman Z and Podolsky DK, 1993, Enhanced colonic nitric oxide generation and nitric oxide synthase activity in ulcerative colitis and Crohn's disease. *Gut.* **36:** 718-723.

Ravi R, Mookerjee B, Bhujwalla ZM, Sutter CH, Artemov D, Zeng Q, Dillehay LE, Madan A, Semenza GL and Bedi A, 2000, Regulation of tumor angiogenesis by p53-induced degradation of hypoxia-inducible factor 1alpha. *Genes Dev.* **14:** 34-44.

Ring P, Johansson K, Hoyhtya M, Ribin K and Lindmark G, 1997, Expression of tissue inhibitor of metalloproteinases TIMP-2 in human colorectal cancer—a predictor of tumor stage. *Br J Cancer.* **76:** 805-811.

Robinson SC, Scott KA and Balkwill FR, 2002, Chemokine stimulation of monocyte matrix metalloproteinase-9 required endogeneous TNF-alpha. *Eur J Immunol.* **32:** 404-412.

Robinson SC, Scott KA, Wilson JL, Thompson RG, Proudfoot AEI and Balkwill F, 2003, A chemokine receptor antagonist inhibits experimental breast tumor growth. *Cancer Res.* **63:** 8360-8365.

Roeb E, Dietrich CG, Winograd R, Arndt M, Breuer B, Fass J, Schumpelick V and Matern S, 2001, Activity and cellular origin of gelatinases in patients with colon and rectal carcinoma differential acivity of matrix metalloproteinase-9. *Cancer.* **92:** 2680-2691.

Rollins BJ, 1997, Chemokines. *Blood.* **90:** 909-928.

Rubin JB, Kung AL, Klein RS, Chan JA, Sun YP, Schmidt K, Kieran MW, Luster AD and Segal RA, 2003, A small-molecule antagonist of CXCR4 inhibits intracranial growth of primary brain tumors. *Proc Natl Acad Sci U S A.* **100:** 13513-13518.

Ruehlmann JM, Xiang R, Niethammer AG, Ba Y, Pertl U, Dolman CS, Gillies SD and Reisfeld RA, 2001, MIG (CXCL9) chemokine gene therapy combines with antibody-cytokine fusion protein to suppress growth and dissemination of murine colon carcinoma. *Cancer Res.* **61:** 8498-8503.

Sato H, Takino T, Okada Y, Cao J, Shinagawa A, Yamamoto E and Seiki M, 1994, A matrix metalloproteinase expressed on the surface of invasive tumor cells. *Nature.* **370:** 61-65.

Schadendorf D, Moller A, Algermissen B, Worm M, Sticherling M and Czarnetzki BM, 1993, IL-8 produced by human malignant melanoma cells in vitro is an essential autocrine growth factor. *J Immunol.* **151:** 2667-2675.

Schimanski CC, Schwald S, Simiantonaki N, Jayasinghe C, Gonner U, Wilsberg V, Junginger T, Berger MR, Galle PR and Moehler M, 2005, Effect of chemokine receptors CXCR4 and CCR7 on the metastatic behavior of human colorectal cancer. *Clin Cancer Res.* **11:** 1743-1750.

Schonbeck U, Mach F and Libby P, 1998, Generation of biologically active IL-1 beta by matrix metalloproteinases: a novel caspase-1-independent pathway of IL-1 beta processing. *J Immunol.* **161:** 3340-3346.

Scotton CJ, Wilson JL, Scott KA, Stamp G, Wilbanks GD, Fricker S, Bridger G and Balkwill F, 2002, Multiple actions of the chemokine CXCL12 on epithelial tumor cells in human ovarian cancer. *Cancer Res.* **62:** 5930-5938.

Semenza GL, 2003, Targeting HIF-1 for cancer therapy. *Nat Rev Cancer.* **3:** 721-732.

Shepherd FA, Giaccone G, Seymour L, Debruyne C, Bezak A, Hirsh V, Smylie M, Rubin S, Martins H, Lamont A, Krzakowski M, Sadura A, Zee B, 2002, Prospective, randomized, double-blind, placebo-controlled trial of marimastat after response to first-line chemotherapy in patients with samll-cell lung cancer: A trial of the National Cancer Institute of Canada-Clinical Trials Group and the European Organization for Research and Treatment of Cancer. *J Clin Oncol.* **20:** 4434-4439.

Shibuta K, Begum NA, Mori M, Shimoda K, Akiyoshi T and Barnard GF, 1997, Reduced expression of the CXC chemokine hIRH/SDF-1alpha mRNA in hepatoma and digestive tract cancer. *Int J Cancer.* **73:** 656-662.

Shiozawa J, Ito M, Nakayama T, Nadashima M, Kohno S and Sekine I, 2000, Expression of matrix metalloproteinase-1 in human colorectal carcinoma. *Modern Pathol.* **13:** 925-933.

Sis B, Sagol O, Kupelioglu A, Sokmen S, Terzi C, Fuzun M, Ozer E and Bishop P, 2004, Prognostic significance of matrix metalloproteinase-2, cathepsin D, and tenascin-C expression in colorectal carcinoma. *Pathol Res Pract.* **200:** 379-387.

Smith MC, Luker KE, Garbow JR, Prior JL, Jackson E, Piwnica-Worms D and Luker GD, 2004, CXCR4 regulates growth of both primary and metastatic breast cancer. *Cancer Res.* **64:** 8604-8612.

Sparano JA, Bernardo P, Gradishar WJ, Ingle JN, Zucker S and Davidson NE, 2002, Randomized phase III trial of marimastat versus placebo in patients with metastatic breast cancer who have responding or stable disease after first-line chemotherapy: An Eastern Cooperative Oncology Group Trial (E2196). *Am Soc Clin Oncol Meeting on Molecular Therapeutics* (oral presentation).

Sparano JA, Bernardo P, Stephenson P, Gradishar WJ, Ingle JN, Zucker S and Davidson NE, 2004, RAndomized phase III trial of marimastat versus placebo in patients with metastatic breast cancer who have responding or stable disease after first-line chemotherapy: Eastern Cooperative Oncology Grouop trial E2196. *J Clin Oncol.* **22:** 4683-4690.

Staller P, Sulitkove J, Lisztwan J, Moch H, Oakeley EJ and Krek W, 2003, Chemokine CXCR4 downregulated by von Hippel-Lindau tumour suppressor pVHL. *Nature.* **425:** 307-311.

Sternlicht MD, Lochter A, Sympson CJ, Huey B, Rougie, JP, Gray JW, Pinkel B, Bissell M J. and Werb Z, 1999, The stromal proteinase MMP3/stromelysin-1 promotes mammary carcinogenesis. *Cell.* **98:** 351-358.

Sternlicht MD and Werb Z, 2001, How matrix metalloproteinases regulate cell behavior. *Annu Rev Cell Dev Biol.* **17:** 463-516.

Stoker W and Bode W, 1995, Structural features of a superfamily of zinc-endopeptidases: the metzincins. *Curr Opin Str Biol.* **5:** 383-390.

Streiter RM, Belperio JA, Phillips RJ and Keane MP, 2004, CXC chemokines in angiogenesis of cancer. *Sem Cancer Biol.* **14:** 195-200.

Su LK, Kinzler KW, Vogelstein B, Preisinger AC, Moser AR, Luongo C, Gould KA and Dove WF, 1992, Multiple intestinal neoplasia caused by a mutation in the murine homolog of the APC gene. *Science.* **256:** 668-670.

Sun YX, Schneider A, Jung Y, Wang J, Dai J, Wang J, Cook K, Osman NI, Koh-Paige AJ, Shim H, Pienta KJ, Keller ET, McCauley LK, Taichman RS, 2005, Skeletal localization and neutralization of the SDF-1 (CXCL12)/CXCR4 axis blocks prostate cancer metastasis and growth in osseous sites in vivo. *J Bone Min Res.* **20:** 318-329.

Sun YX, Wang J, Shelburne CE, Lopatin DE, Chinnaiyan AM, Rubin MA, Pienta KJ and Taichman RS, 2003, Expression of CXCR4 and CXCL12 (SDF-1) in human prostate cancers (Pca) in vivo. *J Cell Biochem* **89:** 462-473.

Sunami E, Tsuno N, Osada T, Saito S, Kitayama J, Tomozawa S, Tsuruo T, Shibata Y, Muto T and Nagawa H, 2000, MMP-1 is a prognostic marker for hematogenous metastasis of colorectal cancer. *Oncologist.* **5:** 108-114.

Sunami E, Tusuno NH, Kitayama J, Saito S, Osada T, Yamguchi H, Tomozawa S, Tsuruo T, Shibata Y and Nagawa H, 2002, Decreased synthesis of matrix metalloproteinase-7 and adhesion to the extracellular matrix proteins of human colon cancer cells treated withtroglitazone. *Surg Today.* **32:** 343-350.

Taichman RS, Cooper C, Keller ET, Pienta KJ, Taichman NS and McCauley LK, 2002, Use of the stromal cell-derived factor-1/CXCR4 pathway in prostate cancer metastasis to bone. *Cancer Res.* **62:** 1832-1837.

Takamori H, Oades ZG, Hoch OC, Burger M and Schraufstatter IU, 2000, Autocrine growth effect of IL-8 and GROalpha on a human pancreatic cancer cell line, Capan-1. *Pancreas.* **21:** 52-56.

Takanami I, 2003, Overexpression of CCR7 mRNA in nonsmall cell lung cancer: correlation with lymph node metastasis. *Int J Cancer.* **105:** 186-189.

Takeuchi T, Hisanaga M, Nagao M, Ikeda N, Fujii H, Koyama F, Mukogawa T, Matsumoto H, Kondo S, Takahashi C, Noda M, Nakajima Y, 2004, The membrane-anchored matrix metalloproteinase (MMP) regulator RECK in combination with MMP-9 serves as an informative prognostic indicator for colorectal cancer. *Clin Cancer Res.* **10:** 5572-5579.

Tam EM, Morrison CJ, Wu YI, Stack MS and Overall CM, 2004, Membrane protease proteomics: isotope-coded affinity tag MS identification of undescribed MT1-matrix metalloproteinase substrates. *Proc Natl Acad Sci U S A.* **101:** 6917-6922.

Tavor S, Petit I, Porozov S, Avigdor A, Dar A, Leider-Trejo L, Shemtov N, Deutsch V, Naparstek E, Nagler A, Lapidot T, 2004, CXCR4 regulates migration and development of human acute myelogenous leukemia stem cells in transplanted NOD/SCID mice. *Cancer Res.* **64:** 2817-2824.

Toomey D, Harmey J, Condron C, Kay E and Bouchier-Hayes D, 1999, Phenotyping of immune cell infiltrates in breast and colorectal tumours. *Immunol Invest.* **28:** 29-41.

Tutton MG, George ML, Eccles SA, Burton S, Swift RI and Abulafi AM, 2003, Use of plasma MMP-2 and MMP-9 levels as a surrogate for tumour expression in colorectal cancer patients. *Int J Cancer.* **107:** 541-550.

Vaday GG, Franitza S, Schor H, Hecht I, Brill A, Cahalon L, Hershkoviz R and Lider O, 2001, Combinatorial signals by inflammatory cytokines and chemokines mediate leukocyte interactions with extracellular matrix. *J Leukoc Biol.* **69:** 885-892.

Vaday GG, Peehl DM, Kadam PA and Lawrence DM, 2005, Expression of CCL5 (RANTES) and CCR5 in prostate cancer. *Prostate.* in press.

Van Damme J, Struyf S and Opdenakker G, 2004, Chemokine-protease interactions in cancer. *Sem Cancer Biol.* **14:** 201-208.

Van den Steen PE, Proost P, Wuyts A, Van Damme J and Opdenakker G, 2000, Neutrophil gelatinase B potentiates interleukin-8 tenfold by aminoterminal processing, whereas it degrades CTAP-III, PF-4, and GRO-alpha and leaves RANTES and MCP-2 intact. *Blood.* **96:** 2673-2681.

Van den Stehen PE, Wuyts A, Husson SJ, Proost P, Van Damme J and Opdenakker G, 2003, Gelatinase B/MMP-9 and neutrophil collagenase/MMP-8 process the chemokines human GCP-2/CXCL6, ENA-78/CXCL5 andn mouse GCP-2/LIX and modulate their physiological activities. *Eur J Biochem.* **270:** 3739-3749.

Vargo-Gogola T, Fingleton B, Crawford HC and Matrisian LM, 2002, Matrilysin (matrix metalloproteinase-7) selects for apoptosis-resistant mammary cells in vivo. *Cancer Res.* **62:** 5559-5563.

Wang H, Nemoto-Sasaki Y, Kondo T, Akiyama M and Mukaida N, 2003, Potential involvement of monocyte chemoattractant protein (MCP)-1/CCL2 in IL-4-mediated tumor immunity through inducing dendritic cell migration into the draining lymph nodes. *Int Immunopharmacol.* **3:** 627-642.

Wang J, Xi L, Hunt JL, Gooding W, Whiteside TL, Chen Z, Godfrey TE and Ferris RL, 2004a, Expression pattern of chemokine receptor 6 (CCR6) and CCR7 in squamous cell carcinoma of the head and neck identifies a novel metastatic phenotype. *Cancer Res.* **64:** 1861-1866.

Wang W-H, Huang JQ, Zheng GF, Lam SK, Karlberg J and Wong BC-Y, 2004b, Non-steroidal anti-inflammatory drug use and the risk of gastric cancer: a systematic review and meta-analysis. *J Natl Cancer Inst.* **95:** 1784-1791.

Wilson CL, Heppner KJ, Labosky PA, Hogan BLM and Matrisian L, 1997, Intestinal tumorigenesis is suppressed in mice lacking the metalloproteinase matrilysin. *Proc Natl Acad Sci U S A.* **94:** 1402-1407.

Witty JP, McDonnell S, Newell KJ, Cannon P, Navre M, Tressler RJ and Matrisian L, 1994, Modulation of matrilysisn levels in colon carcinoma cell lines affects tumorigenicity in vivo. *Cancer Res.* **54:** 4805-4812.

Woessner JF, 1991, Matrix metalloproteinases and their inhibitors in connective tissue remodeling. *FASEB J.* **5:** 2145-2154.

Xu E, Lai M, Lv B, Xing X, Huang Q and Xia X, 2004, A single nucleotide polymorphism in the matrix metalloproteinase-2 promoter is associated with colorectal cancer. *Biochem Biophys Res Commun.* **324:** 999-1003.

Yang SK, Choi MS, Kim OH, Myung SJ, Jung HY, Hong WS, Kim JH and Min YI, 2002, The increased expression of an array of C-X-C and C-C chemokines in the colonic mucosa of patients with ulcerative colitis: regulation by corticosteroids. *Am J Gastroenterol.* **97:** 126-132.

Yang W, Aril S, Gorrin-Rivas M, Mori A, Onodera H and Imamura M, 2001, Human macrophage metalloelastase gene expression in colorectal carcinoma and its clinicopathologic significance. *Cancer.* **91:** 1277-1283.

Yu Q and Stamenkovic I, 2000, Cell surface-localized matrix metalloproteinase-9 proteolytically activates TGF-β and promotes tumor invasion and angiogenesis. *Genes Dev.* **14:** 163-176.

Zeelenberg IS, Ruuls-Van Stalle L and Roos E, 2003, The chemokine receptor CXCR4 is required for outgrowth of colon carcinoma micrometastases. *Cancer Res.* **63:** 3833-3839.

Zeng ZS, Huang Y, Cohen AM and Guillem JG, 1996, Prediction of colorectal cancer relapse and survival via tissue RNA levels of matrix metalloproteinase-9. *J Clin Oncol* **14:** 3133-40.

Zhong H, De Marzo AM, Laughner R, Lim M, Hilton DA, Zagzag D, Buechler P, Isaacs WB, Semenza GL and Simons JW, 1999, Overexpression of hypoxia-inducible factor 1 alpha in common human cancers and their metastases. *Cancer Res.* **59:** 5830-5835.

Zinzindohoue F, Lecomte T, Ferraz JM, Houllier AM, Cugnenc PH, Berger A, Blons H and Laurent-Puig P, 2005, Prognostic significance of MMP-1 and MMP-3 fucntional promoter polymorphisms in colorectal cancer. *Clin Cancer Res.* **11:** 594-599.

Zlotnik A and Yoshie O, 2000, Chemokines: a new classification system and their role in immunity. *Immunity.* **12:** 121-127.

Zucker S, Cao J and Molloy CJ, 2002, Role of matrix metalloproteinases and plasminogen activators in cancer and metastaasis: Therapeutic strategies. *In:*Anticancer Drug Development. Eds. BC Baguley and DJ Kerr. Academic Press. San Diego, CA pp. 91-122.

Zucker S, Hymowitz M, Rollo EE, Mann R, Conner CE, Cao J, Foda H, Tompkins DC and Toole B, 2001, Tumorigenic potential of extracellular matrix metalloproteinase induce (EMMPRIN). *Am J Pathol.* **158:** 1921-1928.

Zucker S, Lysik RM, DiMassimo BI, Zarrabi HM, Moll UM, Grimson R, Tickle SP and Docherty AJP, 1995, Plasma assay of gelatinase B:Tissue Inhibitor of Metalloproteinase (TIMP) complexes in cancer. *Cancer.* **76:** 700-708.

Chapter 12

Angiotensin-Converting Enzyme (ACE) in Gut Inflammation

Fernando Magro
Gastroenterology Department and Institute of Pharmacology and Therapeutics, Faculty of Medicine, 4200-319 Porto, Portugal

1. INFLAMMATORY BOWEL DISEASE AS A MODEL OF INFLAMMATION

Inflammatory bowel disease (IBD) is a chronic relapsing disease and affects all parts of the gastrointestinal (GI) tract. The major clinical features of the disease include diarrhoea, abdominal pain, weight loss and bleeding. The two main forms of idiopathic IBD, Crohn's disease (DC) and ulcerative colitis (UC) can be distinguished by clinical, radiological, endoscopic and pathologic features. In CD the lesions extend throughout the GI and in UC are limited to colon. In UC the endoscopic lesions have a continuous involvement and in DC the wall is discontinuous affected, that is, in the same endoscopic area ulcers are surrounding by normal endoscopic mucosa. The inflammatory process in UC is confined to the inner lining of the gut (mucosa and submucosa) and is characterized by crypt abscesses and ulcerations. Unlike UC, in DC the inflammatory process extends throughout the bowel wall (transmural) and is characterized by the presence of granulomas and fistulae.

Mucosal inflammation is almost always mediated by one of two pathways (Bouma *et al* 2003): T_H1- cell response or T_H2-cell response. The T_H1- cell response is associated with increased secretion of IL-12, IFN-γ and/or TNF-α and T_H2-cell response is associated with increased secretion of IL-4, IL-5 and/or IL-13 (Strober *et al* 2002). This dual type of response is shown in the TNBS and oxazolone colitis. In the former the TNBS induces an IL-12-mediated T_H1 – cell response characterized by transmural cellular infiltration associated with granulomas, in some cases, and can be abrogated with

U. Lendeckel and Nigel M. Hooper (eds.), Proteases in Gastrointestinal Tissue, 301-314.

antibodies specific for IL-12 (Neurath *et al* 1995). In the later the oxazolone induces inflammation characterized by superficial cellular infiltration associated with a greater infiltration of neutrophils (Boirivant *et al* 1998). This mucosal inflammation results from the induction of natural-killer T (NKT) cells producing IL-13 (Heller *et al* 2002). Also a large number of mice with different genetic defects develop spontaneous mucosal inflammation reinforcing the importance of inflammation in IBD. That is, colitis can be induced by different ways: due to defective induction of regulatory cells ($CD4^{+}CD45RB^{hi}$) (Powrie *et al* 1993), regulatory cell defects (IL-10-deficient mice, TGF-β-deficient mice) (Shull *et al* 1992; Kuhn *et al* 1993) or increased effector-cell responses (Stat4 transgenic mice, G-protein subunit α1,2-deficient mice) (Rudolph *et al* 1995; Wirtz *et al* 1999).

The data support the evidence that CD is a T_H1- mediated inflammation. Various immunohistochemical studies indicate that in situ IL-12 is over-produced by macrophages (Monteleone *et al* 1997) and macrophages that are isolated from the inflammatory lesions of patients with CD produce increased amounts of IL-12 ex-vivo (Liu Z *et al* 1999). In addition, nuclear extracts of T cells from tissues of patients with CD contain increased amounts of activated STAT4, which is indicative of IL-12 signalling (Neurath *et al* 2002; Parrello *et al* 2000). Also T cells from CD patients produce markedly amounts of IFN-γ and markedly decreased of IL-4, T_H2 cytokine, compared with controls (Parronchi *et al* 1997; Fuss *et al* 1996). UC, T_H2- mediated inflammation, is associated with antibodies production (IgG1 and IgG4) and increased secretion of IL-5 (Fuss *et al* 1996; Kett *et al* 1987).

A rate-limiting step in the pathophysiology of IBD is the activation and recruitment of leukocytes. Tissue trafficking of leukocytes is orchestrated by a coordinated expression of chemokines and adhesion molecules. In fact, when the endothelial cells are activated they display surface markers such as P-selectin, E-selectin, intercellular adhesion molecule-1 (ICAM-1), vascular cell adhesion molecule-1 (VCAM-1) and integrins. The adhesion of leukocytes to the endothelium is initiated by weak interactions that produce a characteristic rolling motion of the leukocytes on the endothelial surface (Ley *et al* 1995; Lasky *et al* 1995). P-selectin, acting in cooperation with L-selectin, is implicated in the mediation of these initial interactions (True *et al* 1990). The selectins family is composed of three distinct carbohydrate receptors expressed by endothelial cells (E-selectin), leukocytes (L-selectin), or platelets and endothelium (P-selectin). E-selectin initiates the so-called rolling of leukocytes on the endothelial surface, with subsequent expression of intercellular adhesion molecule-1 (ICAM-1) and vascular cell adhesion molecule-1 (VCAM-1) on the endothelium (Springer 1990). ICAM-1 and VCAM-1 appear to be particularly important for the firm attachment and transendothelial migration of leukocytes. ICAM-1 promotes the initial interaction between macrophages and T-cells during immune activation

(Nielsen *et al* 1994) and the enhanced expression of VCAM-1 may facilitate the transmigration of monocytes and $CD4^+$ memory/effector cells, since these cells express VLA-4, the ligand for VCAM-1 (Horgam *et al* 1992).

Soluble isoforms of E-selectin, P-selectin, ICAM-1 and VCAM-1 have been found in the plasma of normal individuals (Patel *et al* 1995), probably arising from proteolytic cleavage of the surface-expressed molecule (Gearing *et al* 1993). E-selectin is substantially lost from the surface of endothelial cells within 24 hours, and circulating P-selectin appears to be slightly smaller than native P-selectin. An alternatively spliced mRNA encoding a form of human P-selectin, lacking the transmembrane anchoring domain, has been reported for both megakaryocytes and endothelial cells (Gearing *et al* 1993), and evidence suggests that the majority of circulating soluble P-selectin originate in this manner.

Patel R *et al* (Patel *et al* 1995) in 83 IBD patients showed that the plasma levels of sICAM and sE-S were significantly higher in those with active UC and CD than those in controls and inactive disease. Nielsen *et al* (Nielsen *et al* 1994) also found higher levels of s-ICAM in IBD patients (n = 58) than in patients in remission and controls. However, in 93 IBD patients, Goke M *et al* (Goke *et al* 1997) did not find any relation between disease activity and the increased serum levels of sE-S, sP-S, s-ICAM and s-VCAM.

We stratified 218 patients ((145 with Crohn's disease (CD) and 73 with ulcerative colitis (UC)) into three categories of activity - clinical remission, biochemical evidence of inflammation (biologically active patients) and clinical evidence of activity. Patients with biochemical evidence of inflammation were considered because they represent a group with sub-clinical activity. This categorization help to show that in inactive IBD patients the serum levels of selectins and immunoglobulin superfamily molecules were lower than those found in controls (Magro *et al* 2004). The low serum levels of adhesion molecules in periods of remission in IBD patients suggest continuous leukocytic activation. This theory is in accordance with chemiluminescent response of neutrophils from IBD patients (Faden *et al* 1985). Moreover, low serum levels of L-selectin were found mainly in patients with inflammatory vascular discords or connective tissue diseases associated with vasculitis due to counter receptor-bearing cells.

2. ANGIOTENSIN, ACE AND BRADYKININ AS AGENTS OF INFLAMMATION

Angiotensinogen is the circulating protein substrate from which renin cleaves angiotensin I. In humans, the concentration of angiotensinogen in the circulation is less than Km of the renin-angiotensinogen reaction and is therefore an important determinant of the rate of formation of angiotensin. Angiotensin I has little or no biologic activity. Angiotensin-converting enzyme (ACE) is a dipeptidyl carboxypeptidase that catalyzes the cleavage of dipeptides from the carboxyl terminal of certain peptides. The most important substrates are angiotensin I which is converts to angiotensin II, and bradykinin, which is inactivated (Nadel 1996). It also cleaves enkephalins and substance P (SP) (Nadel 1996) (Figure 1). The aim somatic ACE activity is associated with tissues such as the luminal side of the vascular endothelium or the renal epithelium. A soluble form of the enzyme that circulates in the plasma is also released after proteolytic cleavage of extracellular ACE (Beldent *et al* 1993). A polymorphic marker, which correlates with circulant ACE, has been described (45). The marker consists of the presence (*Insertion*) or absence (*Deletion*) of a 287 bp repeat sequence (Tiret *et al* 1992). The *Insertion/ Insertion* genotype has the lowest circulant ACE levels while the *DD* genotype has the highest. The serum ACE level tend to be higher according to ACE genotype in order II, <ID<DD (Furuya *et al* 1996). In the physiological point of view the activity of ACE is very interesting because the levels of three important substances are directly modulated for it, namely angiotensin II, bradykinin and SP (Figure 1).

The Ang II acts via two receptors: AT1 and AT2. AT1 receptors have a high affinity for losartan and a low affinity for PD 123177, while AT2 receptors have a high affinity to PD 123177. Most of the known actions of Ang II are mediated by AT1 receptor, a G protein-coupled receptor (Dinh *et al* 2001). Dendritic cells (DC) have mRNA expression of angiotensinogen, renin-binding protein, ACE, and angiotensin II/vasopressin receptor (Lapteva *et al* 2001). It was found that Ang II-induced leukocyte rolling is mainly mediated by P-selectin and that firm adhesion is LFA-1-dependent in colonic venules. Moreover, this P-selectin-mediated rolling was found to be a precondition for the subsequent firm adhesion of leukocytes to the vascular endothelium in response to Ang II (Riaz *et al* 2004). In animal model, New Zealand White rabbits, Ang II was implicated in the recruitment of monocytes into the vessel wall (Hernandez-Presa *et al* 1997) and Schieffer *et al* (Schieffer *et al* 2004) showed that AT1-receptor blockade enhances serum levels of IL-10 and reduce metalloprotease-9 protein/activity in patients with angiographically documented coronary artery disease. Moreover, the AT1-receptor blockade specifically reduced thromboxane A2-dependent effects in platelets; an effect that has not been reported for ACE inhibitors. Furthermore, stimulation of monocytes with Ang II causes the activation of NF-kB and subsequent increases the TNF-α production (Ruiz-Ortega *et al* 2000). Ang II increases the family member of PYRIN-containing Apafl-like proteins in DC cells (Lapteva *et al* 2002). The family of PYRIN-containing Apafl-like proteins participates in inflammatory signalling by regulating the activation of NF-kB and cytokine processing (Wnag *et al* 2002).

By activating in neurokinin 1 receptors (NK-1R), SP is capable of inducing a number of inflammatory responses including plasma extravasation, leukocyte activation, endothelial cell adhesion molecules expression, cytokine production, and mast cell activation (Quartara *et al* 2002). In addition, there is increasing evidence that SP is capable, directly or indirectly, of acting on T lymphocytes (Payan *et al* 1984; Lai *et al* 1982). Moreover, human and murine lymphocytes express NK-1R an SP augments the mitogen-and-Ag-induced proliferation and IL-2 secretion of T Lymphocytes. Also SP is capable of directly inducing T cell IFN-γ that is known to suppress IL-4 and the development of a Th2 cell phenotype. A recent in vitro study demonstrated that the addition of a specific NK1-R antagonist partly reduced T cell proliferation during the interaction with syngenic or allogenic DC cells and in the absence of DC cells, proliferation of T cells induced by direct CD3/CD28 ligation, was partly dependent on signalling thought NK1-R, revealing an autocrine effect of SP.

Bradykinin (BK) is a powerful mediator capable of promoting symptoms of inflammation, including vasodilatation, plasma extravasion, and pain by the activating bradykinin receptors (B-R), in particular B2-R (Hall 1992). Activation of B2-R on sensory nerves triggers the release of neuropeptides such as SP and calcitonin gene-related peptide, which results in amplification of neurogenic inflammation (Geppetti 1993). Moreover, bradykinin is a potent vasodilator and exerts its action by stimulation of endothelial receptors to release prostacyclin and NO (Linz *et al* 1995).

An interesting fact is the relationship between ACE and thrombotic mediators. ACE is associated with stimulation of the production of plasminogen activator inhibitor-1 (PAI-1) (Nishimura *et al* 1999). Elevated levels of PAI-1 have been implicated in the pathogenesis of thromboembolic diseases (Vaughn 1997). Enhancing the activity of PAI-1 can result in a reduction in the breakdown of fibrin strands and thus an acceleration of thrombus formation (Moriyama *et al* 1997).

ACE inhibitors (captopril, enalapril and cilazapril) suppress the synthesis of TNF and IL-1 in mononuclear cells (Fukuzawa *et al* 1997). Moreover, captopril reduces the level of tissue factor expression in endotoxin-stimulated mononuclear leukocytes (Napolene *et al* 2000) and significantly inhibited LPS-induced production of TNF-α, IL-12 and IL-18 (Lapteva *et al* 2002).The immunomodulatory actions of captopril have been explained by several mechanisms, including anti-proliferation, anti-oxidant activity, inhibition of metalloproteases, and elevation of prostaglandin synthesis. The inhibitory properties of captopril may be related to the presence of thiol groups in the captopril structure as well as the indirect suppression of expression of the gene encoding ACE.

3. ANGIOTENSIN, ACE, BRADYKININ AND SP IN MODELS OF INFLAMMATION

In a mouse model of ischemia/reperfusion (I/R) in the colon it was found that gene expression of ACE was up-regulated, the plasma levels of Ang II were increased and captopril (an ACE inhibitor) reduced leukocyte responses (64% reduction). Moreover, it was found that inhibition of AT1 receptor attenuated I/R inflammation (Riaz *et al* 2004). In granulomatous response to *Schistosoma mansoni* the SQ 14225, an inhibitor of ACE, partially inhibited the granulomatous response to Schistosoma eggs and the pathological manifestations associated (Weinstock *et al* 1981). Also chronic captopril treatment improved portal pressure, body and liver weight, and produced sustained granulomatous response in Schistosoma – infected mice (Weinstock *et al* 1981). In experimental colitis the prophylactic administration of captopril was effective in preventing colonic fibrosis in TNBS-induced colitis. The antifibrotic action of captopril could be due to the blockage of TGB-β overexpression, and/or to a direct down-regulation of TGB-β transcript (Wengrower *et al* 2004). In pancreatic inflammation model lisinopril alleviated chronic pancreatitis and fibrosis in male WBN/kob rats and suppressed the expression of TGB-β1 mRNA, preventing pancreatic stellate cell activation (Kuno *et al* 2003). Furthermore, the degree of TNBS colitis in angiotensinogen gene knockout mice was impaired as well as the expression of proinflammatory cytokines - IL-1beta and Interferon-gamma. As opposite, the expression of IL-4 and IL-10 in the colon of Ag-/Ag- mice was increased. Also subcutaneous infusion of losartan suppressed colitis and the production of proinflammatory cytokines (IL-1β and IFN-γ) (Inokochi *et al* 2005).

The icatibant, a bradykinin B2 receptor antagonist, significantly suppressed shortening of the large intestine, the onset of diarrhoea, and worsening of the general health in dextran sulphate sodium-induced colitis in mice (a model of UC). Moreover, in kininogen deficient rats the severity of colitis was decreased as well as the severity of colitis. Also the FR173657, an active B2 antagonist, decreased the inflammation, putting in evidence the role of endogenous kinins generated from the kallikrein-kinin system (Kamata *et al* 2002). The mutation Ser511Asn increases the susceptibility to inflammation by increasing the cleavage of high molecular weight kininogen in rats genetically susceptible (Isordia-Salas *et al* 2003). Moreover, a specific plasma kallikrein inhibitor modulated chronic granulomatous enterocolitis and systemic inflammation in genetically susceptible Lewis rats (Stadnicki *et al* 1998).

Substantial evidence supports a role of SP in the pathophysiology of colitis (Mantyh *et al* 1988). Stucchi *et al* (Stucci *et al* 2000) showed that the early administration of neurokinin 1 receptor (NK-1R) antagonist (NK-1RA) is efficacious in reducing experimentally induced colitis. Also in the treatment of ileal pouch inflammation the intraperitoneal administration of NK-1RA antagonist (CJ-12,255) diminished the physical signs of clinical pouchitis and the rise in MPO levels were prevented (Stucci *et al* 2003). Weistoch *et al* showed that SP regulates Th1-type of colitis in IL-10 Knockout mice and the NK-1R antagonist reverses ongoing intestinal inflammation (Weinstock *et al* 2003).

4. ANGIOTENSIN, ACE, BRADYKININ AND SP IN IBD

An increase in SP receptor binding sites was reported by Mantyh *et al* (Mantyh *et al* 1995) in small blood vessels, lymphoid aggregates, and enteric neurones of the small and large bowel of patients with CD and UC. In a subsequent study, the same group showed that whereas the ectopic expression of NK-1R in UC is confined to active disease. In DC up-regulation of NK-1R was evident in positive and negative samples of the small and large bowel (Mantyh *et al* 1995). Renzi *et al* showed that in normal human intestine NK-1R and NK-2R are expressed in multiple cell types and both receptors are up-regulated in patients with CD and UC (Renzi *et al* 2000). Moreover, they found direct evidence of NK-1R up-regulation on inflammatory cells of the lamina propria, as well as on epithelial cells lining the mucosal surface and crypts. Up-regulated expression of NK-1R may have important implications in the pathophysiology of IBD. NK-1R expression on lamina propria inflammatory cells and in the endothelium of submucosal venulas may participate in the margination and extravascular migration of granulocytes, lymphocytes, and monocytes into inflamed tissues.

Stadnicki *et al* (Stadnicki *et al* 2003) showed that in human intestinal tissue kallikrein is in the goblet cells of normal and inflamed colon and in macrophages of IBD patients. The plasma cells on the border of the granuloma contain large amounts of kallikrein. This observation emphasizes the close relationship between the immune response and the kallikrein-kinin system. Kallikrein and the intestinal kallistatin levels were significantly decreased in inflamed intestinal tissue. Stadnicki *et al* (Stadnicki *et al* 2005) using specific immunostaining and image quantification, observed in the normal tissue B2R and the inducible B1R. In general, in the normal condition B1R is present in most tissue only in minimal amounts but is induced during inflammatory process. The same group found in inflamed active IBD tissue significantly higher B1R protein levels than in the controls and also observed co-localization of kallistatin as well as kinin receptor proteins in the endothelium of intestinal vessel and in the macrophages forming granulomas (Stadnicki *et al* 2005).

Jaszewski *et al* (Jaszewski *et al* 1990) found that in colonic mucosa the levels of angiotensin I and II were greater in patients with CD than in controls and these levels were also higher in Crohn's colitis than in UC. The mucosal levels of angiotensin I and II correlated well with the degree of macroscopic inflammation.

The significance of serum ACE levels in patients with CD and UC has been controversial. Physiologically sex and age affect the serum ACE level. The serum ACE levels in men are higher than that in women and the levels decrease with age. Nunes-Gornes *et al* (Nunes-Gornes *et al* 1981) reported that only serum ACE levels of patients receiving steroids were decreased and they concluded that the decreased of serum ACE levels was due to the administration of steroids. Silverstein *et al* (Silverstein *et al* 1981) found that enzyme activity tended to be depressed in Crohn's ileitis and colitis, but not in Crohn's ileocolitis and UC. They concluded that granulomatous inflammation in Crohn's disease differs from that in sarcoidosis, in which striking elevation of angiotensin-converting enzyme is present in granulomatous tissue and frequently in serum. D'Onofrio et al. determined the serum ACE activity and found that it was depressed in active Crohn's disease compared to either controls subjects or patients with inactive disease (D`onofrio *et al* 1984). Sommer et al. (Sommer *et al* 1986) showed that serum ACE was significantly lowered in active Crohn's disease and in UC as long as the ileum or cecum was affected. Also Takeuchi *et al* (Takeuchi *et al* 1992), found decreased ACE levels in Crohn's disease compared with healthy controls and significant negative regression between ACE and CDAI was observed. Matsuda *et al* (Matsuda *et al* 2001) showed significantly decreased ACE levels in patients with CD with steroid therapy whose genotype was II, and in those with UC whose genotype was DD, but even among patients without steroid treatment. The serum ACE levels were significantly lower in patients with IBD than in controls for each genotype.

A polymorphism marker of ACE, which correlates with circulant levels, consists of the presence (insertion) or absence (deletion) of a 287 bp repeat sequence. Those with insertion/insertion genotypes have the lowest circulant levels. The PAI-1 is the fast-acting inhibitor of tissue plasminogen activator (t-PA). Assays in vivo of promoter activity demonstrated that under conditions of cytokine stimulations, as those found in IBD, the 4G allele has significant more activity than the 5G allele. In our patients the allelic frequencies of ACE Del and PAI-1 4G were higher in IBD patients than in reference population (Magro *et al* 2003) (Table 1).

In conclusion, the ACE is an essential step in kinin-kallikrein system, Angiotensin and SP. There is evidence of the involvement of this enzyme in the inflammatory process, experimental colitis and IBD, and a new target is open for new therapies.

Table 1: Allelic frequency in Inflammatory Bowel disease (n = 116) and reference population (n = 141) of ACE *Del* and PAI-1 *4G*

	Crohn's disease	Ulcerative colitis	Reference population	P*
ACE *Del*	0.58	0.50	0.19	0.001
PAI-1 *4G*	0.46	0.49	0.15	0.001

*Comparison between Crohn's disease, Ulcerative colitis and reference population using Chi-square test with a significant threshold of 5%

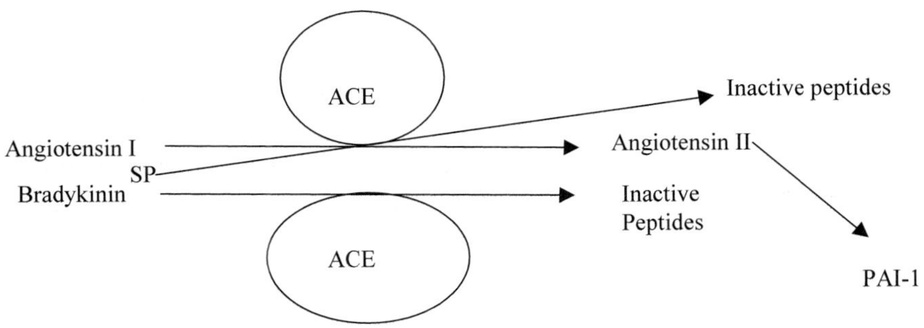

Figure 1: Central role of angiotensin converting enzyme (ACE).

REFERENCES

Beldent V, Michaud A, Wei L, Chauvet MT, Corvol P, 1993, Proteolytic release of human angiotensin-converting enzyme: localization of the cleavage site. *J Biol Chem.* **268:** 26428.

Boirivant T, Fuss IJ, Chu A, Strober W, 1998, Oxazolone colitis: a murine model of T helper cell type 2 colitis treatable with antibodies to interleukin 4. *J Exp Med.* **188:**129-139.

Bouma G, Strober W, 2003, The immunological and genetic basis of inflammatory bowel disease. *Nat Immunol Rev.* **3:** 521-533.

Dinh DT, Frauman AG, Johnston CI, Fabiani ME, 2001, Angiotensin receptors: distribution, signalling and function. *Clin Sci.* **100:** 481-492.

D'onofrio GM, Levitt S, Ilett KF, 1984, Serum angiotensin converting enzyme in Crohn's disease, ulcerative colitis and peptic ulceration. *Aust N Z Med.* **14:** 27-30.

Faden H, Rossi TM, 1985, Chemiluminescent response of neutrophils from patients with inflammatory bowel disease. *Dig Dis Sci.* **30:**139-42.

Fukuzawa M, Satoh J, sagara G, Muto Y, Muto S, Nishimura S, Miyaguchi S, Qiang Y, Sakata T, Nakazawa T, Ikehata F, Ohta S, Toyota T, 1997, Angiotensin converting enzyme inhibitors suppress production of tumor necrosis factor-alpha in vitro and in vivo. *Immunopharmacol.* **36:** 49-55.

Furuya K, Yamaguchi E, Kawakami Y, 1996, Delectionpolymorphism in the angiotensin I converting enzyme (ACE) gene as a genetic facor for sarcoidosis. *Thorax.* **51:** 777-780.

Fuss IJ, Neurath M, Boirivant M, Klein JS, de la Motte C, Strong SA, Fiocchi C, Strober W, 1996, Disparate CD4+ lamina propria (LP) lymphokine secretion profiles in inflammatory bowel disease. Crohn's disease LP cells manifest increased secretion of IFN-gamma, whereas ulcerative colitis LP cells manifest increased secretion of IL-5. *J Immunol.* **157:** 1261-1270.

Gearing AJ, Newman W, 1993, Circulating adhesion molecules in disease. *Immunol Today.* **14:** 506-512.

Geppetti P, 1993, Sensory neuropeptide release by bradykinin:mechanisms and pathophysiological implications. *Regul Pept.* **47:** 1-23.

Goke M, Hoffmann JC, Evers J, Kruger H, Manns MP, 1997, Elevated serum concentrations of soluble selectin and immunoglobulin type adhesion molecules in patients with inflammatory bowel disease. *J Gastroenterol Hepatol.* **32:** 480-486.

Hall JM, 1992, Bradykinin receptors:pharmacological properties and biological roles. *Pharmacol Ther.* **56:**131-190.

Heller F, Fuss IJ, Nieuwenhuis EE, Blumberg RS, Strober W, 2002, Oxazolone colitis, a Th2 colitis model resembling ulcerative colitis, is mediated by IL-13-producing NK-T_cells. *Immunity.* **17:** 629-638.

Hernandez-Presa M, Bustos C, Ortego M, Tunon J, Renedo G, Ruiz-Ortega M, Egido J, 1997, Angiotensin-converting enzyme inhibition prevents arterial nuclear factor-Kappa B activation, monocyte chemoattractant protein-1 expression, and macrophage infiltration in a rabbit model of early-accelerated atherosclerosis. *Circulation.* **95:** 1532-1541.

Horgan KJ, Luce GE, Tanaka Y, Schweighoffer T, Shimizu Y, Sharrow SO, Shaw S, 1992, Differential expression of VLA-alpha 4 and VLA-beta 1 discriminates multiple subsets of CD4+CD45R0+ "memory" T cells. *J Immunol.* **149:** 4072-4077.

Inokuchi Y, Morohashi T, Kawana I, Nagashima Y, Kihara M, umemura S, 2005, Ameloration of 2,4,6-trinitrobenzene sulphonic acid induced colitis in angiotensinogen gene knockout mice. *Gut.* **54:** 349-356.

Isordia-Salas I, Pixley RA, Parekh H, Kunapuli SP, Li F, Stadnicki A, Lin YS, Sartor B, Colman RW, 2003, The mutation Ser511Asn leads to N-glycosylation and increases the cleavage of high molecular weight kininogen in rats genetically susceptible to inflammation. *Blood.* **102:** 2835-2842.

Jaszewski R, Tolia V, Ehrinpresis MN, Bodzin JH, Paleman RR, Korlipara R, Weinstock JV, 1995, Increased colonic mucosal angiotensin I and II concentrations in Crohn's colitis. *Gastroenterol.* **98:** 1543-1548.

Kamata K, Hayashi I, Mizuguchi Y, Arai K, Saeki T, Ohno T, Saigenji K, Majima M, 2002, Suppression of dextran sulfate sodium-induced colitis in kininogen-deficient rats and non-peptide B2 receptor antagonist-treated rats. *Jpn J Pharmacol.* **90:** 59-66.

Kett K, Rognum TO, Brandtzaeg P, 1987, Mucosal subclass distribution of immunoglobulin G-producing cells is different in ulcerative colitis and Crohn's disease. *Gastroenterol.* **93:** 919-924.

Kuhn R, Lohler J, Rennick D, Rajewsky K, Muller W, 1993, Interleukin-10-deficient mice develop chronic enterocolitis. *Cell.* **75:** 263-274.

Kuno A, Yamada T, Masuda K, Ogawa K, Sogawa M, Nakamura S, Nakawaza T, Ohara H, Nomura T, Joh T, Shirai T, Itoh M, 2003, Angiotensin-converting enzyme inibitor attenuates pancreatic inflammation and fibrosis in male Witar Boo/Kobori rats. *Gastroenterol.* **124:** 1010-1019.

Lai JP, Douglas SD, Ho WZ, 1998, Human lymphocytes express substance P and its receptor. *J Neuroimmunol.* **86:** 80-86.

Lapteva NM, Nieda M, Ando K, Ide Y, Hatta-Ohashi G, Dymshits Y, Ishikawa T, Juji K, Tokunaga K, 2001, Expression of renin-angiotensin system genes in immature and mature dendritic cells identified using human cDNA microarray. *Biochem Biophys Res Commun.* **285:** 1059-1065.

Lapteva NM, Ide K, Nieda M, Ando Y, Hstts-ohashi Y, Minami M, Dymshits G, Egawa K, Juji T, Tokunaga K, 2002, Activation and suppression of renin-angiotensin system in human dendritic cells. *Biochem Biophys Res Comm.* **296:** 194-200.

Lasky LA, 1995, Selectin-carbohydrate interactions and the initiation of the inflammatory response. *Annu Rev Biochem.* **64:** 113-139.

Ley K, Tedder TF, 1995, Leukocyte interactions with vascular endothelium. New insights into selectin-mediated attachment and rolling. *J Immunol.* **155:** 525-528.

Linz W, Wiemer G, Gohlke p, Unger T, Scholkens BA, 1995, Contribution of kinins to the cardiovascular actions of angiotensin-converting enzyme inhibitors. *Pharmacol Rev.* **47:** 25-49.

Liu Z, Colpaert S, D'Haens GR, Kasran A, de Boer M, Rutgeerts p, Geboes K, Ceuppens JL, 1999, Hyperexpression of CD40 ligand (CD154) in inflammatory bowel disease and its contribution to pathogenic cytokine production. *J Immunol.* **163:** 4049-4057.

Magro F, Dinis-Ribeiro M, Araujo FM, Pereira P, Fraga MC, Cunha-Ribeiro LM, Tome-Ribeiro A, 2003, High prevalence of combined thrombophilic abnormalities in patients with inflammatory bowel disease. *Eur J Gastroenterol Hepatol.* **15:** 1157-1163.

Magro F, Araujo F, Pereira P, Meireles E, Diniz-Ribeiro M, Velosom FT, 2004, Soluble selectins, sICAM, sVCAM, and angiogenic proteins in different activity groups of patients with inflammatory bowel disease. *Dig Dis Sci.* **49:** 1265-1274.

Mantyh PM, Mantyh CR, Gates T, Vigna SR, Maggio JE, 1988, Receptor binding sites for substance P and substance K in the canine gastrointestinal tract and their possible role in the inflammatory bowel disease. *Neurosci.* **25:** 817-837.

Mantyh CR, Vigna SR, Bollingger RR, Mantyh PM, Maggio JE, Pappas TN, 1995, Differential expression of substance P receptors in patients with Crohn's disease and ulcerative colitis. *Gastroenterol.* **109:** 850-860.

Matsuda T, Suzuki M, Furuya MD, Masutani MD, Kawakami Y, 2001, Serum angiotensin I-Converting enzyme is reduced in Crohn's disease and ulcerative colitis irrespective of genotype. *Am J Gastroenterol.* **96:** 2705-2710.

Monteleone G, Biancone L, Marasco R, Morrone G, Marasco O, Luzza F, Pallone F, 1997, Interleukin 12 is expressed and actively released by Crohn's disease intestinal lamina propria mononuclear cells. *Gastroenterol.* **112:** 1169-1178.

Moriyama Y, Ogawa H, S. O, Takazoe K, Honda Y, Hirashima O, Arai H, Sakamoto T, Sumida H, Suefuji H, Kaikita K, H. Y, 1997, Captopril reduced plasminogen activator inhibitor activity in patients with acute myocardial infarction. *Jpn Circ J.* **61:** 308-314.

Nadel J, 1996, Peptidase modulation of neurogenic inflammation. In Neurogenic inflammation. P.Geppetti and P. Holzer, eds. *CRC Press, Boca Raton, FL.* 115-127.

Napolene E, Di Santo A, Camera E, Tremoli R, Lorenzey R, 2000, Angiotensin-converting enzyme inhibitors downregulate tissue factor synthesis in monocytes. *Cir Res.* **86:** 139-143.

Neurath MF, Weigmann B, Finotto S, Glickman J, Nieuwenhuis EE, Iijima H, Mizoguchi A, Mizoguchi E, Mudter J, Galle PR, Bhan AK, Autschbach F, Sullivan BM, Szabo SJ, Glimcher LH, Blumberg RS, 2002, The transcription factor T-bet regulates mucosal T cell activation in experimental colitis and Crohn's disease. *J Exp Med.* **159:** 1129-1143.

Neurath MF, Fuss I, kelsall BL, Stuber E, Strober W, 1995, Antibodies to interleukin-12 abrogate established experimental colitis in mice. *J Exp Med* **182:** 1281-1290.

Nielsen OH, Langholz E, Hendel J, J. B, 1994, Circulating soluble intercellular adhesion molecule-1 (sICAM-1) in active inflammatory bowel disease. *Dig Dis Sci.* **39:** 1918-1923.

Nishimura H, Tsuji H, Masuda H, Kasahara T, Yoshizumi M, Sugano T, Kimura S, Kawano H, Kunieda Y, Yano S, Nakagawa K, Kitamura H, Nakahara Y, Sawada S, Nakagawa M, 1999, The effects of angiotensin metabolites on the regulation of coagulation and fibrinolysis in cultured rat aortic endothelial cells. *Thromb Haemost.* **82:** 1516-1521.

Nunes-Gornes JF, Tewksbury DA, 1981, Serum angiotensin-converting-enzyme (sACE) in Crohn's disease. *Am J Gastroenterol.* **75:** 384-385.

Parrello T, Monteleone G, Cucchiara S, Monteleone I, Sebkova L, Doldo P, Luzza F, Pallone F, 2000, Upregulation of the IL-12 receptor beta 2 chain in Crohn's disease. *J Immunol.* **165:** 7234-7239.

Parronchi P, Romagnani P, Annunziato F, Sampognaro S, Becchio A, Giannarini L, Maggi E, Pupilli C, Tonelli F, Romagnani S, 1997, Type 1 T-helper cell predominance and interleukin-12 expression in the gut of patients with Crohn's disease. *Am J Pathol.* **150:** 823-832.

Patel RT, Pall AA, Adu D, Keighley MR, 1995, Circulating soluble adhesion molecules in inflammatory bowel disease. *Eur J Gastroenterol Hepatol.* **7:** 1037-1041.

Payan DGDR, Brewster A, Missirian-Bastian A, Goetzl J, 1984, Substance P recognition by a subset of human T lymphocytes. *J Clin Invest.* **74:** 1532.

Powrie F, Leaach MW, Mauze S, Caddle LB, Coffman RL, 1993, Phenotypically distinct subsets of CD4+ T cells induce or protect from chronic inestinal inflammation in C.B-17 scid mice. *Int Immunol.* **5:** 1461-1471.

Quartara L, Maggi AC, 1998, The tachykinin NK1 receptor. Part II:Distribution and pathophysiological roles. *Neuropeptides.* **32:** 1-49.

Renzi D, Pellegrini B, Tonelli F, Surrenti C, Calbro A, 2000, Substance p (Neurokinin-1) and Neurokinin A (NeuroKinin-2) receptor gene and protein expression in the healthy and inflamed human intestine. *Am J Pathol.* **157:** 1511-1522.

Riaz AA, Wang Y, Schramm R, Sato T, Menger MD, Jeppsson B, Thorlacius H, 2004, Role of angiotensin II in ischemia/reperfusioon-induced leukocyte-endothelium interactions in the colon. *FASEB J.* **18:** 881-883.

Rudolph U, Finegold MJ, Rich SS, Harriman GR, Srinivasan Y, Brabet P, Boulay G, Bradley A, L. B, 1995, Ulcerative colitis and adenocarcinoma of the colon in G alpha i2-deficient mice. *Nature Genet.* **10:** 143-150.

Ruiz-Ortega M, Lorenzo M, Ruperez S, Konig S, Wittig B, Egido J, 2000, Angiotensin II activates nuclear transcription factor kB through AT1 and AT2 in vascular smooth muscle cells: molecular mechanisms. *Circ Res.* **86:** 1266-1272.

Schieffer B, Bunte C, Witte J, Hoeper K, Boger RH, Schwedhelm E, Drexler H, 2004, Comparative effects of AT1-Antagonism and Markers of inflammation and platelet aggregation in patiensts with coronary artery disease. *J Am Coll Cardiol* **44:** 362-368.

Shull MM, Ormsby I, Kier AB, Pawlowski S, Diebold RJ, Yin M, Allen R, Sidman C, Proetzel G, Calvin D, 1992, Targeted disruption of the mouse transforming growth factor-beta 1 gene results in multifocal inflammatory disease. *Nature.* **359:** 693-699.

Silverstein E, Fierst SM, Simon MR, Weinstock JV, Friedland J, 1981, Angiotensin-converting enzyme in Crohn's disease and ulcerative colitis. *Am J Clin Pathol.* **75:** 175-178.

Sommer H, Schweisfurth H, Schulz M, 1986, Serum angiotensin-I-Converting enzyme and carboxypeptidase N in Crohn's disease and ulcerative colitis. *Enzyme.* **35:** 181-188.

Springer TA, 1990, Adhesion receptors of the immune system. *Nature.* **346:** 425-434.

Stadnicki A, Sartor RB, Janardham R, Majluf-Cruz A, Kettner CA, Adam AA, Colman RW, 1998, Specific inhibition of plasma kallikrein modulates chronic granulomatous intestinal and systemic inflammation in genetically susceptible rats. *FASEB J.* **9:** 325-333.

Stadnicki A, Mazurek U, Gonciarz M, Plewka D, Nowaczyk G, Orchel J, Pastucha E, Plewka A, Wilczok T, Colman RW, 2003, Immunolocalization and expression of kallistatin and tissue kallikrein in human inflammatory bowel disease. *Dig Dis Sci.* **48:** 615-623.

Stadnicki A, Pastucha E, Nowaczyk G, Mazurek U, Plewka A, Machnick G, Wilczok T, Colman RW, 2005, Immunolocalization and expression of kinin B1R receptors in human inflammatory bowel disease. *Am J Physiol Gastrointest Liver Physiol.* **289:** G361-366.

Strober W, Fuss I, Blumberg RS, 2002, The immunology of mucosal models of inflammation. *Annu Rev Immunol.* **20:** 495-549.

Stucchi AF, Shofer S, Leeman S, Materne O, Beer E, McClung J, Shebani K, Moore F, O'Brien M, Becker JM, 2000, Nk-1 antagonist reduces colonic inflammation and oxidative stress in dextran sulfate-induced colitis in rats. *Am J Gastrointest Liver Physiol.* **279:** G1298-G1306.

Stucchi AF, Shebani KO, Leeman SE, Wang A-C, Reed KL, Fruin AB, Gower AC, McClung JP, Andry AD, O'Brien MJ, Pothoulakis C, Becker JM, 2003, A neurokinin 1 receptor antagonist reduces an ongoing ileal pouch inflammation and the response to a subsequent inflammatory stimulus. *Am J Physiol Gastrointest Liver Physiol.* **285:** G1259-G1267.

Takeuchi N, Fukushima T, Sugita A, Tsuchiya S, 1992, Angiotensin-converting-enzyme (ACE) in Crohn's disease. *Nippon Shokakibyo Gakkai Zasshi.* **89:** 596-600.

Tiret L, Rigat B, Visvikis S, Breda C, Corvol P, Cambien F, Soubrier F, 1992, Evidence, from combined segregation and linkage analysis, that a variant of the angiotensin I-converting enzyme (ACE) gene controls plasma ACE levels. *Am J Hum Genet.* **51:** 197-205.

True DD, Singer MS, Lasky LA, Rosen SD, 1990, Requirement for sialic acid on the endothelial ligand of a lymphocyte homing receptor. *J Cell Biol.* **111:** 2757-64.

Vaughn DE, 1997, The renin angiotensin system and fibrinolysis. *Am J Cardiol.* **82:**12-16.

Wang L, Manji JM, Grenier A, Garawi A, Merriam S, Lora JM, Geddes BJ, Briskin M, Distefano JB, 2002, PYPAF7: a novel PYRIN-containing APaf1-like protein that regulates activation of NF-kB and caspase-1-dependent cytokine processing. *J Biol Chem.* **17:** 17.

Weinstock JV, Ehrinpreis MN, Boros DL, J.B. G, 1981, Effect of SQ 14225, an inhibitor of angiotensin I-converting enzyme, on the granulomatous response to Schistosoma mansoni eggs in mice. *J Clin Invest.* **67:** 931-936.

Weinstock JV, Boros DL, 1981, Alteration of the granulomatous response in murine schistosomiasis by the chronic administration of captopril, an inhibitor of angiotensin-converting enzyme. *Gastroenterol.* **1981:** 953-958.

Weinstock JV, Blum A, Metwali A, Elliott D, Bunnett N, Arsenescu R, 2003. Substance P regulates Th1-type colitis in IL-10 Knockout mice. *J Immunol.* **171:** 3762-3767.

Wengrower D, Zannieli G, Pappo O, Latella G, Sestieri M, Villanova A, Faitelson Y, Pines M, Goldin E, 2004, Prevention of fibrosis in experimental colitisby captopril: the role of TGF-beta1. *Inflamm Bowel Dis.* **10:** 536-545.

Wirtz S, Finotto S, Kanzler S, Lohse AW, Blessing M, Lehr HA, Galle PR, Neurath MF, 1999, Cutting edge: chronic intestinal inflammation in STAT-4 transgenic mice: Characterization of disease and adoptive transfer by TNF-plus IFN-gamma-producing CD4+ T cells that respond to bacterial antigens. *J Immunol.* **162:** 1884-1888.

Chapter 13

Intestinal Apical Protein Transport in Health and Disease

[2]Stephan von Hörsten, [1]Michael Krahn, [1]Nadine Frerker, [3]Anja Gemeinhardt, [1]Dennis Schwab, [1]Silvia Slesiona, [1]Hassan Naim, and [1]Marwan Alfalah
[1]Department of Physiological Chemistry, School of Veterinary Medicine Hannover; [2]Department of Functional and Applied Anatomy, Hannover Medical School, Hannover; [3]Institute of Physiological Chemistry, Faculty of Veterinary Medicine, University of Leipzig, Leipzig, Germany

1. INTRODUCTION

Epithelial transport is essential for the maintenance and propagation of life. In this course we will explore the possible role of epithelial cells in the controlled and directional passage of ions, nutrients, and water across the barriers along the alimentary, renal, respiratory or reproductive systems. The importance of a very strictly regulated transport through epithelial cells can be appreciated by considering the possible pathological consequences due to disregulated transport events. Completely different diseased may be related to transport defects. Examples are the infectious diarrhoea (it accounts for more than five million child-deaths per year in developing countries), which is caused by an excess in the secretion of intestinal fluids. On the other hand, the cystic fibrosis, the most common genetic disease in the developed world, may be the pathogenic evidence of the inability of epithelial tissues to secrete any fluid. As a result, possible malnutrition, infertility and respiratory failure represent the main sever pathological effects developing into death.

The common features of the transport in epithelial cells and the technologies available for their study will be first presented. This preliminary overview will be followed by a more detailed description of the role of epithelial cells in the gastrointestinal tract. Particular emphasis will be placed on the understanding of the cellular transport mechanisms that are required for a

U. Lendeckel and Nigel M. Hooper (eds.), Proteases in Gastrointestinal Tissue, 315-338.

normal physiological function of these systems. Our comprehension in this respect has been improved by investigating disease-models. Some of them will be highlighted.

The brush border membrane of intestinal epithelial cells contains a large number of enzymes capable of degrading carbohydrates, peptides and proteins. Major advances have been made over the last few years in our knowledge of the number of enzymes involved, their biochemical characteristics, their biogenesis and, most recently through new methods in molecular biology and their molecular architecture. The disaccharidases of the brush border membrane in human small intestinal cells illustrates their intracellular transport to the cell surface. Defects in these enzymes have only been found in the disaccharidases sucrase-isomaltase (SI), lactase-phlorizin hydrolase (LPH) and trehalase (Jacob *et al* 2000; Spodsberg *et al* 2001; Ritz *et al* 2003). In this chapter we present defect in another intestinal proteins, dipeptide peptidase IV(DPPIV) A peptide hydrolase has at one time been postulated as representing the possible primary defect in celiac disease. Due to the considerable overlap in substrate specificity of the brush border membrane peptide hydrolases (Sterchi and Woodley, 1980) it seems unlikely that the absence of one could lead to a serious condition such as celiac disease. In this chapter we present what is currently known about the structure and the biogenesis of dipeptid peptidase IVand sucrase-isomaltase, with particular reference to human tissue. The chapter is divided into three sections. The first describes the methods employed in investigating the molecular forms, the biosynthesis and the post-translational processing of human brush border membrane Proteins. In the second section the structure, function and biosynthesis of disaccharidases in normal tissue are summarized. The final section deals with the application of these methods to the study of disaccharidase deficiencies and the results obtained.

1.1 Polarized epithelial cell

Each tissue or organ in the mammalian body has a specialised function, reflected in its anatomy and metabolic activity. Polarized epithelial cells for example are organized into sheets occurring on the body surface and forming a layer that covers most of internal body cavities of mammalian (e.g. respiratory, urinary, reproduction, and digestive systems) called epithelium. The most important function of epithelial cells is to provide protection and regionalization to the body, and regulate the molecular composition of and exchange between, the compartments that they separate. (Lombardi *et al* 1985).

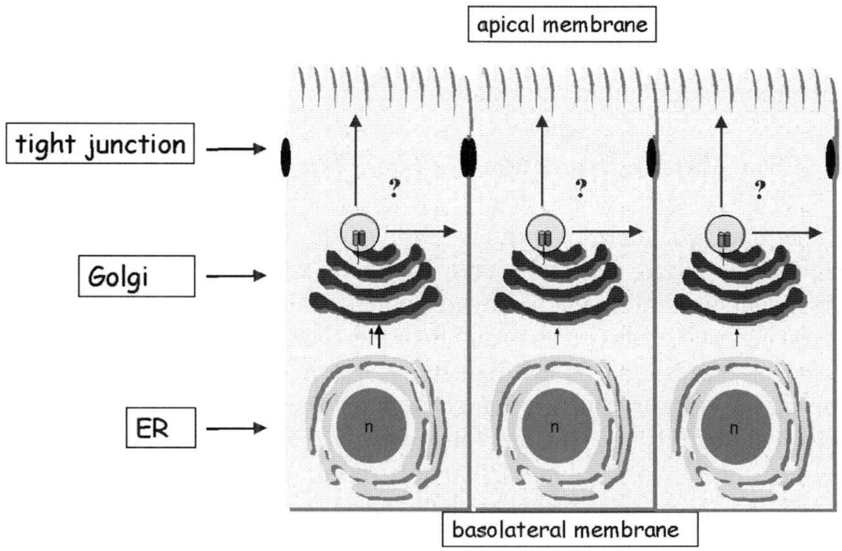

Figure 1: Schematic diagram of polarized epithelial cell.

Many functions of epithelial cells, neuronal cells and certain cells of the immune system depend on the maintenance of characteristically polarized phenotype, polarity also is fundamental to understanding tissue morphogenesis, neural transmission and aspects of the immune response (Mellman *et al* 1993). These highly specialised cellular functions require a unique structural und functional organization of the cell. First, specialized cell adhesion complexes and cytoskeleton organization are required to maintain cell-to-cell adhesion and cell attachment to extracellular matrix (ECM) (Yeaman *et al* 1999). Second, the plasma membrane of these highly differentiated cells is divided into two structurally and functionally distinct membrane domains commonly called apical and basolateral domains. Each domain is comprises of a distinct subset of proteins and lipids composition whose biological function may critically depend upon their localization in the correct surface domain (Aroeti *et al* 1998). The apical membrane domain, often covered with finger like projections called microvilli which faces the external milieu of the organism, whereas the basolateral domain is in contact with neighbouring cell and the internal milieu, facing the mesenchymal space and blood supply (Dragsten *et al* 1981). Both domains are separated by tight junctions that encircle the apex of the cell and seal neighbouring cells to each other. Neuronal cells also have distinct membrane domains, axonal matodendritic. Certain polarity feature are shared between epithelial cells and neurons (Dotti and Simons, 1990), which derive embryologically from epithelial cells during embryonic development, epithelial and neuronal cell phenotypes are acquired de novo, by expression of new genes (e.g. of neuron from epithelial cells and trophoplast epithelium from unpolarized morula blastomeres).

1.2 Polarized sorting

The understanding of protein synthesis and how plasma membrane proteins are sorted and transported to distinct organelles or to the same plasma domains in different polarized epithelial cells is still the most fascinating process and one of the greatest and exciting challenges in biochemistry. This process requires that the delivered proteins have to have intrinsic information in their structure which is interpreted by the sorting machinery of the cell that is responsible for sorting to the correct final destination (Mellman *et al* 1993; Matter 2000). In recent years sorting signals which defined the target destination and the mechanisms that guide proteins to proper membrane domains have been extensively studied. A series of signal sequences and/or structures are characterised (Brewer and Roth, 1991). In a typical mammalian cell we find a great number of different types of proteins. In general, most of these proteins are synthesised on ribosomes in the cytosol. A few proteins are synthesized on the ribosomes of mitochondria and chloroplast (in plants). But the transport from this point diverges into two main routes. In the first one, the nascent protein is released into cytosol after its synthesis has been completed. Some of these proteins have specific uptake signal sequences which direct them by delivering from cytosol to the final destination (e.g. mitochondria, peroxysome or nucleus) (Rothman 1990), while others with out specific sorting signals remain in the cytosol as permanent cytosolic proteins (Sabatini *et al* 1988). The great part of nascent proteins which are destined for lysosome, secretion or integration in the plasma membrane, take the second main route which was defined by Palade called the secertory pathway (Palade 1975). In this pathway all nascent proteins possess a signal sequence, a stretch of at least 6 hydrophobic amino acids, that mediates the intergration of nascent protein into the ER (Rapoport 1991). Some of these proteins either retained there. The majority is transported onward by vesicular transport (Rodriguez-Boulan and Powell, 1992) or by tubular structure (Presley *et al* 1997) to the cis-golgi network (CGN) up to trans-golgi network (TGN). Secretory and membrane-bound proteins undergo several structurally and posttranslationally modification reactions in the different cellular compartments before being delivered to their final intended destination. This includes signal sequence cleavage and attachment of mannose-rich carbohydrate chains in ER (Gilmore 1993), converting and modification of N-glycans and addition of O-glycans as well as proteolytic cleavage in Golgi complex (Naim *et al* 1991). In TGN where apical and basolateral proteins in polarized cells, as in contrast to non polarised cells, sorted into different cellular membrane domains or secreted into exterior milieu by virtue of specific sorting signals or motifs contained in their primary, secondary or tertiary structures (Matter 2000; Caplan 1997). They were then incorporated selectively into structurally distinct apical and basolateral vesicular carriers for delivery to their specific final destination (Mostov *et al* 1992). Targeting and delivery of proteins to the basolateral membrane occurs directly from TGN to that domain in most epithelial cell types like the LDL receptor and lysosomal membrane glycoprotein (Igp120) (Mostov 1991). On the other hand, delivery of proteins to the apical membrane domain varies. According to cell and protein type they are transported to their final destination along at least two different routes. I.e. a direct route from TGN (e.g. membrane proteins responsible for catalysing dietary carbohydrates, like sucrase-isomaltase (SI) which is delivered directly from TGN to the apical plasma membrane domain of intestinal epithelial cells (Rodriguez-Boulan and Powell, 1992; Alfalah *et al* 1999). And an indirect route from TGN to basolateral surface followed by transcytosis to the apical domain, like IgA and its polymeric immunoglobulin receptor pIgR, as well as dipeptidyl peptidase IV (DPPIV) (Casanova *et al* 1991). In some polarized cells, such as hepatocytes, transcytosis is the most common pathway for apical delivery (Bartles *et al* 1987).These finding suggest that sorting of plasma membrane proteins in polarized epithelial cells occurs from two sorting centres, the TGN and the endosomes. It has been proposed that both centres may share a similar sorting mechanism (Apodaca *et al* 1991).

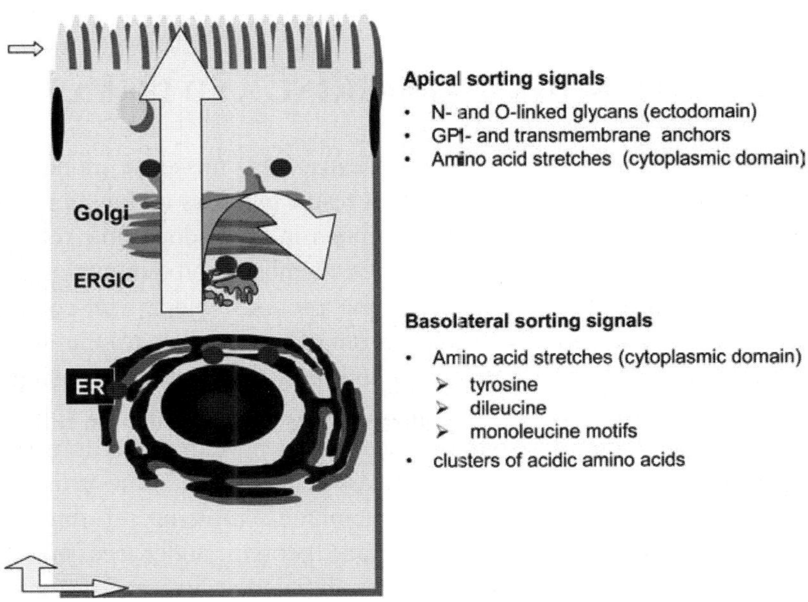

Figure 2: Schematic diagram of sorting signals.

1.3 Intestinal epithelial cells as cell model

The epithelial cells that line our small intestine are a highly polarized cells with regard to the function, structure and biochemical composition of their surface membrane domain (Lloyd *et al* 1992; Matter 2000). These kinds of cells are an excellent model to study and analyse for various reasons. Firstly, to study the biogenesis and trafficking of membrane proteins and lipids to the appropriate cell surface domain (Matter *et al* 1990). Secondly, they also provide a good experimental system to study endocytosis and transepithelial transport from basolateral to apical membranes for some proteins like polymeric immunoglobulin receptors pIgR (Apodaca *et al* 1991; Bomsel and Mostov, 1991) and DPP IV (Hauri *et al* 1985). Thirdly, the major constituents of the apical microvillar membrane of the intestinal epithelium are digestive hydrolases, including peptidases and disaccharidases, like sucrase-isomaltase, lactase-phlorizin hydrolase and dipeptidyl peptidase IV (Hauri *et al* 1985; Naim 2001). The presence of these proteins make the intestinal epithelium a valuable model to study the biosynthesis of brush border hydrolases as well as the structure and function of these highly interesting membrane proteins. Finally, the dramatic change during differentiation from relatively non polar progenitor to high polarized cell is extremely useful for studying the cell differentiation and the development of intestinal cell polarity and the various mechanisms which contribute to generating and maintaining their characteristically polarized feature (Lesuffleur *et al* 1991).

2. PROTEIN MISTRAFFICKING AND DISEASE

A surprising number of diseases are caused by missense mutations in genes encoding membrane proteins which result in a loss of function due to the misfolding and mistrafficking of the protein in the endoplasmic reticulum. We seek to elucidate the molecular bases for membrane protein misfolding by carrying out studies of purified membrane proteins under well-controlled conditions and by correlating results from these studies to the folding/ misfolding of the same proteins *in vivo* and *in vitro*. We are purposing two systems. The first involves the Human sucrase-isomaltase (SI). SI appears to be an ideal model system for studies of membrane protein misfolding as well as mistrafficking, like a number of disease-related membrane proteins. A second project involves the integral membrane protein, rat dipeptidyl-peptidase IV (CD26). This transmembrane protein undergoes mutation-prompted misfolding which results in a deficiency in enzyme activity. defective intracellular transport, secretion and sorting of proteins, as well as loss of function. These studies employ a wide range of techniques spanning the territory between molecular biophysics/biochemistry to cellular/molecular biology. Ultimately, we hope to use the information derived from these studies to develop novel therapeutics based on the avoidance or correction of misfolding and Protein mistrafficking.

2.1 Sucrase-isomaltase

SI is an apical type II integral membrane disaccharidase that is found exclusively in enterocytes of adult (Naim *et al* 1988a) intestine and is expressed in a complex pattern along the intestinal crypt-villus axis. Sucrase-isomaltase is an integral protein of the small intestine brush border membrane responsible for catalyzing the hydrolysis of dietary sucrose and some of the products of starch digestion. The glycoprotein comprises two subunits that are highly homologous and are thought to be derived from the same ancestral gene These two subunits are associated with each other by strong noncovalent, ionic interactions (Naim *et al* 1988a,b). SI is synthesized in the rough ER as a single chain mannose-rich precursor comprising both subunits (pro-SIh, 210 kD) (Naim *et al* 1988b). It is transported to the golgi apparatus at a relatively slow rate and does not form homodimers before ER exit (Matter and Hauri, 1991) The strong homologies between the two main domains suggest that quasi-dimers or pseudo-dimers are formed, (Jascur *et al* 1991) which are presumably sufficient for acquisition of transport competence. After modification of the N-linked glycans and *O*-glycosylation, SI is sorted to the apical membrane and cleaved in situ by lumenal pancreatic proteases to its two active subunits sucrase and isomaltase (Naim *et al* 1988b; Hauri *et al* 1979).

2.2 Congenital sucrase-isomaltase deficiency

Congenital sucrase-isomaltase deficiency (CSID) is an autosomal recessive human intestinal disorder hat is clinically characterized by fermentative diarrhea, abdominal pain, and cramps upon ingestion of sugar. The symptoms are the consequence of absent or drastically reduced enzymatic activities of sucrase and isomaltase, the components of the intestinal integral membrane glycoprotein sucrase-isomaltase (SI). Several known phenotypes of CSID result from an altered posttranslational processing of SI. SI deficiency is an example of a disease in which mutation results in transport-incompetent molecules. (Hauri *et al* 1979; Ritz *et al* 2003). By studies at the subcellular and protein level with monoclonal antibodies against sucrase-isomaltase (Naim *et al* 1988a), at least 4 phenotypes were identified: one in which sucrase-isomaltase accumulated intracellularly, probably in the endoplasmic reticulum, as a membrane-associated high-mannose precursor; one in which the intracellular transport of the enzyme was apparently blocked in the Golgi apparatus; and one in which catalytically altered enzyme was transported to the cell surface. In all patients, electrophoretically normal or near-normal high-mannose sucrase-isomaltase was demonstrated. one in which pro-SI undergoes an unusual intracellular cleavage that eliminates its transmembrane domain (Jacob *et al* 2000) Apparently, different mutations in the sucrase-isomaltase gene lead to the synthesis of transport-incompetent or functionally altered enzyme. We found that the deficiency was the consequence of a defect in intracellular transport. Spodsberg *et al* (2001) demonstrated a severe defect in intracellular sorting of the enzyme. Congenital sucrase-isomaltase deficiency is an example of a disease in which mutation results in transport-incompetent molecules (Figure 3. A, B). Ritz *et al* (2003) noted that sucrase-isomaltase (SI) is not transported to the brush border membrane but accumulates as a mannose-rich precursor in the endoplasmic reticulum (ER), the ER-golgi intermediate compartment and the cis-golgi, where it is finally degraded (Figure 3. C).

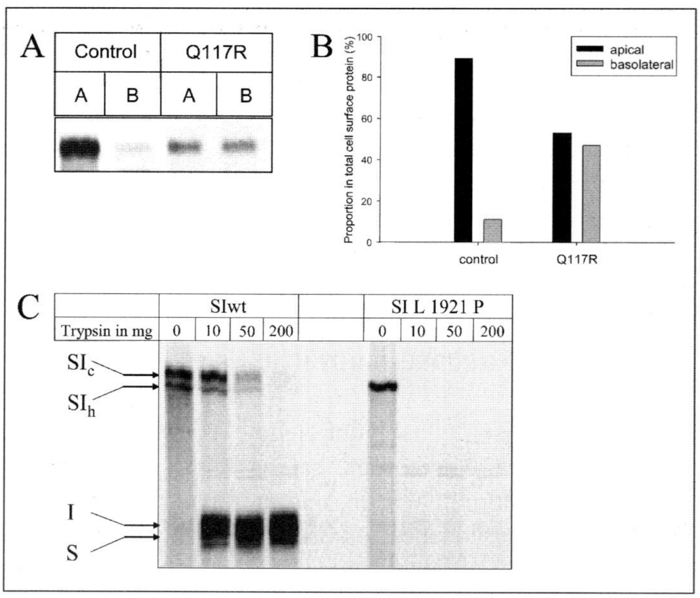

Figure 3: Polarized expression of mutant SI in MDCK cells. *A*, MDCK cells expressing wild type (*WT*) and mutant SI were grown on transmembrane filters, labeled with [^{35}S]methionine for 4 h followed by cell-surface immunoprecipitation of SI from the apical (*panel a*) or basolateral (*panel b*) membranes. The immunoprecipitates were subjected to SDS-PAGE. *A*, quantification of the proportions of complex glycosylated SI shown in *B*. Trypsine sensitivity of pro-SI_{L620P} molecule. Transiently transfected COS-1 cells were biosynthetically labelled with ^{35}S-methionine for 4 h. Detergent extracted were treated with 0, 10, 20, 50 and 200 mg/ml trypsine for 40 min at 37°C prior the cell lysis an immunoprecipitated with anti-SI. The precipitates were analysed by SDS-PAGE. Trypsin sensitivity of the C.

3. APICAL INTESTINAL DIPEPTIDYL PEPTIDASE IV

Dipeptidyl peptidase IV (DPPIV) is a 110 kD trans-membrane serine protease, also known as CD26, or adenosine desaminase binding protein (ADAbp) with ubiquitous expression. DPPIV has numerous functions including involvement in T-cell activation, cell adhesion, digestion of proline containing peptides in the kidney and intestines, HIV infection, apoptosis and regulation of tumorigenicity in certain melanoma cells. Constitutively it is expressed on numerous epithelial cell types (Lendeckel *et al* 2002; Weihofen *et al* 2004) DPPIV is efficiently sorted to the apical membrane of the small intestinal epithelial cells (Aertgeerts *et al* 2004; Fan *et al* 1997).

Fundamental functions of columnar epithelial cells are maintained through the segregation of particular membrane proteins and lipids to the two domains, basolateral and apical and thus characterize the structural and functional polarity of these cells. Proteins destined for these surfaces possess various types of structures or motifs that are recognized by specific sorting mechanisms in the *trans*-golgi network (TGN) and are subsequently delivered via separate vesicles to the correct surface domain (Kojima *et al* 1992; Elbein *et al* 1983). The failure to sort proteins to the correct domain often results in pathological conditions (Fransen *et al* 1991; Moolenaar *et al* 1997). Sorting is therefore a critical mechanism by which the function of sorted proteins is maintained.

In this part we investigate the role of glycans in sorting of a heavily *N*- and *O*-glycosylated glycoprotein, dipeptidyl peptidase IV. This protein is usually sorted with high fidelity to the apical membrane of intestinal cells (Matter *et al* 1990). By virtue of its convenient structural features DPPIV serves as an exquisite protein model for analyses aimed at elucidating the sorting behavior and sorting signals of proteins. DPPIV is a type II membrane glycoprotein that is synthesized with an uncleavable signal sequence that functions as a membrane anchoring domain (Misumi *et al* 1992; Fan *et al* 1997). Processing of the 100 kDa mannose-rich DPPIV species to the 124 kDa complex glycosylated mature form includes an extensive *O*-glycosylation event, mainly in a Ser/Thr-rich stalk domain adjacent to the membrane anchor (Naim *et al* 1999). After maturation in the Golgi apparatus, DPPIV is transported to the apical membrane, either directly from the TGN or along the transcytotic pathway through the basolateral membrane (Matter *et al* 1990). In Caco-2 cells at least 85% of newly synthesized DPPIV is expressed at the apical membrane and in steady state determinations and in pulse-chase experiments DPPIV is entirely found at the apical membrane after prolonged chase periods (Matter *et al* 1990). These observations indicate that the transcytotic pathway is not the major sorting event, otherwise substantially more DPPIV would be present at the basolateral membrane.

The identity and location of the sorting signals of DPPIV, as well as the sorting mechanism, have not yet been investigated in great detail. Recent data have proposed *O*-glycosylation to be crucial for apical sorting (Slimane *et al* 2000). A possible role of *N*-linked glycosylation remains undetermined and recent data have excluded sialic acids on *N*-linked glycans being implicated in the sorting event of DPPIV (Aertgeerts *et al* 2004).

We delineate in this chapter the mechanism by which DPPIV is sorted to the apical membrane in Caco-2 cells. We show that *O*-glycans play a role in the sorting event. However, a high sorting fidelity is substantially strengthened by the presence of complex glycosylated but not mannose-rich *N*-linked glycans. Furthermore, DPPIV associates on its way to the brush border membrane with Triton X-100-insoluble cholesterol-rich microdomains, although sphingolipids do not constitute a critical structure of these domains. Inhibition of the processing of N- and O-linked glycosylation results in a random distribution of DPPIV over the apical and basolateral membranes. Previous work from our laboratory (Naim *et al* 1999, Alfalah *et al* 2002) has shown that polarized sorting of DPPIV is not affected when complex N-linked glycosylation was modulated at the site of action of swainsonine, an inhibitor of golgi mannosidase II. Additionally, swainsonine had neither a direct nor an indirect effect on *O*-glycosylation of DPPIV, whereas the size of the *N*-linked glycans was smaller than the normally glycosylated DPPIV species. By contrast dMM which inhibits the processing of the outermost mannose-rich mannoses by mannosidase I has markedly shifted the high polarity of DPPIV to an almost randomly distributed protein on both sides of the membrane. At this stage of investigation the effect was attributed to the absence of *O*-glycans, the processing of which has been indirectly affected by the presence of the unprocessed mannose-rich chains (*see* Naim *et al* 1999 for more details). The sorting pattern of DPPIV was not as drastically altered upon inhibition of *O*-glycosylation by benzyl-GalNAc as it was in the presence of dMM and this is explained as follows. First, only partial *O*-glycosylation occurred in the presence of benzyl-GalNAc but was sufficient to prevent a complete depolarization of the targeting pattern of DPPIV. Second, additional components to *O*-glycans are implicated in the sorting of DPPIV. Possible candidates are mature complex glycosylated *N*-linked glycans. The following observations lend support to this hypothesis. In the presence of dMM the processing of mannose-rich *N*-linked glycans of DPPIV to the mature form does not take place, *O*-glycosylation is impaired, and targeting of DPPIV follows a random pattern. On the other hand, in the presence of swainsonine, which inhibits mannosidase II, an incompletely processed but nevertheless endo H-resistant *N*-linked and *O*-glycosylated DPPIV is correctly sorted to the apical membrane (Naim *et al* 1999; Alfalah *et al* 2002; Jacob *et al* 2000).

Altogether a possible role for complex glycosylated *N*-linked glycans in conjunction with *O*-linked glycans could be hypothesized. To examine this possibility, we labeled cells in the presence of benzyl-GalNAc and swainsonine to affect both *N*- and *O*-linked glycosylation and we analyzed the sorting of DPPIV. Under these conditions DPPIV shifted further to a smaller protein ($DPPIV_{c/benzyl/swa}$) as compared with the glycoforms obtained in the presence of benzyl-GalNAc or swainsonine alone. The sorting behavior of this DPPIV glycoform was next investigated using a pulse-chase protocol of biosynthetically labeled Caco-2 cells.

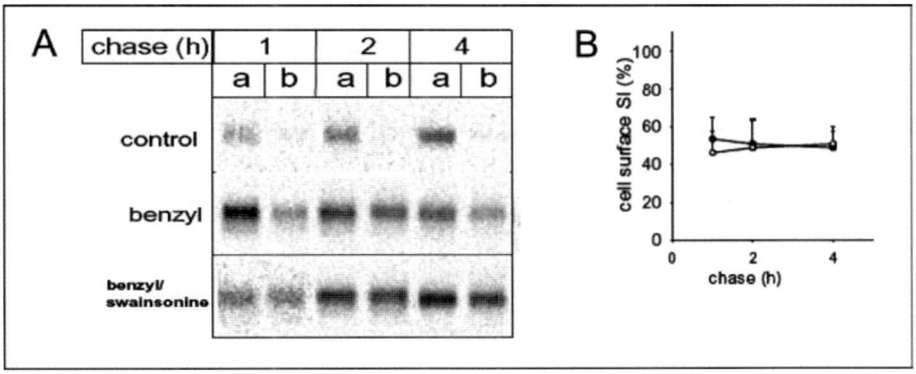

Figure 4: This figure demonstrates that a further alteration in the trafficking of DPPIV as compared with DPPIVc/benzyl has occurred. At 1 h of chase only 55% of DPPIVc/benzyl/swa was located at the apical membrane. With increasing chase DPPIVc/benzyl/swa became almost equally distributed at the apical and basolateral membranes. The results demonstrate that the type and structure of N- and O-linked complex glycans are together critical elements in the apical targeting of DPPIV. It is also obvious that O-linked glycans alone are not sufficient for a sorting of DPPIV with high fidelity to the apical membrane.

3.1 Dipeptidyl-peptidase IV deficiency

Altered and defective intracellular transport, secretion and sorting of proteins, as well as loss of function, are in many cases generated by mutations in the coding regions of the proteins. Such defects are often lethal during early stages of development or lead later on to severe disorders due to disturbances in function. A sequence alteration of DPPIV mRNA by spontaneous mutation has been described by Tsuji *et al* (1992) in Fischer 344 (F344) rat substrains (Charles River breeding colony, Germany and Atsugi breeding colony, Japan). They reported that an exchange from G to A at position 1897 in the open reading frame of DPPIV-mRNA results in a substitution of Glycin by Arginine at amino acid position 633. (DPPIV-G633A). We analysed the effect of this mutation on protein structure, trafficking function and enzymatic activity. The mutated proteins were studied in detail by transfecting the full-length cDNA of DPPIV in mammalian cells. The intracellular distribution, analysed by confocal microscopy using indirect immune-fluorescence, showed that the mutant is retained in the endoplasmic reticulum (ER) whereas wildtype DPPIV is localized in the trans-golgi network, in golgi vesicles and to a high extend on the cell surface.

DPPIV is a type II membrane glycoprotein that is synthesized with an uncleavable signal sequence that functions as a membrane anchoring domain (Misumi *et al* 1992; Fan *et al* 1997; Weihofen *et al* 2004; Lendeckel *et al* 2001). Processing of the 100 kDa mannose-rich DPPIV lead to the 124 kDa complex glycosylated mature form includes an extensive *O*-glycosylation event, mainly in a Ser/Thr-rich stalk domain adjacent to the membrane anchor (Naim *et al* 1999; Alfalah *et al* 2002; Lendeckel *et al* 2001). After maturation in the Golgi apparatus, DPPIV is transported to the apical membrane. This observation is in line with the biochemical data: as described above DDPIV is first expressed as a ~100 kDa mannose-rich precursor protein, which is trimmed and complexly glycosylated during protein maturation in the golgi apparatus, finally resulting in a approximately 124 kDa mature form (Alfalah *et al* 2002).

In case of mutated DPPIV-G633A only the high mannose form can be identified, indicating that the mannose-rich form is expressed but the correct further glycosylation fails. This date is proofed by application of endo-glycosidase H, which is capable to cleave N-linked sugar residues off the mannose-rich precursor form, but not off the complex glycosylated protein. As expected, both high mannose form the wild-type DPPIV, as well as the mutant shift after treatment of endoglycosidase H to a size of about 85 kDa, whereas the upper mature form representing the complex glycosylated form of DPPIV wild type do not effected. The mutant protein is obviously no more able to acquire a sufficient transport competence to be expressed on the membrane but is rapidly degraded in the ER.

The enzymatic activity is nearly totally deficient in plasma and other tissues of F344-rats bearing the described mutation. As mRNA levels are comparable to those of wild-type DPPIV, a structural alteration in the protein itself must be responsible for the lack of activity.

Christallographic structure analyses of DPPIV traced down the affected sequence (Gly^{629} – Trp – Ser – Tyr – Gly^{633}) directly in the catalytic centre of the enzyme with the Ser^{631} as the active amino acid, indicating that enzymatic activity is abolished by the exchange of Glycine to Arginine. This rat substrain accidently lacking any enzymatic activity of DPPIV is an excellent model for studying the *in vivo* role of this peptidase in various physiological function and could furthermore give insights in mechanisms of diseases linked to DPPIV like type II diabetes and chemical induced colitis.

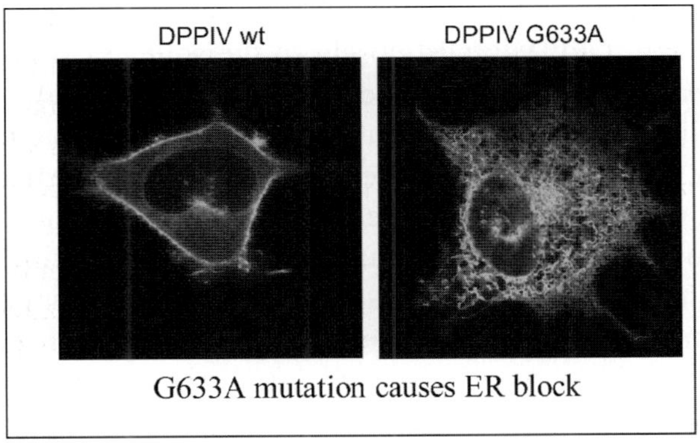

Figure 5: Subcellular localisation of the DPPIV and transiently transfected COS-1 cells. (A) COS-1 cells were transiently transfected with mutated and wild type DPPIV-GFP. Expression of DPPIV-GFP shows ER specific staining by the mutant and in case of the wild type in the plasmamembrane. (B) Biosynthetically labelled transfected COS-1 cells with mutated and wild type DPPIV-GFP.

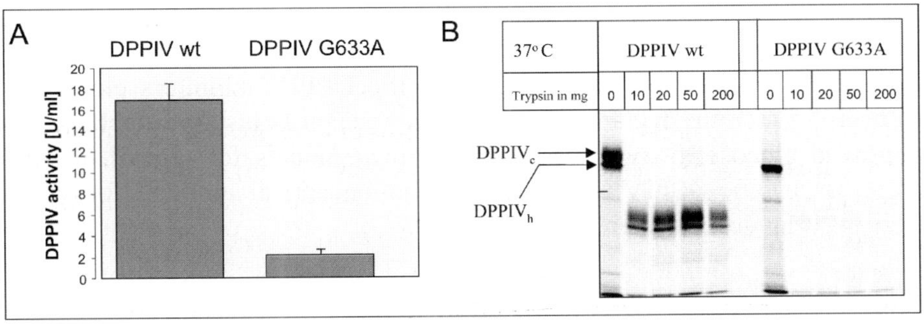

Figure 6: Mutated DPPIV shows deficincy in enzyme activity. (A) Enzyme activity difference between wild type and mutated DBBIV. (B) Trypsine sensitivity of DPPIV molecule. Transiently transfected COS-1 cells were biosynthetically labelled with ^{35}S-methionine for 4 h. Detergent extracted were treated with 0, 10, 20, 50 and 200 mg/ml trypsine for 40 min at 37°C prior the cell lysis an immunoprecipitated with anti-GFP. The precipitates were analysed by SDS-PAGE.

3.2 Peptide truncation by dipeptidyl peptidase IV

Membrane peptidases are a group of ectoenzymes with a broad functional repertoire. In protein metabolism, their importance is well known, especially in peptide degradation and amino acid scavenging at the intestinal and renal brush border. However, they also perform more subtle tasks; not only do they provide or extinguish signals by cleaving exterior peptide mediators, but they also may function as receptors or participate in signal transduction or in adhesion. DPPIV is unique among these peptidases because of its ability to liberate Xaa-Pro and less efficiently Xaa-Ala dipeptides from the N-terminus of regulatory peptides. In addition to, but independent of its serine type catalytic activity, DPPIV binds closely to the soluble extracellular enzyme adenosine deaminase. The *in vivo* expression on epithelial, endothelial and lymphoid cells of DPPIV is compatible with a role as physiological regulator of a number of peptides that serve as biochemical reporters between and within the immune and neuroendocrine system. Surprisingly, not cytokines with a N-terminal Xaa-Pro motif, but a number of chemokines have recently been identified as substrates. Despite DPPIV mediates only a minimal N-terminal truncation, important alterations in chemokine activities and receptor specificities were observed *in vitro* together with modified inflammatory and antiviral responses. Most probably the great flexibility of the N-terminus of a number of chemokines facilitates the accessibility to the catalytic site of DPPIV. Other known substrates which are subject *in vitro* to receptor-specific changes induced by DPPIV truncation include neuropeptides such as substance P, peptide YY and neuropeptide Y. On the other hand, DPPIV mediated cleavage of the N-terminal His-Ala or Tyr-Ala dipeptides from circulating incretin hormones like, glucagon-like peptides (GLP)-1 and -2, gastric inhibitory polypeptide (GIP), all members of the enteroglucagon/GRF superfamily, results in their biological inactivation *in vitro* and *in vivo*. Administration of specific DPPIV inhibitors closes this pathway of incretin degradation and greatly enhances insulin secretion. The improved glucose tolerance in several animal models for type II diabetes points to specific DPPIV inhibition as a pharmaceutical approach for type II diabetes drug development.

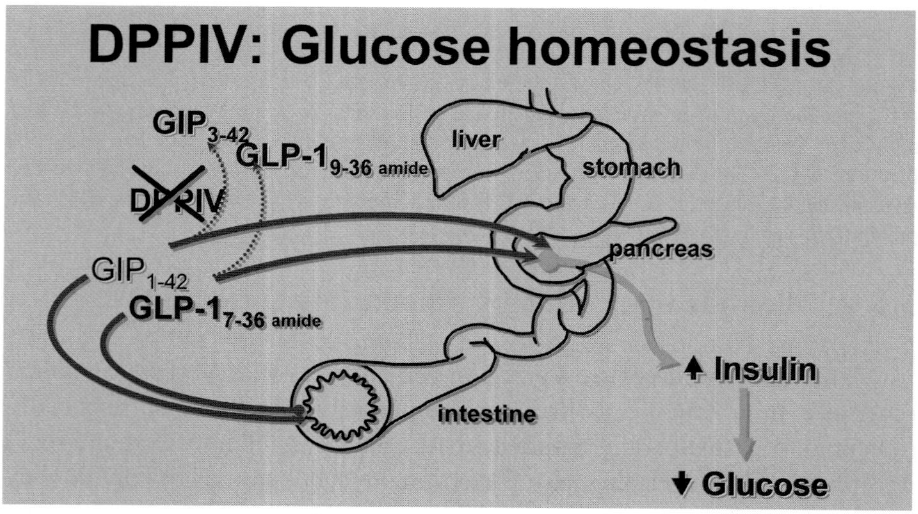

Figure 7: GPI and GLPs are potent substrates for DPPIV.

3.3 DPPIV and diabetes

Type II diabetes is a metabolic disorder caused by insufficient insulin levels in the mammalian organism. During a proceeding development, a defect in insulin activity as well as secretion in contrast to a mostly physiological glucagon function leads to overt hyperglycemia and forces the organism into a state of ketotic metabolism.

It has been found that the glucagon-like peptide 1 (GLP-1) and the glucose-dependent insulinotropic polypeptide (GIP) influence the secretion of insulin in the Langerhanns' isles of the pancreas and therefore are potential control mechanisms of blood insulin levels. GLP-1 and GIP both stimulate insulin secretion. Furthermore, GLP-1 is also capable to stimulate insulin gene expression, whereas secretion of glucagon is inhibited (Holst *et al* 1998). Beside this, proliferation and differentiation of insulin secreting β-cells in the pancreas are strongly enhanced by GLP-1 (Stoffers *et al* 2000; Zhou *et al* 1999) and even apoptosis of β-cells can be inhibited (Buteau *et al* 2004). GLP-1 is secreted by intestinal L-cells in response to food intake as a peptide of 30 amino acids and binds to a specific receptor (GLP-1-R) expressed on the cell surface of β-cells. By means of a stimulatory G-protein, adenylate cyclase is activated resulting in elevated levels of cAMP causing exocytosis of insulin containing vesicles via a variety of signal transducers.

A knockout mouse model missing the GLP-1-receptor showed a significant glucose intolerance (Miyawaki *et al* 1999) strongly suggesting that GLP-1 plays an important role in regulation of blood glucose levels. Similar results have also been found in patients suffering from type 2 diabetes (Vilsboll and Holst, 2004). Therefore, administration of GLP-1 functions has already been found as an antidiabetic approach for type II diabetes (Nauck and Meier, 2005; Deacon 2004; Baggio and Drucker, 2002).

GLPs and GIP are potent substrates for DPPIV and are normally rapidly inactivated by enzymatic cleavage via DPPIV. It has been shown, that specific inactivation of GLP-1 by N-terminal processing occurs in the plasma in the presence of active DPPIV (Marguet *et al* 2000). Incubation of the substrate with plasma lacking DPPIV activity led to unspecific C-terminal cleavage and endo-degradation. GIP was even totally resistant towards degradation when incubated with plasma of DPPIV deficient rats. These facts indicate, that DPPIV is the major enzyme responsible for N-terminal processing of GLP-1 in plasma and probably the exclusive one in case of GIP. A decreased DPPIV enzyme activity therefore should result in a reduced inactivation of GLP-1 and GIP, finally resulting in an increased induction of insulin secretion and a higher glucose clearance in the plasma. Upon this thesis, different groups examined blood glucose levels and glucose tolerance. Marguet *et al* (2000) used a knockout mouse model revealing that the fasting blood concentration of glucose in DPPIV-deficient mice is not different from strains expressing wild type DPPIV. In contrast, during the oral glucose tolerance test, significant lower levels of blood glucose have been detected 30, 60 and 90 minutes after oral glucose application whereas at the critical end point at 120 minutes, both strains exhibited normal concentrations again. Furthermore, they also showed results of blood GLP-1 and Insulin levels being significantly higher during glucose tolerance tests in rats lacking DPPIV activity. Similary results have been found in the DPPIV-deficient Fischer rat strains described above (Pospisilik *et al* 2002).

These findings strongly indicate that mice lacking DPPIV activity exhibit a significant improved glucose tolerance and therefore could be more resistant against diabetes type II than wild type strains. Obviously a lack of enzyme activity of DPPIV leads to a decreased inactivation of GLP-1, which can not completely compensated by other proteases and GIP, resulting in elevated levels of both hormones and insulin. Similar data have been observed by inhibition of DPPIV with valine-pyrrolidide. But as the effect of DPPIV-down regulation on glucose tolerance can also be observed in mice lacking the GLP-1-receptor, there must be more substrates involved in DPPIV-dependent regulation of insulin secretion and activation. GIP could certainly be one, others are not yet known.

New therapeutic approaches for treatment of diabetes type II concentrate on the development of DPPIV inhibitors as rapid degradation of injected GLP-1 and its analogues turned out to be the major problem. One of them, the Probiodrug DPPIV inhibitor isoleucine thiazolidide has been tested on Vancouver diabetic fatty rats during 12 weeks oral application and proofed to improve glucose tolerance, insulin sensitivity and β-cell responsiveness (Pospisilik *et al* 2002).

Valine-pyrrolidide has also been found to prevent inactivation of GLP-1 and GIP by DPPIV (Reimer *et al* 2002). Even more promising, the prolonged Ferring inhibitor, FE 999-011, continuously inhibits plasma DPPIV activity resulting in physiological glucose levels after oral glucose intake in insulin-resistant Zucker obeses rats. Furthermore, the onset of hyperglycaemia in Zucker diabetic fatty rats is significantly delayed (Sudre *et al* 2002).

The most worrying concern about potential side effects of DPPIV inhibitors raised from the fact that DPPIV physiologically cleaves a wide range of hormones and chemokines. Studies in knock out mice and DPPIV-deficient Fischer rats showed that even a total lack of DPPIV does mainly affect glucose metabolism, so far different implications are not reported.

The first clinical study was done with the short-acting Novartis inhibitor, NVP-DPP728 (Ahren *et al* 2002). A two- or three times a day administration during four weeks was capable to reduce both fasting and prandial glucose levels significantly in patient suffering from type II diabetes. Concerns about undesirable side effects seem to be - at least according to this trial - not intimidating, as NVP-DPP728 appeared to be well tolerated and, importantly, hypoglycemia was not reported. Another inhibitor, LAF237, also developed by Novartis, is longer-acting and therefore suitable for once-daily administration. It has been found, that it induces higher baseline and prandial levels of GLP-1. Surprisingly, both inhibitors did not increase insulin levels but, interestingly, glucagon levels were significantly suppressed. Phase III clinical trials are currently in progress, and filing for FDA approval is expected in 2006. Many other companies are in progress with clinical studies as well.

In contrast to GLP-1 analogues, studied DPPIV inhibitors showed the advantage, beside the prolonged half-time, to have no effect on the body weight.

3.4 Dipeptidyl peptidase and intestinal disease

The gastrointestinal mucosal epithelium contains a diverse number of specialized enteroendocrine cells that synthesize and secrete peptide hormones, frequently in a nutrient-dependent manner. Following secretion into circulation, gut-derived hormones may act in an endocrine manner by binding to receptors in tissues such as pancreas and liver, leading to the activation of signal transduction pathways and downstream physiological events (Ware *et al* 1999; Kirk *et al* 1997). Consistent with their location in the intestinal mucosal epithelium, enteroendocrine peptides may function in part to regulate gastrointestinal motility and nutrient digestion and absorption. For example, gastrin promotes acid secretion, whereas secretin inhibits acid secretion and promotes pancreatic exocrine secretion. Peptide hormones are structurally related to secretin. The GLP-2 administration to mice or rats promotes stimulation of crypt cell proliferation and inhibition of enterocyte apoptosis resulting in hyperplasia of the small bowel villous epithelium (Ware *et al* 1999; Kirk *et al* 1997). GLP-2 also exerts trophic effects in animal models of both small and large bowel injury such as experimental small bowel resection or chemically induced colitis (Kirk *et al* 1997; Adrian 2005). In addition to stimulation of epithelial proliferation, GLP-2 also acutely regulates gastric emptying and exerts rapid metabolic effects promting stimulation of intestinal hexose transport within 30 min following intravenous GLP-2 infusion (Tsuji *et al* 1992; Kimball *et al* 2004).

Inflammatory bowel diseases (IBD) such as ulcerative colitis, Crohn's disease and celiac disease are characterized by diminished intestinal barrier function, erosive loss of intestinal mucosa, inflammatory infiltrates in the submucosa and mucosa and dysregulated cytokine including interferon-γ and T-helper cell profiles. There is evidence to suggest that proteases play a role in the submucosa and mucosa, and dysregulated cytokine including interferon-γ and T-helper cell profiles.

The dextran sulphatic sodium (DSS) model of experimental colitis in rodents provides pathology similar to human colitis, which is characterized by a discontinuous pattern of mucosal epithelial damage in the distal colon, shrinkage in colon length and increases in the wet colonic tissue weight, infiltration of inflammatory cells and diarrhoea (Kimball *et al* 2004). This disease carries a risk of colorectal cancer that is 30 times greater than that of the general population with the incidence rising steadily with increasing duration and extent of disease.

We analysed the effects of DSS in the synthesis and cell surface delivery of sucrase-isomaltase (SI), dipeptidylpeptidase IV (DPPIV) and aminopeptidase N (APN) in the DSS mice model. The animals were treated with 2% DSS in drinking water for seven days. The animal devolpe an acute colonic inflammation with typical clinical colitis signs including abdominal cramping, weight loss, and loose, bloody stool. Although remission of symptoms is common, the disease will usually recur (Podolsky 1991; Glickman 1994; Bohe 1987; Bohe *et al* 1986). Control animals got normal water.

Our data shown there was a rapid decline in sucrase activity, while DPPIV and APN were unaffected over a 7-day treatment period. Quaroni *et al* (1993) shows that Intracellular degradation and reduced cell-surface expression of sucrase-isomaltase in cultured Caco cells at 42,5°C while DPPIV and APN were unaffected over a 3-day period (Quaroni *et al* 1993). The body reacted with fever to the inflammation. This could effect the protein transport. Interferon-gamma (IFN-γ) was part of the regulation of aminopeptidase N. IFN-γ was produced by T cells of the immune system. More T-helper cells then normal were in inflammantory tissue, so more IFN-γ was emitted and the ANP concentration increased (Gabrilovac *et al* 2005). It was also described that the brush border APN concentration became higher in changed colontissue (Young *et al* 1992).

4. CONCLUSION

The failure to sort proteins to the correct domain often results in pathological conditions. Sorting is therefore a critical mechanism by which the function of sorted proteins is maintained. It is clear that some type of apical sorting signal must exist, and that proteins are not transported to the apical surface by default simply because they lack a basolateral targeting signal. Current concepts have proposed either N-linked or O-linked glycans affect as sorting signals for apical proteins. This study demonstrates for the first time and in two different cell lines that complex N- as well as O-linked glycans constitute the basis of an apical sorting signal. The sorting of human intestinal DPPIV to the microvillar membrane in Caco-2 and HT-29 cells requires the concerted action of both types of glycosylation. Faulty and defective intracellular delivery, secretion and polarization, as well as loss of function of membrane proteins can lead to serious diseases such as cystic fibrosis and renal cystic diseases. An exception to this are mutations in intestinal brush border hydrolases that lead to mild diseases. Congenital sucrase-isomaltase deficiency is an example of a disease in which mutant phenotypes generate transport-incompetent molecules. We have now evaluated the biological effects of altered and defective intracellular transport, secretion and sorting of DPPIV, as well as loss of function. DPPIV plays a major role in regulation of physiological processes including immune, inflammatory, CNS and endocrine functions. DPPIV plays an important role in maintaining glucose homeostasis. These studies reveal that DPPIV helps regulate plasma glucose levels by controlling the activity of the incretins glucagon-like peptide 1 (GLP-1) and glucose-dependent insulinotropic polypeptide (GIP). Inhibition of DPPIV in wild-type and diabetic mice leads to increased levels of unprocessed GLP-1 and GIP in circulation, enhanced insulin secretion and improved glucose tolerance. Selective inhibitors of DPPIV, as well as the experment in DPPIV negative rat improve plasma glucose levels in human type II diabetics whereas GLP-2 exerts trophic effects on intestinal mucosal epithelia. Although GLP-1 actions are preserved in diseases such as diabetes, GLP-2 action has not been extensively studied in the setting of intestinal disease. GLP-2 significantly reduced cytokine induction, bacteremia, enhanced epithelial proliferation and reduced apoptosis in the crypt compartment and enhances repair of damaged intestinal tissue.

REFERENCES

Adrian TE, 2005, Importance of gut hormones in gastrointestinal, metabolic, and malignant diseases. *Curr Opin Endocrinol Diab*. **12:** 80-88.

Aertgeerts K, Ye S, Tennant MG, Kraus ML, Rogers J, Sang B-C, Skene RJ, Webb DR, Prasad GS, 2004, Crystal structure of human dipeptidyl peptidase IV in complex with a decapeptide reveals details on substrate specificity and tetrahedral intermediate formation *Prot Sci.* **13**: 412-421.

Ahren B, Simonsson E, Larsson H, Landin-Olsson M, Torgeirsson H, Jansson PA, Sandqvist M, Bavenholm P, Efendic S, Eriksson JW, Dickinson S, Holmes D, 2002, Inhibition of dipeptidyl peptidase IV improves metabolic control over a 4-week study period in type 2 diabetes. *Diabetes Care*. **25:** 869-875.

Alfalah M, Jacob R, Preuss U, Zimmer KP, Naim H, and Naim HY, 1999, O-linked glycans mediate apical sorting of human intestinal sucrase-isomaltase through association with lipid rafts. *Curr Biol.* **9:** 593-596.

Alfalah M, Jacob R, Naim HY, 2002, Intestinal dipeptidyl peptidase IV is efficiently sorted to the apical membrane through the concerted action of N- and O-glycans as well as association with lipid microdomains. *J Biol Chem.* **277:** 10683-10690.

Apodaca G, Bomsel M, Arden J, Breitfeld PP, Tang K, and Mostov KE, 1991, The polymeric immunoglobulin receptor. A model protein to study transcytosis. *J Clin Invest.* **87:** 1877-1882.

Aroeti B, Okhrimenko H, Reich V, and Orzech E, 1998, Polarized trafficking of plasma membrane proteins: emerging roles for coats, SNAREs, GTPases and their link to the cytoskeleton. *Biochim Biophys Acta.* **1376:** 57-90.

Baggio LL, Drucker DJ, 2002, Harnessing the therapeutic potential of glucagon-like peptide-1: a critical review. *Treat Endocrinol.* **1:** 117-125.

Bartles JR, Feracci HM, Stieger B, and Hubbard AL, 1987, J Cell Biol. 105: 1241-1251.

Bohe M, Genell S, Ohlsson K, 1986, Protease inhibitors in plasma and faecal extracts from patients with active inflammatory bowel disease. *Scand J Gastroenterol.* **21:** 598-604.

Bohe M, 1987, Pancreatic and granulocytic endoproteases in faecal extracts from patients with active ulcerative colitis. *Scand J Gastroenterol.* **22:** 59-64.

Bomsel M, and Mostov K, 1991, *Curr Opin Cell Biol.* **3:** 647-653.

Boonacker E, Van Noorden CJF, 2003, The multifunctional or moonlighting protein CD26/DPPIV. *Eur J Cell Biol.* **82**: 53-73.

Brewer CB and Roth MG, 1991, A single amino acid change in the cytoplasmic domain alters the polarized delivery of influenza virus hemagglutinin. *J Cell Biol.* **114:** 413-421.

Buteau J, El-Assaad W, Rhodes CJ, Rosenberg L, Joly E, Prentki M, 2004, Glucagon-like peptide-1 prevents beta cell glucolipotoxicity. *Diabetologia.* **47:** 806-815.

Caplan MJ, 1997, Membrane polarity in epithelial cells: protein sorting and establishment of polarized domains. *Am J Physiol.* **272:** F425-F429.

Casanova JE, Mishumi Y, Ikehara Y, Hubbard AL, and Mostov KE, 1991, *J Biol Chem.* **266:** 24428-24432.

Deacon CF, 2004, Therapeutic strategies based on glucagon-like peptide 1. *Diabetes.* **53:** 2181-2189.

Delzenne NM, Cani PD, Daubioul C, Neyrinck AM, 2005, Impact of inulin and oligofructose on gastrointestinal peptides. *Brit J Nut.* **93**: 157-161.

Dotti CG, and Simons K, 1990, Polarized sorting of viral glycoproteins to the axon and dendrites of hippocampal neurons in culture. *Cell.* **62:** 63-72.

Dragsten PR, Blumenthal R, and Handler JS, 1981, Membrane asymmetry in epithelia: is the tight junction a barrier to diffusion in the plasma membrane? *Nature.* **294:** 718-722.

Elbein AD, Pan YT, Solf R, and Vosbeck K, 1983, Effect of swainsonine, an inhibitor of glycoprotein processing, on cultured mammalian cells. *J Cell Physiol.* **115:** 265-275.

Fan H, Meng W, Kilian C, Grams S, and Reutter W, 1997, Domain-specific N-glycosylation of the membrane glycoprotein dipeptidylpeptidase IV (CD26) influences its subcellular trafficking, biological stability, enzyme activity and protein folding. *Eur J Biochem.* **46:** 243-251.

Fischer KD, Dhanvantari S, Drucker DJ, and Brubaker PL, 1997, Intestinal growth is associated with elevated levels of glucagon-like peptide 2 in diabetic rats. *Am J Physiol Endocrinol Metab.* **273:** E815-E820.

Fransen JA, Hauri HP, Ginsel LA, and Naim HY, 1991, Naturally occurring mutations in intestinal sucrase-isomaltase provide evidence for the existence of an intracellular sorting signal in the isomaltase subunit. *J Cell Biol.* **115:** 45-57.

Gabrilovac J, Breljak D, Cupic B, Ambriovic-Ristov A; 2005, Regulation of aminopeptidas N (EC 3.4.11.2; APN; CD13) by interferon-gamma an the HL-60 cell line. *Life Sci.* **76:** 2681-2697.

Gilmore R, 1993, Protein translocation across the endoplasmic reticulum: a tunnel with toll booths at entry and exit. *Cell.* **75:** 589-592.

Glickman RM, 1994, Inflammatory Bowel disease : Ulcerative colitis and Crohn's disease. *In* Harrison's Principles of Internal Medicine. KJ Isselbacher *et al* (eds). New York, McGraw-Hill, 1403-1417.

Hauri HP, Sterchi EE, Bienz D, Fransen JA, and Marxer A, 1985, Expression and intracellular transport of microvillus membrane hydrolases in human intestinal epithelial cells. *J Cell Biol.* **101:** 838-851.

Hauri HP, Quaroni A, and Isselbacher KJ, 1979, Biogenesis of intestinal plasma membrane: posttranslational route and cleavage of sucrase-isomaltase. *Proc Natl Acad Sci U S A.* **76:** 5183-5186.

Hauri HP, Sterchi EE, Bienz D, Fransen JA, and Marxer A, 1985, Expression and intracellular transport of microvillus membrane hydrolases in human intestinal epithelial cells. *J Cell Biol.* **101:** 838-851.

Hegen M, Kameoka J, Dong RP, Morimoto C, and Schlossman SF, 1997, Structure of CD26 (dipeptidyl peptidase IV) and function in human T cell activation. *Adv Exp Med Biol.* **421:** 109-116.

Holst JJ, Deacon C, Toft-Nielsen MB, Bjerre-Knudsen L, 1998, On the treatment of diabetes mellitus with glucagon-like peptide-1. *Ann NY Acad Sci.* **865**: 336-343.

Jacob R, Zimmer KP, Schmitz J, Naim HY, 2000, Congenital sucrase-isomaltase deficiency arising from cleavage and secretion of a mutant form of the enzyme. *J Clin Invest.* **106:** 281-287.

Jacob R, Alfalah M, Grunberg J, Obendorf M, Naim HY, 2000, Structural determinants required for apical sorting of an intestinal brush-border membrane protein**.** *J Biol Chem.* **275:** 6566-6572.

Jascur T, Matter K, and Hauri HP, 1991, Oligomerization and intracellular protein transport: dimerization of intestinal dipeptidyl peptidase IV occurs in the Golgi apparatus. *Biochemistry.* **30:** 1908-1915.

Kimball ES, Wallace NH, Scheider CR, D'Andrea MR, Hornby RJ, 2004, Vanilloid receptor 1 antagonists attenuate disease severtiy in dextran sulphate sodium-induced colitis in mice. *Neurogastroenterol Motil.* **16:** 811-818.

Kojima N, Handa K, Newman W, and Hakomori S, 1992, Inhibition of selectin-dependent tumor cell adhesion to endothelial cells and platelets by blocking O-glycosylation of these cells. *Biochem Biophys Res Commun.* **182:**1288-1295.

Lendeckel U, Arndt M, Wrenger S, Nepple K, Huth C, Ansorge S, Klein HU, Goette A, 2001, Expression and activity of ectopeptidases in fibrillating human atria. *J Mol Cell Cardiol.* **33:** 1273-1281.

Lendeckel U, Arndt M, Wolke C, Reinhold D, Kahne T, Ansorge S, 2002, Inhibition of human leukocyte function, alanyl aminopeptidase (APN, CD13) and dipeptidyl peptidase IV (DP IV, CD26) enzymatic activities by aqueous extracts of Cistus incanus L. ssp. Incanus. *J Ethnopharmacol.* **79:** 221-227.

Leof EB, 2000, Growth factor receptor signalling: location, location, location. *Trends Cell Biol.* **10:** 343-348.

Lesuffleur T, Barbat A, Luccioni C, Beaumatin J, Clair M, Kornowski A, Dussaulx E, Dutrillaux B, Zweibaum A, 1991, Dihydrofolate reductase gene amplification-associated shift of differentiation in methotrexate-adapted HT-29 cells. *J Cell Biol.* **115:** 1409-1418.

Lloyd M, Mevissen G, Fischer M, Olsen W, Goodspeed D, Genini M, Boll W, Semenza G, and Mantei N, 1992, Regulation of intestinal lactase in adult hypolactasia. *J Clin Invest.* **89:** 524-529.

Lombardi T, Montesano R, and Orci L, 1985, Polarized plasma membrane domains in cultured endothelial cells. *Exp Cell Res.* **161:** 242-246.

Marguet D, Baggio L, Kobayashi T, Bernard AM, Pierres M, Nielsen PF, Ribel U, Watanabe T, Drucker DJ, Wagtmann N, 2000, Enhanced insulin secretion and improved glucose tolerance in mice lacking CD26. *Proc Natl Acad Sci U S A.* **97:** 6874-6879.

Matter K, Stieger B, Klumperman J, Ginsel L, and Hauri HP, 1990, Endocytosis, recycling, and lysosomal delivery of brush border hydrolases in cultured human intestinal epithelial cells (Caco-2). *J Biol Chem.* **265:** 3503-3512.

Matter K, Brauchbar M, Bucher K, and Hauri HP, 1990, *Cell.* **60:** 429-437.

Matter K, and Hauri HP, 1991, Intracellular transport and conformational maturation of intestinal brush border hydrolases. *Biochemistry.* **30:** 1916-1924.

Matter K, 2000, Epithelial polarity: sorting out the sorters. *Curr Biol.* **10:** R39-R42.

Mellman I, Yamamoto E, Whitney JA, Kim M, Hunziker W, and Matter K, 1993, Molecular sorting in polarized and non-polarized cells: common problems, common solutions. *J Cell Sci.* **17:** 1-7.

Misumi Y, Hayashi Y, Arakawa F, and Ikehara Y, 1992, Molecular cloning and sequence analysis of human dipeptidyl peptidase IV, a serine proteinase on the cell surface. *Biochim Biophys Acta.* **1131:** 333-336.

Miyawaki K, Yamada Y, Yano H, Niwa H, Ban N, Ihara Y, Kubota A, Fujimoto S, Kajikawa M, Kuroe A, Tsuda K, Hashimoto H, Yamashita T, Jomori T, Tashiro F, Miyazaki J, Seino Y, 1999, Glucose intolerance caused by a defect in the entero-insular axis: a study in gastric inhibitory polypeptide receptor knockout mice. *Proc Natl Acad Sci U S A.* **96:** 14843-14847.

Moolenaar CE, Ouwendijk J, Wittpoth M, Wisselaar HA, Hauri HP, Ginsel LA, Naim HY, and Fransen JA, 1997, A mutation in a highly conserved region in brush-border sucrase-isomaltase and lysosomal alpha-glucosidase results in Golgi retention. *J Cell Sci.* **110:** 557–567.

Mostov K, Apodaca G, Aroeti B, and Okamoto C, 1992, Plasma membrane protein sorting in polarized epithelial cells. *J Cell Biol.* **116:** 577-583.

Mostov K, 1991, The polymeric immunoglobulin receptor. *Semin Cell Biol.* **2:** 411-418.

Naim HY, 2001, Structure, function and regulation of intestinal lactase-phlorizin hydrolase and sucrase-isomaltase in health and disease. In Delvin EE. and Lentze MJ, eds. Gastrointestinal Functions, Nestle Nutrition Workshop Series.

Naim HY, Sterchi EE, and Lentze MJ, 1988a, Biosynthesis of the human sucrase-isomaltase complex . Differential O-glycosylation of the sucrase subunit correlates with its position within the enzyme complex. *J Biol Chem.* **263:** 7242-7253.

Naim HY, Roth J, Sterchi E, Lentze M, Milla P, Schmitz J, and Hauri HP, 1988b, Sucrase-isomaltase deficiency in man. Different mutations disrupt intracellular transport, processing and function of an intestinal brush border enzyme. *J Clin Invest.* **82:** 667-679.

Naim HY, Lacey SW, Sambrook JF, and Gething MJ, 1991, Expression of a full-length cDNA coding for human intestinal lactase-phlorizin hydrolase reveals an uncleaved, enzymatically active, and transport-competent protein. *J Biol Chem.* **266:** 12313-12320.

Naim HY, Joberty G, Alfalah M, and Jacob R, 1999, Temporal association of the N- and O-linked glycosylation events and their implication in the polarized sorting of intestinal brush border sucrase-isomaltase, aminopeptidase N, and dipeptidyl peptidase IV. *J Biol Chem.* **274:** 17961-17967.

Nauck MA, Meier JJ, 2005, Glucagon-like peptide 1 and its derivatives in the treatment of diabetes. *Regul Pept.* **128:** 135-148.

Nelson WJ, 1992, Regulation of cell surface polarity from bacteria to mammals. *Science.* **258 :** 948-955.

Palade G, 1975, Intracellular aspects of the process of protein synthesis. *Science.* **189:** 347-358.

Podolsky DK, 1991, Inflammatory bowel disease. *N Engl J Med.* **325:** 928-937, 1008-1016.

Pospisilik JA, Stafford SG, Demuth HU, McIntosh CH, Pederson RA, 2002, Long-term treatment with dipeptidyl peptidase IV inhibitor improves hepatic and peripheral insulin sensitivity in the VDF Zucker rat: a euglycemic-hyperinsulinemic clamp study. *Diabetes.* **51:** 2677-2683.

Presley JF, Cole NB, Schroer TA, Hirschberg K, Zaal KJ, and Lippincott-Schwartz J, 1997, ER-to-Golgi transport visualized in living cells. *Nature.* **389:** 81-85.

Quaroni A, Paul EC, Nichols BL, 1993, Intracellular degradation and reduced cell-surface expression of sucrase-isomaltase in heat-shockes Caco-2 cells. *Biochem J.* **292:** 725-734.

Rapoport TA, 1991, Protein transport across the endoplasmic reticulum membrane: facts, models, mysteries. *FASEB J.* **5:** 2792-2798.

Reimer MK, Holst JJ, Ahren B. 2002 Long-term inhibition of dipeptidyl peptidase IV improves glucose tolerance and preserves islet function in mice. *Eur J Endocrinol.* **146:** 717-727.

Ritz V, Alfalah M, Zimmer K-P, Schmitz J, Jacob R, Naim HY, 2003, Congenital sucrase-isomaltase deficiency arising from a mutant form of sucrase-isomaltase that accumulates in the endoplasmic reticulum. *Gastroenterol.* **125:** 1678-1685.

Rodriguez-Boulan E and Powell SK, 1992, Polarity of epithelial and neuronal cells. *Annu Rev Cell Biol.* **8:** 395-427.

Rothman JE, 1990, Phospholipid transfer market. *Nature.* **347:** 519-520.

Sabatini DD, Ivanov IE, Gottlieb TA, Compton T, Gonzalez A, Beaudry G, and Rindler MJ, 1988, Use of cultured, virus-infected cells to study the biogenesis of polarity of epithelial cells. *Ann Endocrinol. (Paris)* **49:** 270-286.

Sato K, and Dang NH, 2003, CD26: A novel treatment target for T-cell lymphoid malignancies? (Review). *Int J Oncol.* **22:** 481-497.

Slimane TA, Lenoir C, Sapin C, Maurice M, and Trugnan G, 2000, Apical secretion and sialylation of soluble dipeptidyl peptidase IV are two related events. *Exp Cell Res.* **258:** 184-194.

Spodsberg N, Jacob R, Alfalah M, Zimmer KP, Naim HY, 2001, Molecular Basis of Aberrant Apical Protein Transport in an Intestinal Enzyme Disorder. *J Biol Chem.* **276:** 23506-23510.

Sterchi EE, Woodley JF, 1980, Peptide hydrolases of the human small intestinal mucosa: identification of six distinct enzymes in the brush border membrane. *Clin Chim Acta.* **102:** 57-65.

Stoffers DA, Kieffer TJ, Hussain MA, Drucker DJ, Bonner-Weir S, Habener JF, Egan JM, 2000, Insulinotropic glucagon-like peptide 1 agonists stimulate expression of homeodomain protein IDX-1 and increase islet size in mouse pancreas. *Diabetes.* **49**: 741-748.

Sudre B, Broqua P, White RB, Ashworth D, Evans DM, Haigh R, Junien JL, Aubert ML, 2002, Chronic inhibition of circulating dipeptidyl peptidase IV by FE 999011 delays the occurrence of diabetes in male zucker diabetic fatty rats. *Diabetes.* **51:** 1461-1469.

Tsuji E, Misumi Y, Fujiwara T, Takami N, Ogata S, Ikehara Y, 1992, An active-site mutation (Gly633–>Arg) of dipeptidyl peptidase IV causes its retention and rapid degradation in the endoplasmic reticulum. *Biochemistry.* **31:** 11921-11927.

Vilsboll T, Holst JJ, 2004, Incretins, insulin secretion and Type 2 diabetes mellitus. *Diabetologia.* **47:** 357-366.

Wandinger-Ness A, Bennett MK, Antony C, and Simons K, 1990, Distinct transport vesicles mediate the delivery of plasma membrane proteins to the apical and basolateral domains of MDCK cells. *J Cell Biol.* **111:** 987-1000.

Ware JH, Wan XS, Newberne P, and Kennedy AR, 1999, Bowman-Birk Inhibitor Concentrate Reduces Colon Inflammation in Mice with Dextran Sulfate Sodium-Induced Ulcerative Colitis. *Dig Dis Sci.* **44:** 986- 990.

Weihofen WA, Liu J, Reutter W, Saenger W, and Fan H, 2004, Crystal Structure of CD26/Dipeptidyl-peptidase IV in Complex with Adenosine Deaminase Reveals a Highly. amphiphilic interface. *J Biol Chem.* **279:** 43330-43335.

Yamazaki K, Yasuda N, Inoue T, Nagakura T, Kira K, Saeki T, Tanaka I, 2004, The combination of metformin and a dipeptidyl peptidase IV inhibitor prevents 5-fluorouracil-induced reduction of small intestine weight. *Eur J Pharmacol.* **488:** 213-218.

Yeaman C, Grindstaff KK, and Nelson WJ, 1999, New perspectives on mechanisms involved in generating epithelial cell polarity. *Physiol Rev.* **79:** 73-98.

Young GP, Macrae FA, Gibson PR, Alexeyeff M, Whitehead RH; 1992, Brush border hydrolases in normal and neoplastic colonic epithelium. *J Gastroenterol Hepatol.* **7:** 347-354.

Zhou J, Wang X, Pineyro MA, Egan JM, 1999, Glucagon-like peptide 1 and exendin-4 convert pancreatic AR42J cells into glucagon- and insulin-producing cells. *Diabetes.* **48:** 2358-2366.

Index